Rapid Review
Histology and Cell Biology

Rapid Review Series

Series Editor
Edward F. Goljan, MD

Behavioral Science, Second Edition
Vivian M. Stevens, PhD; Susan K. Redwood, PhD; Jackie L. Neel, DO;
Richard H. Bost, PhD; Nancy W. Van Winkle, PhD; Michael H. Pollak, PhD

Biochemistry, Second Edition
John W. Pelley, PhD; Edward F. Goljan, MD

Gross and Developmental Anatomy, Second Edition
N. Anthony Moore, PhD; William A. Roy, PhD, PT

Histology and Cell Biology, Second Edition
E. Robert Burns, PhD; M. Donald Cave, PhD

Microbiology and Immunology, Second Edition
Ken S. Rosenthal, PhD; James S. Tan, MD

Neuroscience
James A. Weyhenmeyer, PhD; Eve A. Gallman, PhD

Pathology, Second Edition
Edward F. Goljan, MD

Pharmacology, Second Edition
Thomas L. Pazdernik, PhD; Laszlo Kerecsen, MD

Physiology
Thomas A. Brown, MD

USMLE Step 2
Michael W. Lawlor, MD, PhD

USMLE Step 3
David Rolston, MD; Craig Nielsen, MD

Rapid Review
Histology and Cell Biology

SECOND EDITION

E. Robert Burns, PhD

Professor, Department of Neurobiology and Developmental Sciences
Charles Hartzell Lutterloh and Charles M. Lutterloh Professor of Medical Education Excellence
(2005–2007)
Course Director, Medical Microscopic Anatomy (1985–2002)
College of Medicine
University of Arkansas for Medical Sciences
Little Rock, Arkansas

M. Donald Cave, PhD

Professor, Department of Neurobiology and Development Sciences
College of Medicine
University of Arkansas for Medical Sciences
Little Rock, Arkansas

Contributor
William D. Meek, PhD

Professor of Anatomy and Cell Biology
Department of Anatomy and Cell Biology
Oklahoma State University Center for Health Sciences
College of Osteopathic Medicine
Tulsa, Oklahoma

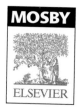

MOSBY
ELSEVIER

1600 John F. Kennedy Blvd.
Suite 1800
Philadelphia, PA 19103-2899

RAPID REVIEW HISTOLOGY AND CELL BIOLOGY, Second Edition   ISBN-10: 0-323-04425-5
Copyright © 2007, 2002 by Mosby, Inc., an affiliate of Elsevier Inc.   ISBN-13: 978-0-323-04425-7

Library of Congress Cataloging-in-Publication Data

Burns, E. Robert.
   Histology and cell biology / E. Robert Burns, M. Donald Cave.—2nd ed.
      p. cm.—(Rapid review)
   Includes index.
   ISBN 0-323-04425-5
      1. Histology—Outlines, syllabi, etc. 2. Cytology—Outlines, syllabi, etc. 3. Physicians—Licenses—
   United States—Examinations—Study guides. I. Cave, M. Donald. II. Title. III. Rapid review series.
   QM553.B84 2007
   611′.018—dc22

                                                          2006041885

Publishing Director: Linda Belfus
Acquisitions Editor: James Merritt
Developmental Editor: Katie DeFrancesco
Design Direction: Steven Stave

Printed in the United States of America.

Last digit is the print number: 9   8   7   6   5   4   3   2   1

To Mary Stuart Lindsey-Burns, the wind beneath my wings
Keith, Sherry, Ayla, and Paul, Jr.—bright lights all
S. Meryl Rose, PhD, Ralph N. Baillif, PhD,
Horace N. Marvin, PhD, John E. Pauly, PhD,
and Lawrence E. Scheving, PhD—mentors still at it

ERB

To the memory of Edith Krugelis MacRae, PhD, 1919–1995,
an outstanding teacher of histology and cell biology at the
University of Illinois College of Medicine and the University of
North Carolina School of Medicine

MDC

To our medical students for constantly challenging us

ERB and MDC

Series Preface

The First Editions of the *Rapid Review Series* have received high critical acclaim from students studying for the United States Medical Licensing Examination (USMLE) Step 1 and high ratings in *First Aid for the USMLE Step 1*. The Second Editions continue to be invaluable resources for time-pressed students. As a result of reader feedback, we have improved upon an already successful formula. We have created a learning system, including a print and electronic package, that is easier to use and more concise than other review products on the market.

SPECIAL FEATURES

Book

- **Outline format:** Concise, high-yield subject matter is presented in a study-friendly format.
- **High-yield margin notes:** Key content that is most likely to appear on the exam is reinforced in the margin notes.
- **Visual elements:** Abundant two-color schematics, black and white images, and summary tables enhance your study experience.
- **Two-color design:** Colored text and headings make studying more efficient and pleasing.
- **Two practice examinations:** Two sets of 50 USMLE Step 1–type clinically oriented, multiple-choice questions (including images where necessary) and complete discussions (rationales) for all options are included.

New! Online Study and Testing Tool

- **350 USMLE Step 1–type MCQs:** Clinically oriented, multiple-choice questions that mimic the current board format are presented. These include images where necessary, and complete rationales for

all answer options. All the questions from the book are included so you can study them in the most effective mode for you!
- **Test mode:** Select from randomized 50-question sets or by subject topics for an exam-like review session. This mode features a 60-minute timer to simulate the actual exam, a detailed assessment report that can be printed or saved to your hard drive, and direct links to all or only incorrect questions. The links include your answer, the correct answer, and full rationales for all answer options, so you can fully analyze your test session and learn from your mistakes.
- **Study mode:** Like the test mode, in the study mode you can select from randomized 50-question sets or by subject topics to create a dynamic study session. This mode features unlimited attempts at each question, instant feedback (either on selection of the correct answer or when using the "Show Answer" feature), complete rationales for all answer options, and a detailed progress report that can be printed or saved to your hard drive.
- **Online access:** Online access allows you to study from an internet-enabled computer wherever and whenever it is convenient. This access is activated through registration on www.studentconsult.com with the pincode printed inside the front cover.

Student Consult

- **Full online access:** You can access the complete text and illustrations of this book on www.studentconsult.com.
- **Save content to your PDA:** Through our unique Pocket Consult platform, you can clip selected text and illustrations and save them to your PDA for study on the fly!
- **Free content:** An interactive community center with a wealth of additional valuable resources is available.

Acknowledgment of Reviewers

The publisher expresses sincere thanks to the medical students and faculty who provided many useful comments and suggestions for improving both the text and the questions. Our publishing program will continue to benefit from the combined insight and experience provided by your reviews. For always encouraging us to focus on our target, the USMLE Step 1, we thank the following:

Michael W. Lawlor, Loyola University Chicago Stritch School of Medicine

Kelly Liang, Jefferson Medical College

Kimberly Liang, Jefferson Medical College

Christopher Lupold, Jefferson Medical College

Tracey A. McCarthy, Loyola University Chicago Stritch School of Medicine

Mrugeshkumar K. Shah, MD, MPH, Tulane School of Medicine, Harvard Medical School/Spaulding Rehabilitation Hospital

John K. Su, MPH, Boston University School of Medicine

Acknowledgments

The authors wish to acknowledge the professionalism and the patience of Susan Kelly, managing editor, for helping us complete this project. We thank Katie DeFrancesco for her efficiency in helping us produce the Second Edition. We thank Ruth Steyn, PhD, for her editing skills. Matt Chansky's expertise as an illustrator will be appreciated by every reader. Thanks to the medical students and the resident physician who reviewed the manuscript and the questions—you offered excellent constructive criticism by always focusing the work on the target, the USMLE Step 1.

E. Robert Burns, PhD
M. Donald Cave, PhD

Contents

Cell Surface

I. Introduction: Levels of Anatomic Organization
   A. Cells
      1. Major cellular components
         a. The nucleus contains the genetic material (deoxyribonucleic acid; DNA) and is surrounded by a double membrane.
         b. The cytoplasm consists of a fluid portion (cytosol), various membrane-bound organelles, inclusions, and cytoskeletal elements.
         c. The plasma membrane (plasmalemma) constitutes the outer boundary of a cell, enclosing the cellular contents and separating them from the external environment.
            - In all cells, the plasma membrane also functions in regulating the intracellular environment and in cell-to-cell communication.
      2. Essential cell functions that enable life
         a. Replication (cells arise only from pre-existing cells)
         b. Regulation of the intracellular environment
         c. Synthesis of proteins and numerous other molecules
         d. Harnessing and transformation of energy
         e. Differentiation and specialization
         f. Interaction to form larger units
   B. Higher levels of organization
      1. Tissues: aggregations of cells and their products specialized to perform a particular function or functions; classified into four major types:
         a. Epithelial tissue

      b. Connective tissue
      c. Nervous tissue
      d. Muscle tissue

   2. Organ: a group of tissues that forms a structural unit and performs a specific function or functions

   3. Organ system: a group of interconnected or interdependent organs that together perform a specific function or functions

   4. Organism: a group of systems interacting to form a living economy

  C. Dimensions of biologic structures and their component molecules are summarized in Figure 1-1.

II. Structure of the Plasmalemma

  A. Trilaminar appearance in cell sections

    • Transmission electron microscopy of cell sections shows the plasma membrane having two electron-dense outer layers (each 3 nm thick) that are separated by a less dense central layer (3.5 nm thick).

    1. The external (exoplasmic) surface faces the cell exterior.

    2. The internal (protoplasmic) surface faces the cytoplasm.

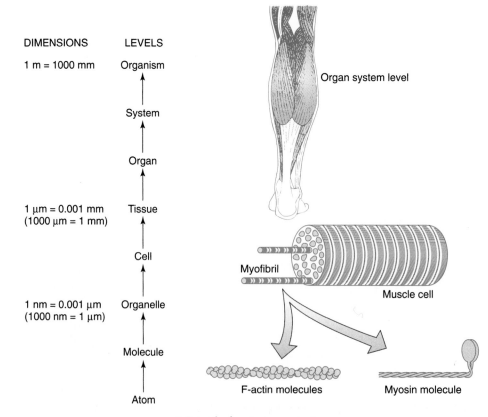

DIMENSIONS   LEVELS

1 m = 1000 mm   Organism

System

Organ

1 μm = 0.001 mm   Tissue
(1000 μm = 1 mm)

Cell

1 nm = 0.001 μm   Organelle
(1000 nm = 1 μm)

Molecule

Atom

Organ system level

Myofibril

Muscle cell

F-actin molecules

Myosin molecule

1-1: Levels of anatomic organization.

B. Lipid bilayer
- The basic structural unit of nearly all cellular membranes is a bimolecular lipid "sheet" composed primarily of phospholipids (Fig. 1-2).
1. Phospholipids are highly amphipathic molecules, containing a hydrophilic "head" group and long hydrophobic "tails" composed of fatty acids.
    - In membranes, phospholipids are arranged as two sheets (leaflets) with their hydrophilic head groups facing outward and their hydrophobic tails facing inward.
    a. Phosphatidylcholine (lecithin) and sphingomyelin are present primarily in the outer leaflet.
    b. Phosphatidylethanolamine and phosphatidylserine are present primarily in the inner leaflet.
2. Cholesterol, located in both leaflets of the plasma membrane, helps to stabilize membrane structure.
3. Glycolipids have their lipid end inserted into the outer leaflet of the plasma membrane, with their carbohydrate moieties extending into the extracellular space.
C. Membrane proteins
- According to the fluid-mosaic model, proteins in cellular membranes "float" and move laterally within the lipid bilayer, which acts as a two-dimensional fluid.
- Proteins can associate with the lipid bilayer in various ways (Fig. 1-3).
1. Extrinsic (peripheral) proteins are present at membrane surfaces but do not penetrate the lipid bilayer.
    - Composed primarily of hydrophilic amino acids, extrinsic proteins are held in place by noncovalent interactions with other membrane proteins, lipids, or oligosaccharides.

In cells without oxygen, activation of membrane phospholipase by Ca^{2+} leads to irreversible cell injury.

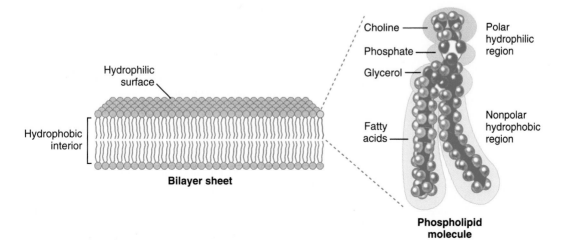

Choline — Polar hydrophilic region
Phosphate —
Glycerol —

Hydrophilic surface

Hydrophobic interior

Fatty acids — Nonpolar hydrophobic region

Bilayer sheet

Phospholipid molecule

1-2: *Structure of the phospholipid bilayer. The hydrophilic heads of the phospholipid molecules face outward, toward the aqueous surroundings.*

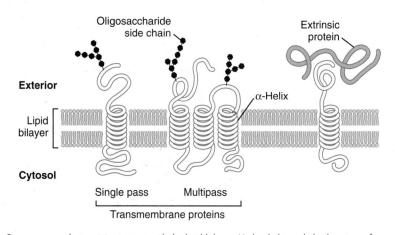

1-3: *Common ways that proteins interact with the lipid bilayer. Hydrophobic, α-helical regions of transmembrane proteins are embedded in the interior of the bilayer. These proteins usually are glycoproteins with oligosaccharide residues covalently attached to the external domain. Extrinsic proteins associate noncovalently with either the external or the cytosolic domain of transmembrane proteins.*

      2. Transmembrane intrinsic (integral) proteins span the entire lipid bilayer and generally have covalently linked carbohydrate residues, which always project into the extracellular space.

         a. Regions rich in hydrophobic amino acids interact with the nonpolar interior of the lipid bilayer.

           (1) In single-pass proteins, the polypeptide chain crosses the membrane once.

           (2) In multipass proteins, the polypeptide chain crosses the membrane more than once.

         b. Regions rich in hydrophilic amino acids extend beyond the membrane surfaces, forming cytosolic and exoplasmic domains.

      3. Lipid-anchored intrinsic proteins have a covalently attached lipid group that tethers them to one or the other of the bilayer leaflets.

   D. Fluidity of membranes

      1. Lateral movement

         • Phospholipids, glycolipids, and some intrinsic proteins diffuse laterally within the individual leaflets of a membrane.

      2. Exchange (flip-flop) between leaflets

         a. Lipids and proteins do not move spontaneously between the inner and outer leaflets of the lipid bilayer.

         b. Phospholipids, which are synthesized in the cytosolic leaflet of the endoplasmic reticulum (ER) membrane, can flip-flop to the other leaflet with the aid of ER-bound enzymes called "phospholipid translocators," or "flippases."

      3. Factors affecting membrane fluidity

         a. Temperature: Fluidity increases as the temperature rises.

         b. Phospholipid type: Shorter fatty acid tails and the presence of double bonds increase fluidity.

    c. Cholesterol content: Fluidity decreases as membrane cholesterol increases (e.g., as a result of ethanol intake).
      • A decrease in fluidity reduces the permeability of membranes to small molecules, such as water.

  E. Uniformity of cellular membranes
    1. A trilaminar appearance and lipid bilayer molecular organization are characteristic of internal cellular membranes (e.g., nuclear, mitochondrial, and ER membranes) as well as of the plasma membrane.
    2. Different cellular membranes have different lipid and protein composition.
      • Organelle-specific membrane proteins confer unique functions on certain organelles.
    3. Membrane "flow" refers to the ready exchange of membranes that occurs between cellular compartments.
      a. Plasma membrane → endocytic vesicle
      b. Membrane of the secretory vesicle → plasma membrane
      c. ER → transfer vesicle → Golgi complex → lysosome

  F. Glycocalyx
    • A carbohydrate-rich layer, also known as the "cell coat," the glycocalyx covers the external surface of the plasma membrane of many cells.
    • In contrast to the plasma membrane, the glycocalyx exhibits extensive variation in thickness, fuzziness, and general appearance in different cell types.
    1. Components of the glycocalyx
      a. Membrane glycolipids and transmembrane glycoproteins (exoplasmic domains)
      b. Extrinsic membrane glycoproteins
      c. Proteoglycans attached to the cell surface
    2. Functions of the glycocalyx
      • Depending on the cell type and tissue, the glycocalyx may assist in the following:
      a. Control of cell permeability by permitting passage of water and small molecules, but not large molecules
      b. Protection and lubrication of the cell surface
      c. Cell–cell recognition and interaction (e.g., in lymphocyte recirculation and sperm–egg interaction)
      d. Localization of extracellular enzymes to the cell surface

III. Movement of Molecules and Ions across Membranes (Fig. 1-4)
    • Various multipass transmembrane proteins, called "transport proteins," mediate the passage of most molecules and all ions across the plasma membrane (and internal membranes).
  A. Passive transport: movement of molecules or ions across the membrane down their concentration or electrochemical gradient; no energy required
    • Transport proteins exhibit a high degree of specificity for the transported molecule or ion and undergo conformational changes during the transport process.

The fluidity of the cellular membranes affects their functions: Temperature and cholesterol content increase fluidity.

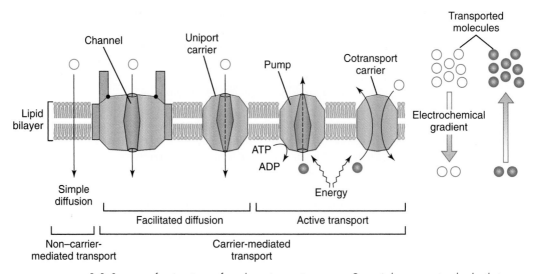

1-4: *Summary of various types of membrane-transport processes. Open circles represent molecules that are moving down their electrochemical gradient. Solid circles represent molecules that are moving against their electrochemical gradient. Such active transport requires an input of energy. ADP, adenosine diphosphate; ATP, adenosine triphosphate.*

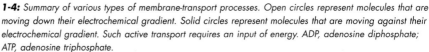

1. Simple diffusion occurs without the aid of transport proteins.
   - Small hydrophobic molecules and small uncharged polar molecules (e.g., H_2O, CO_2, O_2, ethanol) readily diffuse through the lipid bilayer membranes.
2. Facilitated diffusion is mediated by channel proteins and certain carrier proteins.
   a. Channel proteins form hydrophilic pores that extend across the membrane. When the pores are "open," solutes (primarily ions) flow through them.
   b. Uniport carrier proteins, commonly termed "permeases," transport a single solute (e.g., glucose, a particular amino acid) across the membrane in one direction.

B. Active transport: protein-mediated movement of molecules or ions across the membrane against their concentration or electrochemical gradient; energy required
   1. Adenosine triphosphate (ATP)-powered pumps have binding sites for ATP in their cytosolic domains and couple ATP hydrolysis to the transport of ions and small molecules against their gradient.
      - The Na^+/K^+ pump moves three Na^+ ions out of and two K^+ ions into the cell, both against their electrochemical gradients, maintaining their typical gradients across the plasma membrane.
      - A reduction in ATP synthesis (e.g., in cells without adequate oxygen) causes Na^+ to move into cells, leading to cellular swelling (hydropic degeneration).

2. Cotransport carrier proteins couple the energy-releasing transport of one solute (e.g., Na^+) down its gradient to the energy-requiring transport of another solute (e.g., glucose) up its gradient.
   - Na^+/glucose cotransport protein mediates the transport of glucose from the intestinal lumen into epithelial cells.

C. Bulk movement of materials into and out of cells

1. Exocytosis: the release of large quantities of material from cells by a process that involves fusion of the cytosolic surface of the plasma membrane with the cytosolic surface of secretory vesicle membranes

2. Endocytosis: the uptake of large amounts of material into cells by processes that involve fusion of the external surfaces of the plasma membrane
   a. Phagocytosis is a nonselective process whereby large solid particles (e.g., bacteria) are ingested and subsequently degraded.
   b. Pinocytosis is a nonselective process whereby small fluid droplets are ingested.
   c. Receptor-mediated endocytosis is a selective process whereby specific macromolecules (e.g., antigens, low-density lipoprotein, transferrin) are ingested (Fig. 1-5).

D. Disorders involving defective transport

1. Cystic fibrosis is caused by an autosomal recessive mutation in the gene encoding CFTR protein, an ATP-powered Cl^- channel.
   - This genetic defect leads to dysfunction of the exocrine glands in the pancreas, respiratory system, and skin.
   - Common manifestations are excessive sweat with electrolytes (the basis for the sweat chloride test) and excessive amounts of thick mucus in the respiratory tract.

Cystic fibrosis, hereditary hypercholesterolemia, and cystinuria result from defects in membrane transport proteins.

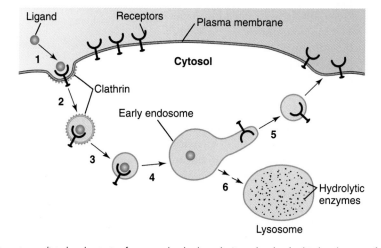

1-5: *Receptor-mediated endocytosis of macromolecular ligands. Ligand molecules bind to their specific cell-surface receptors, which then aggregate over clathrin-coated pits (1). These pits bud off from the membrane (2), forming vesicles that soon shed their coat (3). After uncoated vesicles fuse with endosomes, the low internal pH dissociates the ligand from its receptors (4). The receptors are recycled to the plasma membrane via small vesicles (5), and ligands are moved to lysosomes, where they are enzymatically degraded (6).*

2. Cystinuria, an autosomal recessive disease, results from a defect in the carrier proteins that are needed to reabsorb cystine from the kidney tubules.
    - This condition, marked by excessive excretion of cystine and several other amino acids, may lead to the formation of kidney stones and the presence of hexagonal cystine crystals in the urine.
3. Hereditary hypercholesterolemia, an autosomal dominant disease, occurs in individuals who lack functional receptors for low-density lipoprotein (LDL).
    - LDL, the major carrier of cholesterol in the bloodstream, normally is internalized into cells by receptor-mediated endocytosis.
    - The absence of functional LDL receptors causes high blood levels of cholesterol, which contribute to atherosclerosis and death due to coronary artery disease and stroke at an early age.
4. Tetrodotoxin binds to and inactivates Na^+ channels.
    - When ingested by humans, tetrodotoxin from puffer fish and related fish toxins cause dizziness and tingling around the mouth, which may be followed by ataxia, respiratory failure, and death.

IV. Cell–Cell Communication
- Cells in tissues and organs are continuously bombarded with signaling molecules that carry potentially significant information.
- A cell can respond only to the signaling molecules whose specific protein receptors it produces. The repertoire of receptors that are produced by cells changes during the development and differentiation of various cell types.

A. Sequence of events in cell signaling
1. The release of signaling molecules (ligands) from signaling cells commonly occurs via exocytosis and usually occurs in response to a specific stimulus. Common signaling molecules include
    a. Neurotransmitters
    b. Hormones
    c. Growth factors
    d. Cytokines
2. Binding of a ligand to its specific receptor in a target cell causes receptor activation.
3. Signal transduction from an activated receptor, either directly or indirectly via an intracellular second messenger, leads ultimately to specific cellular responses. Common second messengers include
    a. Cyclic adenosine monophosphate (cAMP)
    b. Cyclic guanosine monophosphate (cGMP)
    c. Inositol 1,4,5-triphosphate (IP$_3$)
    d. 1,2-Diacylglycerol (DAG)
    e. Ca^{2+} ions
    f. Nitric oxide (NO)

B. Types of signaling
1. Autocrine signaling: A response is elicited in the same cell that produces the signaling molecules.

2. Paracrine signaling: A response is elicited in target cells that are in close proximity to the signaling cell.

3. Endocrine signaling: A response is elicited in target cells that are far removed from the signaling cell, with the hormonal signaling molecule carried in the blood.
   - In neuroendocrine signaling, molecules released into the blood from hypothalamic neurosecretory cells act in an endocrine fashion on the anterior pituitary.

C. Classification of receptors (Fig. 1-6)

1. Intracellular receptors are located in the cytoplasm or nucleus and bind lipophilic ligands (e.g., steroid hormones), which diffuse through the plasma membrane.
   a. Ligand binding alters conformation of the receptor, exposing one or more DNA-binding domains in the receptor.

Steroid hormone receptors are located in the cytoplasm or nucleus. Hormone stimulation normally leads to expression of specific target genes.

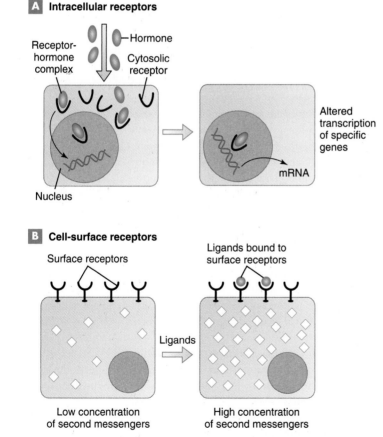

A Intracellular receptors

Receptor-hormone complex — Hormone

Cytosolic receptor

Nucleus

Altered transcription of specific genes

mRNA

B Cell-surface receptors

Surface receptors

Ligands bound to surface receptors

Ligands

Low concentration of second messengers

High concentration of second messengers

1-6: Signaling mediated by two basic types of receptors. **A,** Lipophilic hormones bind to intracellular receptors, forming complexes that stimulate the transcription of specific target genes. **B,** Binding of hydrophilic ligands to cell-surface receptors triggers intracellular signal transduction pathways that commonly involve a second messenger (e.g., cyclic adenosine monophosphate, 1,2-diacylglycerol, Ca^{2+}). Signaling ultimately modulates the activity or expression of specific proteins. mRNA, Messenger ribonucleic acid.

b. The activated ligand–receptor complex binds to the control regions of target genes, activating transcription of these genes.
2. Cell-surface receptors are transmembrane proteins that generally bind hydrophilic ligands. These receptors can be classified into four major types:
   a. Ion-channel receptors: Ligand binding causes the ion channel to open.
      • Examples are nicotinic acetylcholine (ACh) receptors in skeletal muscle cells and receptors for other neurotransmitters (e.g., serotonin, glutamate) in neurons.
   b. Receptors with inherent enzymatic activity: Ligand binding activates the cytosolic catalytic domain of the receptor, which acts as a protein kinase, protein phosphatase, or guanylate cyclase.
      • Examples are insulin receptors and receptors for many growth factors.
   c. Cytokine (tyrosine kinase–linked) receptors: Ligand binding activates tyrosine kinases located in the cytosol.
      • Examples are receptors for cytokines, interferons, human growth hormone, and prolactin.
   d. G protein–linked receptors: Ligand binding leads to the activation of a membrane-associated trimeric G protein, which in turn activates an effector protein that modulates the activity of particular second messengers.
      • Examples are adrenergic receptors, which bind epinephrine and norepinephrine; muscarinic ACh receptor; and receptors for glucagon, thyroid-stimulating hormone (TSH), luteinizing hormone (LH), and adrenocorticotropic hormone (ACTH).
D. Guanosine triphosphate binding proteins—intracellular switches
   • These proteins alternate (switch) between an active state with bound guanosine triphosphate (GTP) and an inactive state with bound guanosine diphosphate (GDP).
   • Examples include trimeric G proteins, which directly interact with G protein–linked receptors, and Ras proteins, which are indirectly coupled to receptors with tyrosine kinase activity.
E. The role of phosphorylation and dephosphorylation in signal transduction
   1. Protein kinases add phosphate groups to specific target proteins, causing conformational changes that modulate protein activity or create docking sites for other proteins.
      • In many signaling pathways, ligand binding to the receptor leads to activation of protein kinases, whose activity transduces the signal.
   2. Protein phosphatases, which remove phosphate groups from specific proteins, oppose the effect of protein kinases.
      • In the absence of ligand binding, the constitutive action of phosphatases inactivates the intracellular signal transduction that is induced by many ligands.
F. Disorders involving defective cell–cell signaling
   1. Mutant Ras proteins are associated with some neoplasms (e.g., colorectal cancer).

Receptors for many hormones, neurotransmitters, and other hydrophilic signaling molecules are transmembrane proteins with ligand-binding sites in their extracellular domain.

- These defective Ras proteins are "turned on" in the absence of normal ligands, leading to neoplastic transformation of cells.
  2. Cholera toxin modifies trimeric G proteins, causing them to remain in the active state in the absence of ligand.
     - Resulting prolonged activation of G proteins → high cAMP levels → movement of water from the blood across the intestinal epithelial cells into the intestinal lumen → massive diarrhea with loss of isotonic fluid
  3. Binding of α-bungarotoxin or curare to nicotinic ACh receptors in skeletal muscle cells leads to paralysis.
  4. Graves' disease is an autoimmune disease in which TSH receptors are stimulated inappropriately by binding of immunoglobulin G (IgG) autoantibodies to the receptor.
     - Manifestations include decreased levels of TSH, enlarged thyroid gland, and hyperthyroidism, leading to symptoms such as exophthalmos (bulging eyes), weight loss, fatigue, hand tremors, and nervousness.

G. Receptor-binding drugs
  1. Agonists bind to and activate receptors, thereby mimicking the action of normal ligands.
  2. Antagonists (e.g., beta blockers) bind to but do not activate receptors, thereby inhibiting the action of normal ligands by competing for binding sites.

V. Specialized Properties of the Plasma Membrane
  - In certain cell types, the plasma membrane has specialized properties that permit it to mediate functions that are not found in other cell types.
  A. Excitability is the ability to respond to stimuli and conduct an action potential.
     - Neurons and muscle cells are the only cells that exhibit excitability.
  B. Specialized attachment areas (cell junctions) are present on cells that are in close contact with other cells.
     1. Morphologic types
        a. Zonula (belt-like) junctions completely encircle cells.
        b. Fascia (sheet-like) junctions form broad areas of contact between cells.
        c. Macula (disk-like) junctions are like "spot welds" on the cell surface.
     2. General functions of cell junctions
        a. Hold cells together into mechanically coherent tissues (adherens and occludens types)
        b. Provide a permeability seal so that tissue as a whole acts as a barrier to diffusion (zonula occludens)
        c. Mediate direct communication between cells so that materials can move from cell to cell without passing through the extracellular space (nexus)
     3. Molecular structure of common cell junctions (Fig. 1-7)
        a. Zonula occludens, or a tight junction, is formed by the interaction of intrinsic membrane proteins (claudins and occludins), thereby fusing the outer leaflets of the plasma membranes of adjacent cells.

Defects in signaling can lead to cancer (abnormal Ras proteins) and Graves' disease (overstimulation of thyroid-stimulating hormone receptors by immunoglobulin G autoantibodies).

Some toxins (e.g., curare) and drugs (e.g., beta blockers) bind to cell-surface receptors and inhibit the action of normal ligands.

Cholera toxin acts on intestinal cells, causing an increase in cyclic adenosine monophosphate, which leads to massive diarrhea.

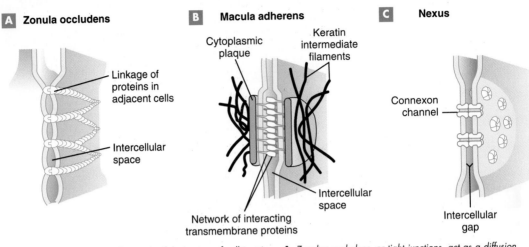

| **A** Zonula occludens | **B** Macula adherens | **C** Nexus |

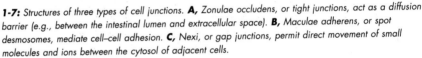

1-7: *Structures of three types of cell junctions. **A,** Zonulae occludens, or tight junctions, act as a diffusion barrier (e.g., between the intestinal lumen and extracellular space). **B,** Maculae adherens, or spot desmosomes, mediate cell–cell adhesion. **C,** Nexi, or gap junctions, permit direct movement of small molecules and ions between the cytosol of adjacent cells.*

   b. Macula adherens, or a spot desmosome, consists of transmembrane proteins that are anchored in cytoplasmic plaques and extend into the intercellular space.
- Adjacent cell membranes are held together by interlocking of the transmembrane proteins (cadherins) into a fibrous network, leaving a substantial space (15 to 35 nm wide) between the membranes.
- Keratin intermediate filaments (tonofibrils) associate with the cytoplasmic plaques (desmoplakins).

   c. Nexus, or a gap junction, is formed by end-to-end association of transmembrane connexon channels in the interacting membranes.
- Six subunits of the protein connexin form each connexon channel.
- Adjacent plasma membranes are separated by a small electron-lucent zone (2 to 3 nm wide) at the gap junctions.

Cytoplasmic Structures

I. Introduction
- The cytoplasm is composed of a fluid phase (cytosol) and three major types of structures: organelles, inclusions, and the cytoskeleton.
  A. Organelles are structural subunits of the cell.
  - Each type of organelle has a characteristic appearance and contains organelle-specific proteins that permit it to carry out specific functions (Fig. 2-1).
  B. Inclusions are particle-like structures that are often transient, insoluble accumulations of metabolites (e.g., glycogen granules, lipid droplets).
  C. The cytoskeleton is a complex collection of macromolecules that provides structural support for the cell and plays a role in cell movement.
  D. Cytosol, the aqueous portion of the cytoplasm in which organelles and inclusions are suspended, contains numerous soluble enzymes.

II. Mitochondria
- In aerobic cells, the mitochondria are the principal sites for the synthesis of adenosine triphosphate (ATP).
  A. Mitochondrial structure (Fig. 2-2)
  - Mitochondria are surrounded by two membranes, which are structurally and functionally distinct.

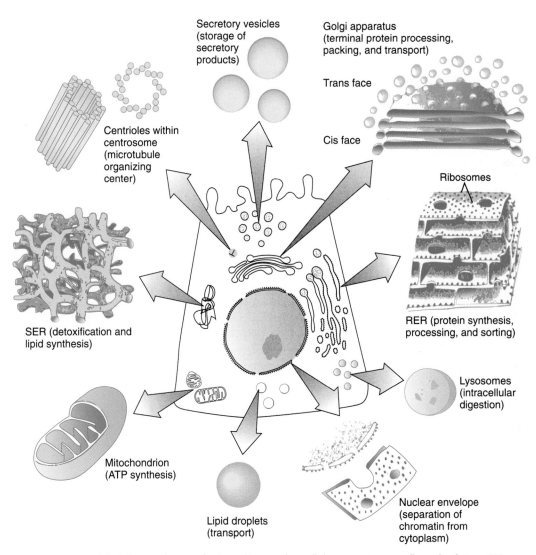

2-1: *Schematic diagram of a "typical" mammalian cell showing major organelles and inclusions. ATP, adenosine triphosphate; RER, rough endoplasmic reticulum; SER, smooth endoplasmic reticulum.*

1. The outer mitochondrial membrane bounds the organelle and is freely permeable to molecules as large as simple sugars.
2. The inner mitochondrial membrane lines the matrix and is relatively impermeable.
   a. Cristae: infoldings of the inner mitochondrial membrane that project into the matrix and are more prominent in metabolically active cells than in quiescent cells
   b. Elementary particles: small particles (9 nm in diameter) that are attached to the inner membrane by a stalk and project into the matrix

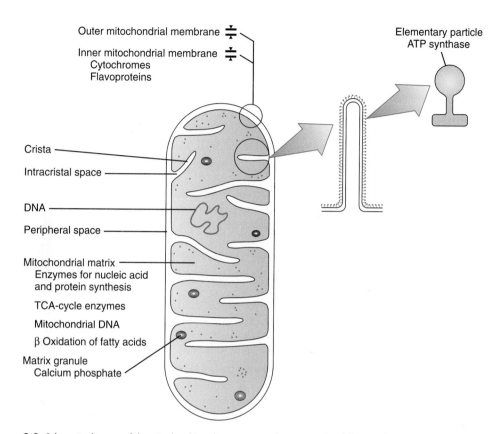

Outer mitochondrial membrane

Inner mitochondrial membrane
Cytochromes
Flavoproteins

Elementary particle
ATP synthase

Crista

Intracristal space

DNA

Peripheral space

Mitochondrial matrix
Enzymes for nucleic acid
and protein synthesis

TCA-cycle enzymes

Mitochondrial DNA

β Oxidation of fatty acids

Matrix granule
Calcium phosphate

2-2: *Schematic diagram of the mitochondrion showing some of its structural and functional components. Both the inner and outer membranes have the typical phospholipid bilayer structure, similar to the plasma membrane. ATP, adenosine triphosphate; DNA, deoxyribonucleic acid; TCA, tricarboxylic acid.*

    3. Membrane-bound compartments in the mitochondrion (see Fig. 2-2)
      a. Peripheral (intermembranous) space
      b. Intracristal space
      c. The matrix region, which contains soluble and insoluble proteins, ribosomes, mitochondrial deoxyribonucleic acid (DNA), and electron-dense granules of calcium phosphate
  B. Mitochondrial ATP production
    1. Location of required enzymes
      a. Tricarboxylic acid (TCA) cycle enzymes are located in the matrix or associated with the inner membrane.
        • These enzymes catalyze the oxidation of acetyl-coenzyme A to CO_2, with generation of reduced coenzymes (NADH and $FADH_2$)
      b. Cytochromes and flavoproteins, which constitute the electron transport system, are localized on the inner membrane.
      c. ATP synthase is localized to the elementary particles associated with the inner membrane.
    2. Mechanisms of mitochondrial ATP production
      • ATP is generated during operation of the TCA cycle.

- Most mitochondrial ATP production involves oxidative phosphorylation via a chemiosmotic coupling mechanism.
  a. As electrons from reduced coenzymes flow through the electron transport system, H^+ ions are pumped from the matrix into the intermembranous space against their electrochemical gradient.
  b. The reverse movement of H^+ ions into the matrix down their electrochemical gradient provides energy for the coupled synthesis of ATP from adenosine diphosphate (ADP) and inorganic phosphate ($P2_i$) by ATP synthase.
C. Biogenesis of mitochondria
  - Mitochondria arise by the division of pre-existing mitochondria (not de novo) and contain their own independent genetic machinery.
  - Most mitochondrial proteins are encoded by nuclear DNA, but a few are encoded by mitochondrial DNA.
  1. Products encoded by mitochondrial DNA
    a. A few subunits of the enzymes required for mitochondrial ATP production
    b. Ribosomal ribonucleic acids (RNAs) and transfer RNAs required for mitochondrial protein synthesis
  2. Synthesis of mitochondrial proteins
    a. Proteins encoded by mitochondrial DNA are synthesized within the mitochondrion on ribosomes assembled within the organelle; these proteins remain with the mitochondria.
    b. Nuclear-encoded mitochondrial proteins are synthesized in the cytosol and imported into the organelle.
  3. Inheritance of mitochondria
    - The ovum contributes most of the mitochondrial DNA to the zygote, whereas the sperm contributes little or none (i.e., maternal inheritance).
D. Diseases associated with defective mitochondria (Box 2-1)

III. Lysosomes
  - Lysosomes function as the digestive system of the cell, degrading many materials taken up by the cell as well as worn-out cellular constituents (e.g., membranes, organelles).
A. Lysosomal enzymes
  1. Acid hydrolases present in the lysosomal lumen are active at acidic pH of approximately 5.0.
    - Examples include acid ribonuclease, acid deoxyribonuclease, acid phosphatase, cathepsins, specific glycosidases, and esterases.
    - These enzymes are inactive if released into the cytoplasm (pH 7.0).
  2. An ATP-powered H^+ pump in the lysosomal membrane pumps H^+ ions into the lysosome, maintaining the acid pH of the lumen.
B. Types of lysosomal activity
  1. Heterophagic function: digestion of materials exogenous to the cell
  2. Autophagic function: digestion of cells and cell components
    - Autolysis: self-destruction of entire cells

HEREDITARY MITOCHONDRIAL DISEASES

Defective mitochondria may exhibit deletions in mitochondrial deoxyribonucleic acid, defects in the enzymes required for the synthesis of adenosine triphosphate, or crystal-like inclusions. These diseases exhibit maternal inheritance. Affected mothers transmit the disease to all of their children, whereas affected fathers do not transmit the disease to any of their children. Tissues with high oxygen demand are most affected by mitochondrial dysfunction.

Mitochondrial encephalomyopathies, which usually present in early adulthood, are characterized by malfunctioning muscle mitochondria and involvement of the central nervous system. Groups of structurally abnormal mitochondria may collect just below the sarcolemma of muscle cells, producing ragged red fibers marked by an irregular contour and staining pattern. There are three common syndromes:

• Kearns-Sayre syndrome: pain in the eyes, degeneration of retinal pigments, progressive weakness of the extraocular muscles, and cardiac conduction defect, which may cause death. Ragged red fibers seen on muscle biopsy.
• MELAS syndrome: mitochondrial encephalomyopathy, lactic acidosis, and stroke-like episodes.
• MERRF syndrome: myoclonus epilepsy with ragged red fibers.

Another mitochondrial disease, Leber's hereditary optic atrophy, is caused by a defect in one of the electron transport complexes. It is characterized by progressive loss of central vision and eventual blindness due to degeneration of the optic nerve. This disease affects more males than females, with onset most commonly occurring in the third decade.

C. Stages in lysosomal digestion (Fig. 2-3)
  1. Endocytic vesicles arise by phagocytosis (phagosome), pinocytosis, or receptor-mediated endocytosis (endosome).
  2. Primary lysosomes arise by budding from the Golgi apparatus.
  3. Secondary lysosomes, the sites where digestion occurs, include two types of digestive vacuoles.
     a. Heterophagic vacuoles, formed by the fusion of primary lysosomes with endocytic vesicles
     b. Autophagic vacuoles, formed by fusion of primary lysosomes with sequestered cellular constituents
  4. Postdigestive secondary lysosomes
     a. Residual bodies: largely indigestible residues of heterophagic and autophagic activity
     b. Lipofuscin granules: large accumulations of lipid-rich material remaining after lysosomal activity in long-lived cells that do not divide

Increased amounts of lipofuscin, an indigestible lipid-rich material within residual bodies, imparts a brown discoloration to tissue. Lipofuscin is sometimes called the "wear and tear" pigment, and the level often is elevated in the elderly.

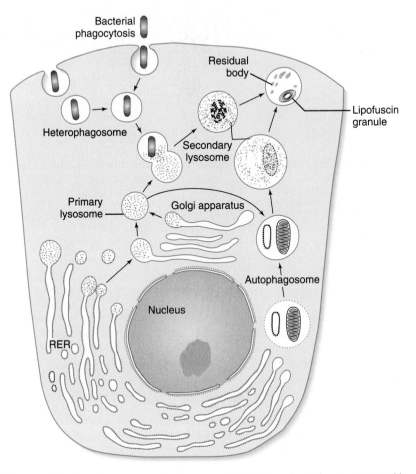

2-3: *Lysosomal digestion of exogenous and endogenous materials. Heterophagic digestion is initiated by phagocytosis of a bacterium (upper left) or by receptor-mediated endocytosis (see Fig. 1-5). Autophagic digestion is initiated by sequestration of cellular components within a membrane (lower right). Residual bodies and lipofuscin granules are remnants remaining after both types of digestion. RER, rough endoplasmic reticulum. (Adapted from Junquiera LC, Carneiro J: Basic Histology, 7th ed. East Norwalk, CT: Appleton-Lange, 1992, p 42.)*

- Lipofuscin is increased in tissues undergoing atrophy and in tissues damaged by free radicals (solutes with unpaired electrons in their outer orbit).

D. Lysosomal storage diseases (Table 2-1)
  - An inherited deficiency of one or more lysosomal enzymes causes accumulation of materials that normally would be degraded. Clinical manifestations can involve multiple tissues and organs.

IV. Peroxisomes
  - Also known as microbodies, peroxisomes are membrane-bound organelles that function in the β-oxidation of long-chain fatty acids and the catabolism of toxic metabolites.

Lysosomal storage diseases (e.g., Tay-Sachs disease, Pompe's disease) result from defective lysosomal enzymes.

TABLE 2-1:
Inherited
Lysosomal Storage
Diseases

Disorder	Accumulated Material	Clinical Features
Mucopolysaccharidosis	Glycosaminoglycans (GAGs) in many tissues and organs	Presence of GAGs in urine Other manifestations depend on which GAGs accumulate (see Box 5-1)
I-cell disease	Many compounds normally degraded in lysosomes (inability to phosphorylate mannose residues that target proteins to lysosomes)	Absence of lysosomal enzymes in lysosomes Severe growth impairment, extreme mental and motor retardation, clear corneas Fibroblasts contain many dark inclusions Onset in young children; fatal
Pompe's disease (type II glycogen storage disease)	Glycogen (deficiency of α-1,4-glycosidase)	Enlarged liver and heart, hypotonia, mental and motor retardation Usually fatal in infants and children In adults, muscle weakness and respiratory problems but usually not fatal
Tay-Sachs disease	Ganglioside in nervous tissue	Doll-like facies, cherry-red macular spot, seizures, hypotonia, early blindness Onset in infancy; death by age 5 years

  A. Peroxisomal enzymes
    1. Oxidases metabolize various substrates, yielding hydrogen peroxide (H_2O_2), which is toxic to cells.
    2. Catalase, present in all peroxisomes, breaks down H_2O_2 to yield H_2O and O_2.
  B. Peroxisomal disorders
    1. Zellweger syndrome (cerebrohepatorenal syndrome) results from the absence of all peroxisomal enzymes in the brain, liver, and kidneys.
      • Clinical manifestations include craniofacial abnormalities, jaundice, hypotonia, hepatomegaly, and polycystic kidneys.
    2. Adrenoleukodystrophy, a sex-linked recessive disease, is marked by impaired peroxisomal oxidation of very long–chain fatty acids, leading to lipid accumulation in the brain, spinal cord, and adrenal glands.
      • Clinical manifestations include mental deterioration (aphasia, apraxia), abnormal adrenal function, and loss of vision.

V. Ribosomes
  • Ribosomes are particle-like ribonucleoprotein complexes that function as the cell's protein-synthesizing machinery.
  A. Structure and function of ribosomes

TABLE 2-2: Ribosomal Subunits

Subunit	Ribosomal Ribonucleic Acid*	Functions
Small (40S)	18	Binds messenger ribonucleic acid and aminoacyl transfer ribonucleic acids Locates AUG start codon
Large (60S)	28S	Binds to small subunit after start codon is located Has peptidyl transferase activity
	5.8S, 5S	

*Each subunit contains one molecule of each ribosomal ribonucleic acid species indicated plus numerous proteins.

- Each ribosome comprises a small and a large subunit, the composition and functions of which differ (Table 2-2).
  1. Ribosome formation: Small (40S) and large (60S) ribosomal subunits exist free in the cytoplasm until they associate with a messenger RNA (mRNA) to form a complete ribosome (80S).
  2. Translation: An 80S ribosome moves along the bound mRNA, adding individual amino acids to the nascent protein chain one at a time.
     a. Codons in the mRNA bound to the small subunit sequentially base-pair with anti-codons in the corresponding activated transfer RNA (tRNA)–amino acid complexes (aminoacyl-tRNAs).
     b. Peptidyl transferase activity of the large subunit sequentially transfers aligned amino acids to the growing peptide chain, and free tRNAs then are released from the ribosome.
  3. Chain termination: Translation ceases when a ribosome encounters a stop codon, causing release of the protein chain and dissociation of the ribosome into its subunits.
  B. Functional states of ribosomes (Fig. 2-4)
  1. Polysomes are extended arrays of individual ribosomes that are all associated with a single strand of mRNA.
     - The length of a polysome and the number of ribosomes composing it reflect the length of the mRNA.
  2. Free polysomes in the cytoplasm carry out synthesis of cytosolic proteins and proteins destined for the nucleus, peroxisomes, and mitochondria.
  3. Polysomes attached to the endoplasmic reticulum (ER) carry out synthesis of all other proteins except those encoded by mitochondrial DNA.

VI. Endoplasmic Reticulum
   - The ER is an anastomosing intracytoplasmic membrane system consisting of vesicular, tubular, and broad cisternal profiles often arranged in regular arrays (see Fig. 2-1).
   - The membranes of the ER are continuous with the nuclear envelope and are highly pleomorphic.
   A. Structural and functional elements of the ER
   1. The rough endoplasmic reticulum (RER) has a studded ("rough") appearance due to ribosomes attached to its outer (cytosolic) surface.

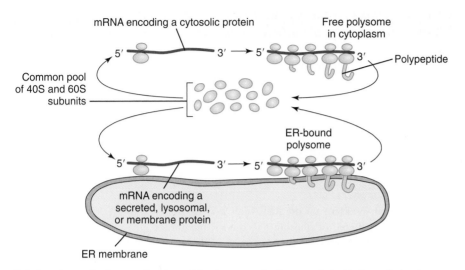

2-4: *Two classes of polysomes. Free (cytosolic) polysomes and polysomes attached to the endoplasmic reticulum (ER) are assembled from a common pool of ribosomal subunits. Each class of polysome synthesizes specific types of proteins. mRNA, messenger ribonucleic acid. (Adapted from Alberts B: Molecular Biology of the Cell, 3rd ed. New York: Garland, 1994, p. 579.)*

- The RER functions in the synthesis and post-translation modification of the following:
    a. Proteins secreted from the cell surface
    b. Soluble luminal enzymes within the ER, Golgi apparatus, and lysosomes
    c. Intrinsic membrane proteins in the plasma membrane and in the ER, Golgi, and lysosomal membranes
  2. The smooth endoplasmic reticulum (SER) shows continuities with the RER but has no attached ribosomes and is not involved in protein synthesis.
B. Functions of the SER
  1. Lipid metabolism
     - The SER is most prominent in lipid-metabolizing cells (see Fig. 4-6). Enzymes localized to the SER catalyze synthesis of the following lipids:
    a. Fatty acids and glycerol
    b. Steroid hormones
    c. Phospholipids and cholesterol, which are incorporated into the cytosolic side of the ER membrane
       - Phospholipid translocases (flippases) transfer some of these to the luminal side of the membrane.
  2. Detoxification by the cytochrome P-450 system
     - In liver cells, SER enzymes in the cytochrome P-450 system modify many toxic substances (e.g., ingested alcohol, pesticide residues, certain drugs), forming less harmful, water-soluble compounds.

The cytochrome P-450 system within the smooth endoplasmic reticulum is important in drug metabolism. Its activity is enhanced by alcohol and barbiturates and inhibited by histamine and proton blockers.

    a. Enhanced by certain drugs (e.g., alcohol, barbiturates, phenytoin), leading to increased metabolism of drugs and increased synthesis of γ-glutamyl transferase

    b. Inhibited by certain drugs (e.g., histamine, proton blockers), leading to drug toxicities

  3. Ca^{2+} storage
- Sequestration and release of Ca^{2+} from the SER is critical in regulating the cytosolic Ca^{2+} level, which mediates various cell functions, including muscle contraction.

  4. Glycogen metabolism
- In liver cells, SER enzymes are involved in the synthesis and breakdown of glycogen.

C. Protein synthesis on the RER (Fig. 2-5)
  1. Attachment of ribosomes to the ER membrane

    a. All proteins synthesized on the ER possess an ER signal sequence (or signal peptide), typically located at the amino-terminal end.

    b. Protein synthesis begins on free polysomes, but once the signal sequence is formed and extruded from a ribosome, it interacts with a signal-recognition particle (SRP) in the cytosol.

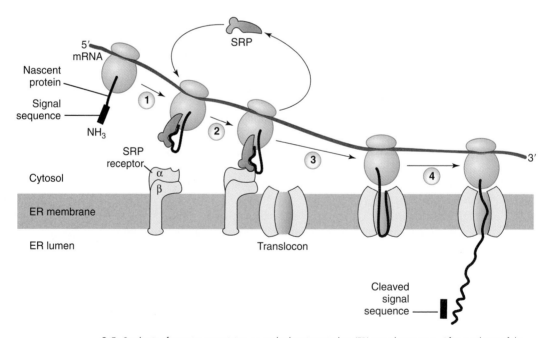

2-5: *Synthesis of proteins containing an endoplasmic reticulum (ER) signal sequence. After synthesis of the signal sequence on a free ribosome in the cytosol, the ribosome becomes attached to the ER membrane with the aid of a signal-recognition particle (SRP) and an SRP receptor (1 and 2). The SRP then dissociates, the ribosome-nascent protein associates with a translocon, and the polypeptide chain enters the open channel in the translocon (3). As translation continues, the elongating polypeptide is translocated into the ER lumen. The signal sequence is subsequently cleaved (4). mRNA, messenger ribonucleic acid. (Adapted from Lodish HA, Berk SL, Zipursky P, Darnell J: Molecular Cell Biology, 4th ed. New York: WH Freeman, 2000, p 698.)*

      c. The SRP–ribosome complex binds transiently to a docking protein in the ER membrane called the *SRP receptor.*

      d. The SRP is released and the ribosome-nascent protein is transferred to a translocator protein complex (translocon) in the ER membrane.

  2. Co-translational translocation

      a. Once the signal sequence is inserted into the transmembrane channel of the translocon, translation of the ER-bound mRNA continues.

      b. The elongating protein chain moves through the translocon channel into the ER lumen.

        (1) Water-soluble proteins: The entire polypeptide chain is translocated into the lumen of the RER; the signal peptide is cleaved off.

        (2) Intrinsic membrane proteins: One or more hydrophobic domains in the polypeptide anchor the protein to the membrane; the signal peptide may or may not be cleaved off.

  3. Glycosylation of proteins

    • Within the RER, a common N-linked oligosaccharide is attached covalently to asparagine residues in nearly all newly synthesized proteins.

  4. Sorting of RER-synthesized proteins

      a. Organelle-specific retention signals direct proteins to their appropriate destinations (default pathways).

      • For example, proteins that are to remain in the ER contain an ER retention signal, which keeps them localized within the ER.

      b. Transfer (transport) vesicles bud off from transitional elements lying between the RER and the SER and fuse with the Golgi apparatus.

      • All RER-synthesized proteins that lack an ER retention signal move to the Golgi apparatus via transfer vesicles.

      c. Recovery pathways

      • Proteins that are not sorted to their proper destinations often can be recovered and resorted via various recovery pathways.

VII. Golgi Apparatus

  • The detailed morphology and intracellular location of the Golgi apparatus vary among cell types.

  A. Structure of the Golgi apparatus

    • In the electron microscope, the Golgi apparatus is visualized as stacks of flattened, disk-shaped saccules bound by a typical trilaminar membrane (see Fig. 2-1).

  1. The cis (immature) face of the Golgi, directed toward the ER, consists of forming cisternae and adjacent transfer vesicles derived from transitional elements of the ER.

  2. The mid-Golgi region consists of a few cisternae between the cis and trans faces.

  3. The trans (mature) face of the Golgi, directed away from the ER, consists of cisternae that bud off to form secretory vesicles and lysosome-bound transfer vesicles.

  B. Functions of the Golgi apparatus

  1. Processing of proteins and lipids delivered from the ER

In the Golgi apparatus, secreted and membrane proteins undergo processing and are sorted to their final destinations.

- Enzymes localized to the cis, medial, or trans portion of the Golgi catalyze specific modifications (Fig. 2-6).
  a. Removal and addition of sugar residues to N-linked oligosaccharides
  b. Formation of O-linked oligosaccharides by sequential addition of sugar residues to serine and threonine residues
  c. Phosphorylation of N-linked oligosaccharides, forming mannose-6-phosphate residues, which target proteins to lysosomes
     - Mannose-6-phosphate receptors in lysosomes segregate these enzymes into lysosome.
  d. Sulfation of the oligosaccharide side chains on proteoglycan core proteins (see Chapter 5)
  e. Proteolytic cleavage of some precursor membrane and secreted proteins, releasing the active proteins
  f. Glycosylation of membrane lipids delivered to the Golgi from the SER
2. Macromolecule sorting from the trans Golgi
  a. After they are processed in the Golgi, proteins and lipids are incorporated into vesicles that bud off from the trans face of the Golgi.
  b. Each vesicle must take up only the appropriate proteins and fuse only with the appropriate target membrane.
3. Distribution of oligosaccharides
  a. The Golgi and RER enzymes that form and modify oligosaccharide side chains are localized to the luminal surface of these organelles.
  b. Thus, oligosaccharides in membrane glycoproteins and glycolipids face the lumen of intracellular organelles, but they become located on the external surface of the plasma membrane during exocytosis.

VIII. Cytoskeleton (Fig. 2-7)
   - The three major components of the cytoskeleton—microtubules, microfilaments, and intermediate filaments—are formed from different proteins, exhibit characteristic structures, and have distinct functions.
   A. Microtubules (see Fig. 2-7A)
      1. Structure and polarity of microtubules
        a. Each microtubule is a hollow cylinder (outer diameter $\approx 24\,nm$) with a rigid wall composed of 13 protofilaments, each of which is a linear polymer of $\alpha\beta$-tubulin dimers.
        b. The plus end is capable of rapid growth by the addition of tubulin dimers, a process that requires guanosine triphosphate (GTP).
        c. The minus end loses dimers but is stabilized in most cells by association with the microtubule organizing center, or centrosome.
      2. Microtubule-associated proteins (MAPs)
        a. Assembly MAPs function primarily to stabilize microtubules, cross-linking them to each other and to other structures.
        b. Motor MAPs (motor proteins) use energy from ATP hydrolysis to walk or slide along microtubules, usually carrying vesicles with them.
          (1) Dyneins move toward the minus end of microtubules.
          (2) Kinesins move toward the plus end of microtubules.

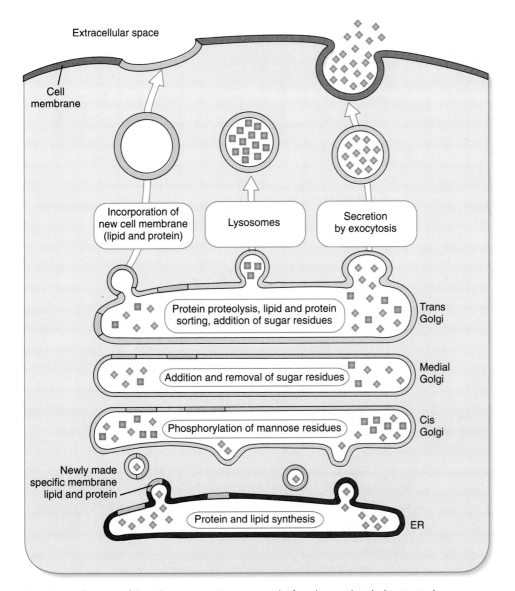

2-6: *Functional regions of the Golgi apparatus. Transport vesicles from the smooth endoplasmic reticulum and rough endoplasmic reticulum fuse with the cis Golgi. This region contains enzymes that phosphorylate mannose residues in the N-linked oligosaccharides of proteins destined for lysosomes. Glycosylation of proteins and membrane lipids occurs in the medial Golgi and is completed in the trans Golgi. Vesicles containing specific macromolecules bud from the trans Golgi and eventually fuse with the corresponding target membranes. ER, endoplasmic reticulum. (Adapted from Stevens A, Lowe JS: Human Histology, 2nd ed. London: Mosby, 1997, p 21.)*

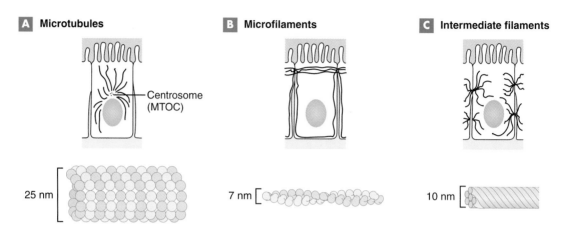

2-7: *Comparison of the three major elements of the cytoskeleton.* **A,** *Microtubules;* **B,** *microfilaments;* **C,** *intermediate filaments. MTOC, microtubule organizing center.*

3. Microtubule-containing structures
   * Microtubules are found in the cytoplasm of all cells radiating from the centrosome, or microtubule organizing center, which regulates their growth.
   * In addition, microtubules are organized into several specialized structures:
   a. The mitotic spindle and centrioles, which are found in most cells
   b. Cilia, flagella, and basal bodies, which have a more limited distribution (see Chapter 4)
      * Immotile cilia syndrome is caused by irregular dynein arms, leading to a loss of ciliary movement. This is characteristic of Kartagener's syndrome, which also is marked by situs inversus (e.g., heart on the right), bronchiectasis, infertility in men and women, and sinusitis.
4. Functions of microtubules
   a. Development and maintenance of cell shape
   b. Intracellular transport of materials within the cytosol
   c. Movement of the cilia, flagella, and chromosomes
B. Microfilaments (see Fig. 2-7B)
   1. Structure and polarity of microfilaments
      a. Globular G-actin monomers polymerize in the presence of ATP to form fibrous F-actin, a threadlike, two-stranded helical filament approximately 6 nm thick.
      b. Monomers are added rapidly to one end (the plus end) and more slowly to the other end (the minus end).
      c. Treadmilling, the continual addition of monomers at the plus end and loss of monomers from the minus end of a microfilament, results in no change in length.

Kartagener's syndrome is associated with irregular dynein arms in the cilia, leading to a loss of ciliary movement.

2. Actin-binding proteins
   - Many functions of microfilaments depend on their association with various proteins. Examples include:
   a. Anchoring proteins (e.g., spectrin in erythrocytes, dystrophin in muscle) link the cortical actin network to the plasma membrane.
      - Spectrin is important in maintaining the biconcave disk shape of red blood cells.
      - Congenital spherocytosis, an autosomal dominant disease, is characterized by a defect in spectrin, leading to the formation of spherocytes and a chronic hemolytic anemia.
   b. Cross-linking proteins (e.g., actinin, filamin) organize actin filaments into fibers, parallel arrays, or networks.
   c. Myosins are motor proteins that slide along actin filaments in muscle and nonmuscle cells, generating movement.
3. Functions of microfilaments
   a. Movement in nonmuscle cells (labile microfilaments)
   b. Contraction of muscle (stable microfilaments)
   c. Support and maintenance of cell shape (cortical actin network)
   d. Control of cell viscosity (sol-gel transformation)
   e. Adhesion to the extracellular matrix and to other cells
C. Intermediate filaments (see Fig. 2-7C)
   - Intermediate filaments primarily provide mechanical support to cells and help organize cells into tissues.
   - Several types of proteins, exhibiting conserved and variable domains, form intermediate filaments.
   1. Structure of intermediate filaments
      a. Protein monomers associate laterally to form dimers with a long coiled-coil central region; additional lateral and end-to-end associations generate ropelike (to 10-nm–thick) filaments.

> In congenital spherocytosis, a defect in spectrin in the cell membrane results in a chronic hemolytic anemia.

> The origin of some tumors can be determined by identifying which intermediate filament proteins they possess. Tumors of epithelial origin contain keratins and lack vimentin. Tumors of muscle origin contain desmin.

TABLE 2-3:
Major Types of Intermediate Filament (IF) Proteins

IF Protein	Location	Function
Desmin	Muscle cells	Helps stabilize sarcomeres
Glial fibrillary acidic protein (glial filaments)	Glial cells of central nervous system	Provides structural support
Keratins	Epithelial cells	Form major part of protective outer layer of skin; assist in cell adhesion by attaching to desmosomes (tonofilaments)
Lamins	Nucleus of all cells	Provide supportive network underneath inner nuclear membrane
Neurofilament proteins	Axons of mature neurons	Form core of axons and determine their diameter
Vimentin	Fibroblasts, leukocytes, and other cells of mesenchymal origin	Supports cellular membranes; associates with microtubules

    b. Unlike microtubules and microfilaments, intermediate filaments do not continually add and lose monomers and thus form much more permanent structures.

2. Distribution of intermediate filaments
   - Several classes of intermediate filaments exhibit cell type–specific distribution, as indicated in Table 2-3.

3

Nucleus and Cell Division

- Structure of chromatin and packing into chromosomes
- Functional elements of chromosomes
- Synthesis and processing of messenger ribonucleic acid
- Role of the nucleolus in the formation of ribosomal subunits
- Cell cycle and its regulation
- Comparison of mitosis and meiosis
- Drug-induced cell-cycle arrest, psoriasis, tumor-suppressor genes, proto-oncogenes, Down syndrome, Turner's syndrome, and other disorders resulting from abnormal cell division

I. Nuclear Structures (Fig. 3-1)
- The nucleus serves as a repository for genetic material (deoxyribonucleic acid [DNA]) and as the site for duplication of DNA and transcription of DNA into ribonucleic acids (RNAs).
  A. Nuclear envelope: a double membrane consisting of two trilaminar membranes with a narrow perinuclear cisterna between them
  1. The outer nuclear membrane is continuous in places with the rough endoplasmic reticulum and is studded with ribosomes on its external surface.
  2. The inner nuclear membrane is separated from the nuclear contents by the nuclear lamina, a fibrous meshwork composed of lamin intermediate filaments.
  3. Nuclear pores are found where the inner and outer membranes fuse.
     - A multiprotein nuclear pore complex associated with each pore actively transports macromolecules in and out of the nucleus.
     - Small, water-soluble molecules can diffuse through aqueous channels in the nuclear pore complex.
  B. Nucleoplasm (karyoplasm): the protoplasm within the nucleus, consisting of a fluid portion, a proteinaceous matrix, and various ribonucleoprotein particles
  C. Nucleolus: a nuclear region not bound by a membrane that is involved in the synthesis of ribosomal RNA (rRNA) and its assembly into ribosomal subunits

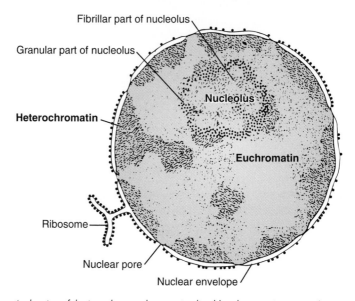

Fibrillar part of nucleolus

Granular part of nucleolus

Nucleolus

Heterochromatin

Euchromatin

Ribosome

Nuclear pore

Nuclear envelope

3-1: *Schematic drawing of the interphase nucleus as visualized by electron microscopy. A narrow space separates the two membranes composing the nuclear envelope. Two types of chromatin are evident: a diffuse form, euchromatin, that is transcriptionally active, and a dense form, heterochromatin, that is largely inactive in transcription. During cell division, the chromatin becomes sufficiently coiled for individual chromosomes to be visible, and the nucleolus disappears. (Adapted from Junquiera LC, Carneiro J: Basic Histology, 7th ed. East Norwalk, CT: Appleton-Lange, 1992, p 51.)*

1. Granular elements are 20- to 30-nm particles representing maturing ribosomal precursors.
2. Fibrillar elements may be intermingled or separated to form a fibrillar core and a granular cortex (the site of rRNA precursor synthesis).

D. Chromatin and chromosomes: the forms in which nuclear DNA exists within cells

- Chromatin is a complex of double-stranded DNA associated with histone proteins.

1. Two forms of isolated chromatin (Fig. 3-2A–C):
   a. In the extended beads-on-a-string form, beadlike nucleosomes are separated by a region of linker DNA.
      (1) The nucleosome core contains two molecules each of the histones H2A, H2B, H3, and H4.
      (2) DNA is wrapped around each nucleosome core approximately two turns.
   b. In the compact 30-nm fiber form, the nucleosomes are packed more closely together in a solenoid arrangement, and a fifth histone (H1) interacts with the DNA between nucleosomes.
2. Metaphase chromosomes
   - Extensive packing of chromatin with the aid of nonhistone scaffold proteins yields highly condensed chromosomes during metaphase (Fig. 3-2D–F).

Antibodies against histones are characteristic of drug-induced lupus.

Antibodies against double-stranded DNA and nuclear protein are characteristic of systemic lupus erythematosus.

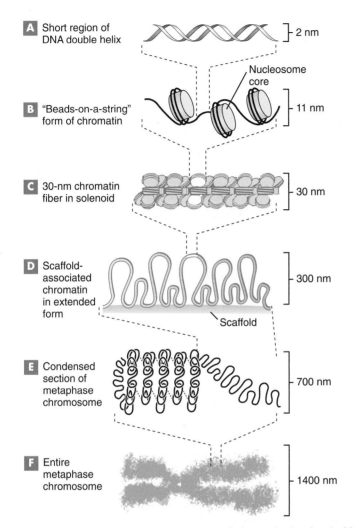

A Short region of DNA double helix — 2 nm

Nucleosome core

B "Beads-on-a-string" form of chromatin — 11 nm

C 30-nm chromatin fiber in solenoid — 30 nm

D Scaffold-associated chromatin in extended form — 300 nm

Scaffold

E Condensed section of metaphase chromosome — 700 nm

F Entire metaphase chromosome — 1400 nm

3-2: *Model of chromatin packing. A nucleosome core is composed of two molecules of each of four types of histone protein with double-stranded deoxyribonucleic acid (DNA) coiled around it twice (**A** and **B**). An additional histone molecule is associated with the surface of each nucleosome (not shown). In interphase chromosomes, long stretches of 30-nm chromatin (**C**) loop out from a protein scaffold (**D**). Further folding of the scaffold yields the highly condensed structure of a metaphase chromosome (**E** and **F**).*

   a. Only during metaphase can chromosomes be visualized as separate structures by light microscopy.
   b. Because the chromosomes are duplicated during the S phase of the cell cycle, a metaphase chromosome is composed of two chromatids, which are attached at a constricted region, the centromere.
   c. Metaphase chromosomes of each species have characteristic sizes, shapes, and banding patterns; the entire set is known as the *karyotype.*
3. Essential functional components of chromosomes
   a. Replication origins: unique protein-binding DNA segments required for replication of DNA in chromosomes

  b. Telomeres: regions at the ends of chromosomes that prevent their shortening during replication
  c. Centromere: region of metaphase chromosomes from which kinetochore fibers extend to the spindle pole; required for proper distribution of chromatids to daughter cells
4. States of chromatin activity (see Fig. 3-1)
  a. Euchromatin: a diffuse, lightly staining form of chromatin that is active in RNA synthesis
    • During interphase, much of the nuclear DNA is present as euchromatin.
  b. Heterochromatin: a condensed, densely staining form of chromatin that is relatively inactive in RNA synthesis
    • Some transcriptionally inactive DNA regions are permanent and present in all cells; others occur in certain tissues or periods of the cell cycle.

II. Transcription of DNA into RNA
  • A gene represents a discrete region of the genome, including a coding region and regulatory sequences, that is required for production of a functional RNA.
  A. Three types of RNA function in protein synthesis.
    1. Messenger RNAs (mRNAs) direct the assembly of amino acids into proteins.
    2. Ribosomal RNAs (rRNAs) form part of ribosomes, the ribonucleoprotein particles on which protein synthesis occurs (see Table 2-2).
    3. Transfer RNAs (tRNAs) carry amino acids to the ribosomes for incorporation into growing proteins.
  B. Synthesis of mRNA occurs outside the nucleolus (Fig. 3-3).
    1. RNA polymerase II catalyzes transcription of protein coding genes into a primary RNA transcript, or pre-mRNA.
    2. Processing to yield functional mRNA entails three basic steps:
      a. 5′ capping: addition of methylated guanine nucleotide to the 5′ end of pre-mRNA
      b. Polyadenylation: addition of multiple adenylate (A) residues at the 3′ end of pre-mRNA
      c. Splicing: removal of noncoding introns and joining of exons by large ribonucleoprotein complexes called *spliceosomes*
  C. Synthesis of rRNA and ribosomal subunits occurs within the nucleolus.
    1. Nucleolar organizer DNA consists of tandem arrays of 45S rRNA genes located on several chromosomes in humans.
    2. RNA polymerase I catalyzes transcription of pre-rRNA genes within the fibrillar regions of the nucleolus, yielding 45S RNA precursors.
    3. Assembly of ribosomal subunits occurs within the granular regions of the nucleolus and involves the following steps (Fig. 3-4):
      a. Packaging of the 45S rRNA precursor with ribosomal proteins imported from the cytoplasm to form ribonucleoprotein particles

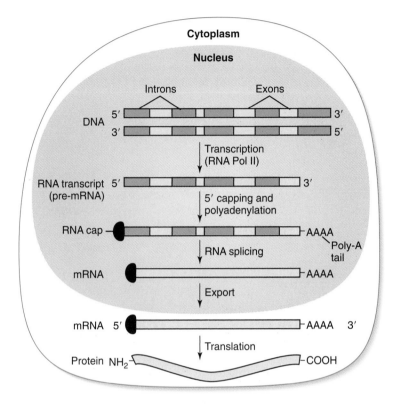

3-3: *Expression of a protein-coding gene. The deoxyribonucleic acid (DNA) sequence, containing coding exons and noncoding introns, is transcribed into a primary ribonucleic acid (RNA) transcript, or pre-messenger RNA (mRNA), by RNA polymerase II (Pol II). Processing of the pre-mRNA yields a functional mRNA, which is translocated through nuclear pores to the cytoplasm, where it is translated into the amino acid sequence of the encoded protein on ribosomes.*

  b. Processing and cleavage of 45S RNA within the ribonucleoprotein particles and addition of 5S RNA that is produced outside the nucleolus
  c. Separation into large (60S) and small (40S) ribosomal subunits and their transport through nuclear pores to the cytoplasm
 D. Differential gene expression, the selective production by a cell of only some of the proteins encoded in the genome, results primarily from regulation of transcription.
   • Different cell types express specific sets of genes related to their unique cellular activities. During development, various genes are turned on and off in highly specific temporal and spatial patterns.
   1. Transcription factors are proteins that bind to regulatory sequences in DNA and modulate the expression of the associated genes.
   2. Reversible modifications to histones (e.g., acetylation, phosphorylation) that lead to more condensed or less condensed packing of chromatin also affect its transcriptional activity.

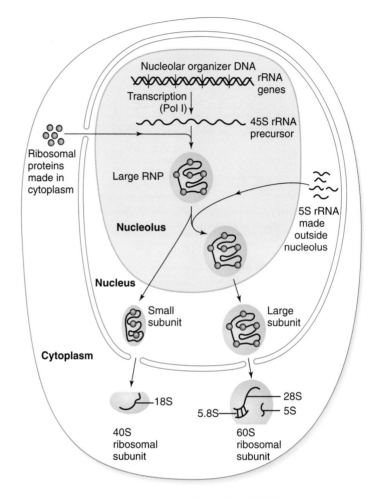

3-4: *Formation of ribosomal subunits. Loops of deoxyribonucleic acid (DNA) containing tandem arrays of 45S ribosomal ribonucleic acid (rRNA) genes function as nucleolar organizers. Transcription of these genes by RNA polymerase I (Pol I) yields the 45S rRNA precursor, which associates with ribosomal and nucleolar proteins into a ribonucleoprotein particle (RNP). Processing involves cleavage of 45S rRNA into 18S, 5.8S, and 28S rRNAs; separation of large and small subunits; and incorporation of 5S rRNA (made outside the nucleolus) into large subunits. Nucleolar proteins involved in processing are recycled within the nucleolus. After their transport to the cytoplasm, large and small subunits associate with each other and with an mRNA molecule to form a functional ribosome.*

III. Cell Cycle

    A. Phases of the cell cycle (Fig. 3-5)

        • The duration of the G_1 phase varies considerably in different cell types, whereas the duration of other phases is relatively constant in different cell types.

        1. G_1 phase: The cell prepares for the S phase.

            a. Cells with a very long G_1 phase, called *resting (quiescent) cells,* are considered to have temporarily exited the cell cycle and entered the G_0 phase.

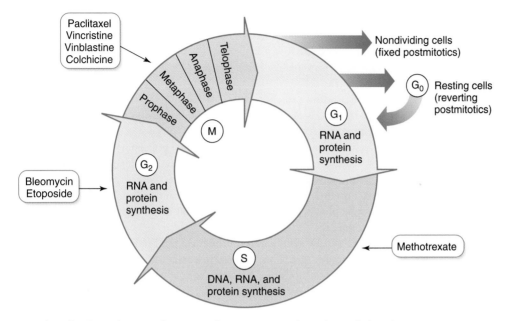

3-5: *The cell cycle in eukaryotic cells. G_1, S, and G_2 constitute interphase, during which synthetic activity takes place. Deoxyribonucleic acid (DNA) synthesis occurs only during the S phase. The major stages of mitosis (M) are indicated. Differentiated cells that no longer divide under any circumstances (e.g., neurons) have left the cycle. Cells that have temporarily stopped dividing (i.e., have very long G_1) but can re-enter the cycle are considered to be resting cells in G_0. Certain drugs arrest cells at the indicated stages of the cell cycle. RNA, ribonucleic acid.*

- Examples are cells of the adrenal cortex, liver cells, and cultured fibroblasts in the absence of growth factors.
  b. Variation in the G_1 phase of neoplastic cells compared with their normal counterparts is primarily responsible for their abnormally long or short cell cycle.
2. S (synthesis) phase: The cell duplicates chromosomal DNA, yielding two chromatids per chromosome.
   a. C amount of DNA is the amount found in the gametes of a species.
   b. Somatic cells have 2C DNA in G_1 and 4C DNA in G_2 after DNA replication.
   c. *Ploidy* refers to the status of the basic chromosome set characteristic of a species and is indicated by *n*.
      (1) Haploid cells = 1*n* = gametes; normal human gametes contain 23 chromosomes.
      (2) Diploid cells = 2*n* = somatic cells; normal human somatic cells contain 46 chromosomes, 23 pairs of homologous chromosomes, with one member of each pair derived from the maternal parent and one from the paternal parent.
3. G_2 phase: The cell prepares for division (e.g., synthesis of tubulin, which is necessary for formation of the mitotic spindle).

4. M (mitotic) phase: Chromatids of duplicated chromosomes segregate toward the spindle poles and the cytoplasm divides (cytokinesis), forming two daughter cells.
   - The M phase generally is the shortest.

B. Regulation of the cell cycle

   1. Cell-cycle control proteins
      - Two major classes of proteins regulate progression through the cell cycle.
      a. Cyclin-dependent protein kinases (Cdks) phosphorylate various target proteins, thereby modulating their activity at different cell-cycle phases.
      b. Cyclins activate Cdks by binding to them.
         - Concentrations of various cyclins rise and fall throughout the cell-cycle phases, leading to the formation of specific cyclin–Cdk complexes.
         (1) Cyclin D, synthesized during early G_1, binds to Cdk4, forming a complex that allows the cell to enter the S phase.
         (2) Cyclin A binds to Cdk1 and Cdk2, forming complexes that allow the cell to progress from the S phase to the G_2 phase and induce the synthesis of cyclin B.
         (3) Cyclin B, synthesized during G_2, binds to Cdk, forming a complex that allows the cell to enter mitosis (M).

   2. Cell-cycle checkpoints
      - Under certain circumstances, arrest of the cell cycle at one of several checkpoints prevents major damage to cells.
      a. G_1 checkpoint: The presence of damaged DNA stops the cycle before entry into the S phase, thus avoiding replication of damaged DNA, which could perpetuate mutations and lead to chromosomal rearrangements.
      b. G_2 checkpoint: The presence of unreplicated or damaged DNA stops the cycle before entry into mitosis.
      c. M checkpoint: Improper spindle formation stops the cycle partway through mitosis, thereby preventing mis-segregation of chromatids to daughter cells.

   3. Role of tumor-suppressor genes in cell-cycle control
      a. Retinoblastoma (Rb) protein, encoded by the *RB* suppressor gene on chromosome 13, inhibits progression from the G_1 phase to the S phase.
         (1) Phosphorylation of Rb protein by an active cyclin D–Cdk4 complex allows the cell to enter the S phase.
         (2) Inactivation of the *RB* suppressor gene accelerates cell entry into the S phase.
      b. The p53 protein, encoded by the *p53* suppressor gene on chromosome 17, is stabilized by damaged DNA, leading to its accumulation.
         (1) Inhibition of cyclin D–Cdk4 activity by p53 protein keeps the cell in G_1 for DNA repair (G_1 arrest) or apoptosis if damage is too extensive.
         (2) Inactivation of the *p53* suppressor gene permits the cell to enter the S phase continuously.

C. Drugs that target the cell cycle (see Fig. 3-5)
- Many antineoplastic drugs reduce cell proliferation by blocking progression through the cell cycle.
1. Colchicine inhibits spindle formation, causing an arrest in metaphase.
   - It is occasionally used in the treatment of gouty arthritis.
2. Vincristine and vinblastine block assembly of the mitotic spindle.
3. Paclitaxel prevents disassembly of the mitotic spindle at the end of mitosis.
4. Fluorouracil (5-FU) and methotrexate, which both inhibit DNA synthesis, primarily inhibit the S phase.
5. Bleomycin and etoposide primarily block the G_2 phase.

D. Classification of cells based on their mitotic activity
- In the adult organism, cells vary with regard to the frequency with which they undergo mitosis.
1. Cells that divide continuously
   a. Vegetative intermitotic cells, or stem cells (e.g., basal cells in the epidermis or intestinal glands, stem cells in the bone marrow)
      - These undifferentiated cells replicate to replace themselves and to provide precursors for specialized cells that are lost or damaged.
   b. Differentiating intermitotic cells (e.g., cells in the spinous layer of the epidermis)
      - These cells, which arise from stem cells, continue to divide as they differentiate into specialized cells.
2. Cells that divide infrequently or not at all
   a. Resting cells, or reverting postmitotics (e.g., liver cells, smooth muscle cells, astrocytes)
      - Most resting cells have exited the cell cycle at G_1, entering the so-called G_0 phase (see Fig. 3-5).
      - These specialized cells require a loss of tissue (trauma) or stimulation by growth factors or hormones to move them into the G_1 phase and resume replication.
   b. Nonreplicators, or fixed postmitotics (e.g., cells in the granulosum or corneum layer of the epidermis, neurons, striated and cardiac muscle cells)
      - These highly specialized cells, which are permanently incapable of cell division, can be replaced only from an appropriate stem cell population.

E. Conditions caused by malfunctioning of the cell cycle
1. Polyploidy results from failure of a cell to undergo cytokinesis (division of the cytoplasm) before it enters the next cell cycle.
   a. Megakaryocytes normally are polyploid.
   b. Many tumor cells are polyploid, one of the many abnormalities of these cells.
2. Psoriasis results from failure of replicating cells of the basal and spinous layers of the epidermis to differentiate into nonreplicating cells of the keratinized layer.
   - Continued proliferation of these cells (hyperplasia) leads to formation of the erythematous plaques characteristic of psoriasis.

Oncogenes (e.g., *ras*, *erbB₂*) can cause the transformation of normal cells into cancer cells. Most oncogenes are mutant, unregulated forms of normal genes encoding proteins that promote cell growth or proliferation.

Tumor-suppressor genes (e.g., *RB*, *p53*) normally encode proteins that inhibit cell proliferation. Inactivating mutations in such genes lead to unrestricted cell growth and the potential for cancer.

A neoplasm, or tumor, is any new, abnormal growth of tissue.

3. Development of many cancers has been associated with mutations in two types of genes that regulate cell growth and proliferation (Box 3-1).
   - Usually, several mutations are required to transform a normal cell into a cancerous cell.
   a. Tumor-suppressor genes (e.g., *RB* and *p53*) encode proteins that normally inhibit cell proliferation.
      - Mutations leading to inactivation of these genes contribute to the development of retinoblastoma, pancreatic and colon cancers, and some breast cancers.
   b. Proto-oncogenes (e.g., *ras* and *erbB₂*) encode proteins that normally promote cell growth and proliferation.
      - Mutations leading to overexpression, amplification, or translocation of these genes contribute to the development of bladder, colon, breast, skin, and lung cancers.

BOX 3-1

PROPERTIES AND CLASSIFICATION OF NEOPLASMS

Benign neoplasms grow relatively slowly, are commonly circular, and are usually encapsulated. Few mitotic figures, which have a normal structure, are seen. The cells are well differentiated, resembling the cell or tissue from which the neoplasm arose.

Malignant neoplasms, or cancers, grow rapidly, are not usually encapsulated, and invade local tissue. Many mitotic figures, with some showing abnormalities (e.g., tripolar metaphase), are seen. The cells are in various stages of dedifferentiation and may change so much (anaplasia) that the cell or tissue of origin cannot be determined. Cancers are categorized as carcinomas or sarcomas.

A carcinoma is any malignant neoplasm that originates in an epithelium (membranous or glandular), regardless of the embryonic germ layer from which the epithelium is derived. For example:

- Squamous cell carcinoma of the epidermis (ectodermal derivative)
- Transitional cell carcinoma of the bladder (mesodermal derivative)
- Adenocarcinoma of the colon (endodermal derivative)
- Carcinoma of the kidney (mesodermal derivative)

A sarcoma is any malignant neoplasm that originates in nonepithelial (mesenchymal) tissue. For example:

- Rhabdomyosarcoma (skeletal muscle origin)
- Leiomyosarcoma (smooth muscle origin)
- Liposarcoma (adipose cell origin)
- Fibrosarcoma (fibroblast origin)
- Osteogenic sarcoma (bone origin)

IV. Mitosis and Meiosis
  A. Mitosis: cell division in which diploid somatic cells give rise to diploid daughter cells (Fig. 3-6A)
      1. Entering mitosis: Each duplicated chromosome = 2 chromatids; the cell contains 92 chromatids = 4C DNA.
      2. At metaphase: Each duplicated chromosome aligns individually along the equatorial plate.
      3. At anaphase: Chromatids of each chromosome are pulled toward opposite spindle poles, leading to equational division.
      4. After mitosis and cytokinesis: Each daughter cell receives 46 chromatids corresponding to 23 pairs of homologous chromosomes = 2C DNA.
      5. During the next S phase: Chromosomes duplicate so that there are 92 chromatids at the beginning of the next mitosis.
  B. Meiosis: a special form of cell division in which diploid developing germ cells give rise to haploid gametes (Fig. 3-6B).
      1. Meiosis I (reductional division)
          a. Pairing of duplicated homologous chromosomes (4C DNA) at the equatorial plate occurs during the first meiotic division.
          b. Crossing over and recombination between maternal and paternal chromatids leads to new combinations of genes on the chromosomes.
          c. The chromatids of each chromosome do not separate during anaphase, and maternally and paternally derived chromosomes are randomly segregated to daughter cells.
          d. Both the number of chromosomes and the DNA content are halved by this reductional division, yielding daughter cells with 23 chromosomes ($1n$), or 46 chromatids = 2C DNA.
      2. Meiosis II (equational division)
          a. Daughter cells from meiosis I soon undergo a second division without any intervening DNA synthesis.
          b. The chromatids separate at anaphase, similar to mitosis.
          c. Each daughter cell (gamete) receives 23 chromosomes (23 chromatids); the haploid chromosome number ($1n$) = 1C DNA.
      3. Fertilization
          • Fusion of the sperm and egg during fertilization restores the diploid chromosome number and 2C DNA in the zygote.
          a. 23 egg chromosomes (1C) + 23 sperm chromosomes (1C) = 46 zygote chromosomes ($2n$, 2C).
          b. DNA synthesis restores the G_2 amount of DNA (4C) before the zygote enters mitosis.
  C. Sex determination (Fig. 3-7)
      1. Human females produce a single type of gamete (ovum) containing 22 autosomes and an X chromosome (23,X).
      2. Human males produce two types of gametes (sperm): One has 22 autosomes and an X chromosome (23,X); the other has 22 autosomes and a Y chromosome (23,Y).
      3. A male offspring results from the fertilization of an ovum by a Y-bearing sperm.

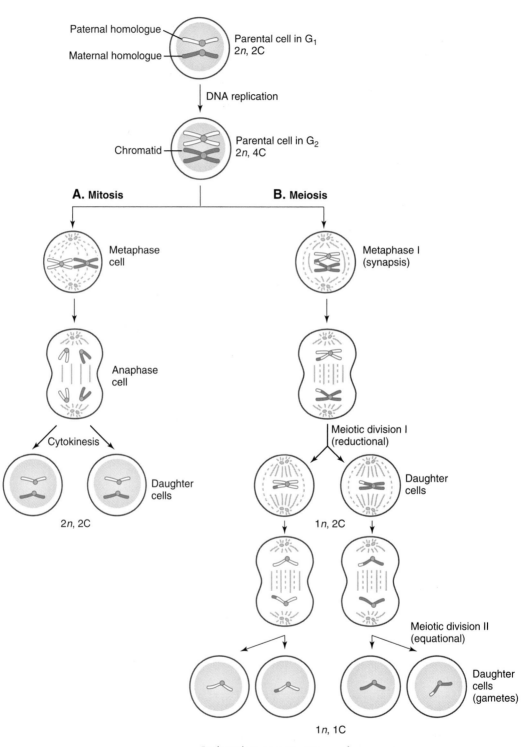

Paternal homologue

Maternal homologue

Parental cell in G_1
$2n$, $2C$

DNA replication

Chromatid

Parental cell in G_2
$2n$, $4C$

A. Mitosis

B. Meiosis

Metaphase
cell

Metaphase I
(synapsis)

Anaphase
cell

Cytokinesis

Meiotic division I
(reductional)

Daughter
cells

Daughter
cells

$2n$, $2C$

$1n$, $2C$

Meiotic division II
(equational)

Daughter
cells
(gametes)

$1n$, $1C$

For legend see opposite page

3-6: *Changes in ploidy and the amount of deoxyribonucleic acid (DNA) per cell during the cell cycle and mitotic or meiotic division. A normal diploid (2n) cell has 2C of nuclear DNA in G_1. During the S phase, the amount of DNA is precisely doubled to 4C.* **A,** *Mitosis occurs in somatic cells. The 4C in a G_1 cell is halved, but the number of chromosomes remains the same (2n) in the daughter cells.* **B,** *Meiosis occurs during the formation of gametes. A diploid germ cell precursor in G_2 with 4C DNA goes through two divisions without intervening DNA synthesis. Meiosis I (reductional division) produces daughter cells (secondary spermatocytes or oocytes) that are haploid (1n) and contain 2C DNA. Meiosis II (equational division) produces gametes (spermatids or ootids), which are haploid (1n) and contain 1C DNA. Because of the recombination at the synapsis of metaphase I and the random segregation of maternal and paternal chromosomes during the first meiotic division, each gamete has a unique genetic constitution.*

⬅ ───

        • The presence of a Y chromosome in the zygote = male phenotype.

    4. A female offspring results from the fertilization of an ovum by an X-bearing sperm.

        • The absence of a Y chromosome in the zygote = female phenotype.

  D. Sex chromatin in females

        • In all somatic cells of females, one of the X chromosomes is permanently in the condensed heterochromatin form, known as a Barr body, which is visible during interphase.

> A Barr body (sex chromatin) is a permanent heterochromatin mass in female cells corresponding to a single, inactive, condensed X chromosome.

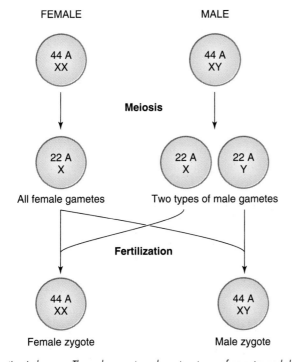

3-7: *Sex determination in humans. The male parent produces two types of gametes and determines the sex of the zygote, which must have a Y chromosome to exhibit the male phenotype. A, autosomes; X and Y, sex chromosomes.*

- The presence or absence of Barr bodies permits identification of the chromosomal sex of an individual, even when the external genitalia are ambiguous. The number of Barr bodies = the number of X chromosomes minus l.

V. Abnormalities of Cell Division

A. Differences in the effects of similar abnormalities

- The clinical manifestations of cell division abnormalities vary depending on whether abnormalities occur during mitosis or meiosis and on which chromosomes are affected.

1. Abnormalities during mitosis result in some somatic cells with the aberration and others that are normal, a condition called *mixoploidy,* or *chromosome mosaicism.*

2. Abnormalities during meiosis produce aberrant gametes. Fertilization of an aberrant gamete with a normal gamete results in offspring in which virtually all of the cells carry the aberration.

B. Major causes of cell division abnormalities

1. Nondisjunction: failure of a single pair of chromosomes (meiosis I) or a single pair of chromatids (meiosis II or mitosis) to separate at cell division

- One daughter cell receives two of the chromosomes or chromatids affected; the other daughter cell receives none.

2. Anaphase lagging: lagging of a chromosome (meiosis I) or a chromatid (meiosis II or mitosis) behind the remainder of the chromosomes so that it is not included in one of the daughter cells

- One daughter cell is normal; the other daughter cell lacks the affected chromosome.

3. Deletion: breaking off of a fragment of a chromosome

- If the fragment lacks a kinetochore, that portion of the chromosome is lost at cell division and is missing from one of the daughter cells.

4. Translocation: Breaking off of a piece of one chromosome and attachment to another chromosome that is not its homologue

C. Specific disorders caused by abnormal meiosis

1. Down syndrome generally results from nondisjunction.

   a. Affected individuals have one extra chromosome 21 (trisomy 21) in all their cells.

   b. Clinical manifestations include mental retardation; atrial septal defect; short stature; an anteroposteriorly flattened skull, with a short, flat-bridged nose; an epicanthal fold; stubby appendages; and a simian crease in the hands.

2. Turner's syndrome results from nondisjunction or anaphase lagging.

   a. Affected individuals lack one sex chromosome (monosomy) in all their cells (most commonly 45,XO, with no Barr bodies).

   b. Clinical manifestations include short stature, undifferentiated gonads, webbing of the neck, aortic coarctation, and sterility.

Nondisjunction during meiosis results in some gametes with an extra copy of one chromosome (e.g., 23) and some gametes lacking that chromosome.

Down syndrome is caused by one extra chromosome 21 (trisomy 21).

Turner's syndrome is caused by the lack of all (45,XO) or a portion of one sex chromosome. It has a female phenotype, with no Barr bodies.

3. Klinefelter's syndrome usually results from nondisjunction.
   a. Affected individuals have an extra X chromosome in all their cells (most commonly 47,XXY, with one Barr body).
   b. Clinical manifestations include tall stature, with disproportionately long arms and legs, small testes; eunuchoid body habitus; gynecomastia; and infertility.
4. Cri du chat syndrome results from a deletion during meiosis.
   a. Affected individuals have a normal number of chromosomes but lack the short arm of chromosome 5 in all their cells.
   b. Clinical manifestations include severe mental deficiency; ventricular septal defect; microcephaly; hypertelorism; and a plaintive, catlike cry.
D. Specific disorders caused by abnormal mitosis
   1. Chronic myelogenous leukemia results from a reciprocal translocation during hematopoiesis in the bone marrow.
      • Blood cells and their precursors contain a shortened chromosome 22 (Philadelphia chromosome) and an abnormal chromosome 9 that carries the *bcr-abl* oncogene formed by the translocation.
   2. Aniridia (absence of the iris) results from deletion of a portion of chromosome 11 during embryonic development of the eye.
      • Individuals with this disorder have a high incidence of Wilms' tumor of the kidney.

Klinefelter's syndrome is caused by an extra X chromosome in males (47,XXY); there is one Barr body.

Philadelphia chromosome is a shortened chromosome 22 (22q⁻) due to translocation with chromosome 9 (9q⁺). It is present in the marrow and blood cells of those with chronic myelogenous leukemia.

Epithelial Tissue

I. Introduction
   A. Major types of epithelia
      1. Membranous epithelia are sheetlike tissues that cover or line the surfaces, cavities, and organs of the body.
      2. Glandular epithelia perform secretory functions and form the parenchyma of glands.
   B. Characteristic properties
      1. Polarity: The cells composing many epithelia have distinct apical, lateral, and basal domains that are structurally and functionally different.
      2. Absence of blood vessels: Epithelia are avascular tissues that receive nourishment from associated vascularized connective tissue.
      3. Separation from the surrounding tissue: The basement membrane separates the epithelia from the underlying connective tissue (see Chapter 5, section V).

II. Classification of Membranous Epithelia (Fig. 4-1 and Table 4-1)
   A. Simple epithelia are composed of a single layer of cells, all of which contact the basement membrane.
   B. Stratified epithelia are composed of multiple layers of cells, with only the cells in the deepest (basal) layer contacting the basement membrane.
   C. The shape of the surface cells is the basis for classifying the epithelia as squamous, cuboidal, or columnar.

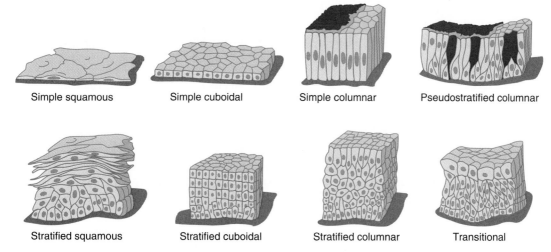

Simple squamous   Simple cuboidal   Simple columnar   Pseudostratified columnar

Stratified squamous   Stratified cuboidal   Stratified columnar   Transitional

4-1: Membranous epithelia. The number of cell layers in an epithelium and the shape of the surface cells provide the basis for classifying epithelia.

TABLE 4-1:
Membranous Epithelia

Type	Surface Layer	Common Locations
Single Layer		
Simple squamous	Flattened cells	Endothelium (lining of blood vessels)
		Mesothelium (lining of peritoneum and pleura)
		Lining of alveoli
		Renal corpuscles
Simple cuboidal	Cuboidal cells	Terminal bronchioles
		Uriniferous tubules
		Ducts of many glands
Simple columnar	Columnar cells	Epithelial lining of stomach and intestines
Pseudostratified columnar	Columnar cells and basal cells (both contact basement membrane)	Epithelial lining of large conducting airways (respiratory epithelium)
Multiple Layers		
Stratified squamous (keratinized, dry, cornified)	Flattened anucleated cells filled with many keratin filaments	Epidermis of skin
Stratified squamous (nonkeratinized, wet, noncornified)	Flattened nucleated cells containing some keratin filaments	Epithelial lining of mouth, esophagus, and vagina
Stratified cuboidal	Cuboidal cells	Ducts of sweat glands
Stratified columnar	Columnar cells	Larger ducts of salivary and mammary glands
Transitional (uroepithelium)	Large, flattened cells when stretched; thicker, dome-shaped cells when relaxed	Lining of ureters and bladder

III. Specialization of the Epithelial Cell Surface
   A. Apical Epithelial Surface
      1. Microvilli are short, nonmotile, fingerlike projections of the plasma membrane ($\approx$1.5 µm long and 0.1 µm in diameter).
         a. A brush, or striated, border is visible by light microscopy and consists of numerous microvilli extending from the apical surface of an epithelium into a lumen.
            • This type of border is prominent in the intestine and the proximal convoluted tubule of the kidney.
         b. Actin microfilaments fill the core of microvilli.
         c. The terminal web, composed of actin containing thin filaments, lies at the base of each microvillus, anchoring it to the cytoskeleton.
      2. Cilia are long, motile processes extending from the cell surface (5 to 15 µm long and 0.2 µm in diameter).
         a. The axoneme, or core, of each cilium has a 9 + 2 pattern consisting of 9 radially arranged doublet microtubules and 2 central singlet microtubules (Fig. 4-2).
         b. A basal body, containing 9 radially arranged triplet microtubules, lies at the base of a cilium and functions to anchor it to the cell.
         c. Beating of the cilia propels the surrounding fluid or particles along the surface in one direction.
            • Dynein side arms, which extend between adjacent doublets, hydrolyze adenosine triphosphate to generate a sliding force that results in a bending movement that is responsible for beating of cilia (Box 4-1).

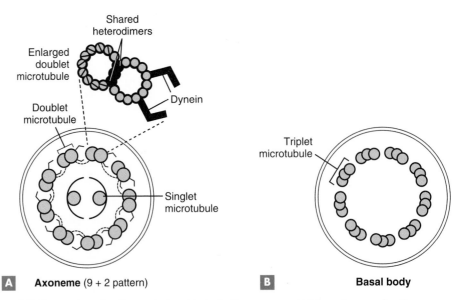

A   **Axoneme** (9 + 2 pattern)   **B**   **Basal body**

4-2: *Cross-sections of a cilium and a basal body.* **A,** *The axoneme, which forms the core of a cilium, contains two central singlet microtubules surrounded by nine doublet microtubules.* **B,** *A basal body, the anchoring structure of a cilium, contains a ring of nine triplet microtubules.*

BOX 4-1

IMMOTILE CILIA SYNDROME

Defects in the dynein arms that affect the ability of cilia to beat cause several hereditary disorders collectively termed *immotile cilia syndrome*. These disorders are characterized by delayed or absent clearance of debris and microbes from the airways, leading to recurrent infection of the lower respiratory tract. Frequently, sperm motility also is impaired.

Kartagener's syndrome involves a combination of situs inversus and immotile cilia syndrome marked by bronchiectasis and sinusitis. It is transmitted as an autosomal dominant trait.

3. Stereocilia are long, nonmotile projections similar in structure to microvilli (not cilia).
   • They are found in the epithelial lining of the epididymis and vas deferens, where they increase the absorptive surface area.
   • They are also present on hair cells of the inner ear, where they have a sensory function (see Chapter 19).
B. Lateral epithelial surfaces (Fig. 4-3)
   1. Junctional complex: three closely associated cell junctions, generally found on the lateral surfaces of columnar epithelial cells

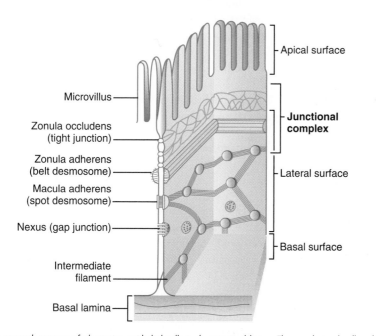

4-3: *The general structure of absorptive epithelial cells in the intestinal lining. These polarized cells exhibit numerous apical, lateral, and basolateral specializations. Also see Figure 1-7.*

a. A zonula occludens, or tight junction, forms a permeability barrier just below the apical surface.

b. A zonula adherens, or belt desmosome, encircles the entire cell periphery, forming a broad region of adhesion just basal to the zonula occludens.

c. Maculae adherens, or spot desmosomes, are disklike adhesive junctions located basal to the zonula adherens.

2. Nexus, or gap junction: protein-lined channel through which ions and small molecules can pass between adjacent cells

C. Basal epithelial surface

1. Hemidesmosomes: specialized adherens junctions in the basal plasmalemma that link cells to the underlying basal lamina (see Chapter 5)

   • Bullous pemphigoid is an autoimmune disease characterized by chronic blisters (bullae) in the skin, mainly on the thighs, arms, and abdomen. It is associated with immunoglobulin G autoantibodies against hemidesmosomes and usually is seen in the elderly.

2. Basal striations: infoldings of the basal plasma membrane found in epithelia engaged in active transport (e.g., proximal and distal convoluted tubules of the kidney, ducts of certain glands)

IV. Glandular Epithelia

   • Glandular epithelial cells are organized into secretory units, which, in some cases, are connected to the surface by ducts.

   • The secretory products synthesized and released by glandular epithelial cells include proteins, steroid hormones, and mucus.

A. Exocrine glands deliver their secretion externally to a surface, either directly or through a duct system.

1. Exocrine glands with ducts are classified in terms of the branching of their ducts (simple, compound) and the shape of their secretory units (tubular, acinar, alveolar) (Fig. 4-4A).

   • These glands include salivary, sebaceous, and glands of the gastrointestinal system as well as the exocrine portions of the pancreas and liver.

2. Exocrine glands without ducts are part of a membranous epithelium (Fig. 4-4B).

   a. Unicellular glands (e.g., goblet cells in the intestinal and respiratory epithelia)

   b. Intraepithelial gland (e.g., urethral glands)

3. Mechanisms of exocrine secretion

   a. Holocrine secretion: Secretory cells in their entirety, along with their contents, are released (e.g., sebaceous gland).

   b. Apocrine secretion: The apical portion of the secretory cells is released with the contents (e.g., mammary gland epithelium).

   c. Merocrine secretion: The contents of secretory granules, or vesicles, are released from the cells by exocytosis (e.g., pancreatic exocrine cell).

B. Endocrine glands, which do not have ducts, deliver their secretions internally into the bloodstream (see Chapter 18).

Bullous pemphigoid (pemphigus vulgaris) is chronic blistering of the skin and mucous membranes resulting from defective adhesion of the epithelia to the underlying matrix.

Glandular epithelial cells release secretory products by holocrine, apocrine, or merocrine secretion.

In exocrine glands, secretory products are released externally to an internal or external surface. These glands may or may not have ducts.

A

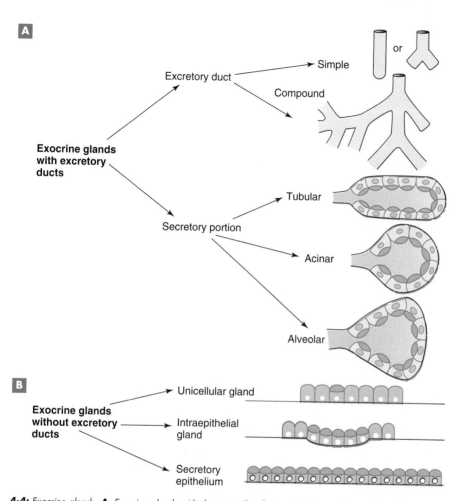

B

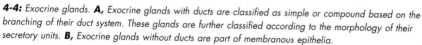

*4-4: Exocrine glands. **A,** Exocrine glands with ducts are classified as simple or compound based on the branching of their duct system. These glands are further classified according to the morphology of their secretory units. **B,** Exocrine glands without ducts are part of membranous epithelia.*

- Scattered hormone-producing cells present in various epithelia (e.g., in the gastrointestinal tract) function as unicellular endocrine glands.
- Most endocrine glands (e.g., thyroid) are multicellular.

In endocrine glands, secretory products are released internally to the bloodstream; no ducts are present.

V. Turnover of Epithelia
- Surface epithelial cells, which constantly undergo cell death or suffer damage, are replaced on a continuous basis.
- Various regulatory mechanisms normally control the generation of replacement cells to balance the loss of cells.
  A. In simple epithelia consisting of relatively nonspecialized cells:
  1. Virtually all the cells either constantly divide and replace themselves (e.g., cuboidal epithelium in bronchioles).
  2. When stimulated by trauma or other signals (e.g., capillary endothelium) (Fig. 4-5A and B) some epithelial cells replicate and divide.

The constant turnover of epithelial cells makes epithelia common sites for tumor development.

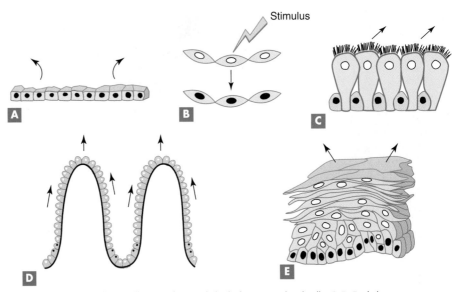

4-5: *Turnover of epithelial cells.* **A** *and* **B,** *Epithelia lacking specialized cells.* **C–E,** *Epithelia containing postmitotic specialized cells and continuously replicating cells. In cells capable of cell division, the nucleus is black; in other cells, the nucleus is white.*

    B. In epithelia containing specialized cells:
- Postmitotic differentiated surface cells, which have lost the ability to divide, are continually sloughed off and are replaced from a population of continuously replicating stem cells.
  1. Pseudostratified epithelium (e.g., respiratory epithelium)
     - Basal cells constantly divide; some of their progeny differentiate into glandular or ciliated cells (Fig. 4-5C).
  2. Gland-containing columnar epithelium (e.g., intestinal epithelium)
     - Cells in the necks of glands constantly divide; some of their progeny differentiate and migrate to the surface, where they replace the surface cells (Fig. 4-5D).
  3. Stratified epithelium (e.g., epidermis, lining of ducts)
     - Basal cells replicate continuously; some of their progeny migrate into the intermediate layers.
     - Cells in the intermediate layers, adjacent to the basal layer, differentiate and migrate to the surface and may continue to replicate and divide.
     - Cells on the surface are postmitotic cells that have lost the ability to replicate or divide.

    C. Replacement of the entire epithelium
- Traumatic loss of all epithelial layers may stimulate cells in associated glands to divide and differentiate into surface epithelial cells.

    D. Epithelial cell tumors
- When normal mechanisms for regulating epithelial turnover fail, tumors can develop (see Box 3-1).

    1. Carcinomas: malignant tumors that arise from membranous epithelia
    2. Adenocarcinomas: malignant tumors that arise from glandular epithelia

VI. Functional Specialization of Epithelial Cells
- The ability of different epithelia to perform various functions depends on their numerous specializations, as illustrated by the following examples:
  A. Protection from injury and abrasion by keratinized (dry) stratified squamous epithelium of the epidermis
    1. The flattened shape of the surface cells provides maximal strength.
    2. Abundant maculae adherens permit strong adhesion between cells.
    3. Keratinized surface cells resist water loss.
  B. Absorption by intestinal epithelial cells (see Fig. 4-3)
    1. The junctional complex maintains the integrity of tissue.
    2. Numerous microvilli (brush border) increase the surface area for absorption.
    3. The filamentous glycocalyx binds digestive enzymes.
    4. Tight junctions (zonulae occludens) act as a diffusion barrier.
    5. Transport proteins in apical and basal membranes mediate the movement of specific substances across surfaces (see Chapter 1, section III).
    6. Polarization of cells permits directed transport of nutrients from the apical (luminal) surface to the basal surface.

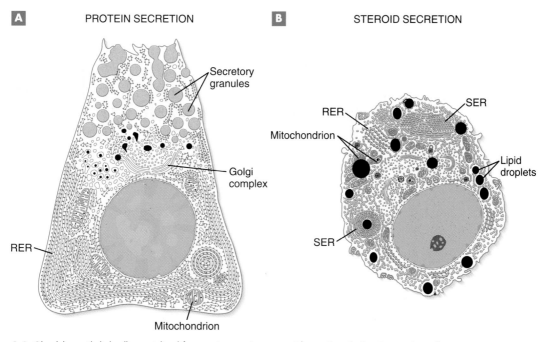

4-6: Glandular epithelial cells specialized for protein secretion or steroid secretion. **A,** Protein-secreting cells exhibit extensive rough endoplasmic reticulum (RER) and a Golgi complex as well as many secretory granules in the apical region. **B,** Steroid-secreting cells exhibit well-developed smooth endoplasmic reticulum (SER) and numerous lipid droplets throughout the cell. All secretory cells possess abundant mitochondria, which produce adenosine triphosphate for synthetic reactions.

C. Transport over the surface of epithelia
   • Beating of cilia on the respiratory epithelium moves debris-filled mucus toward the oral cavity, helping to prevent microorganisms, dust, and other materials from reaching the lungs (see Box 4-1).
D. Transport across the capillary endothelia
   1. A thin, flattened cell shape provides maximal surface area.
   2. A well-developed basal lamina impedes diffusion.
   3. Many pinocytotic vesicles aid in transporting material from one side of the cell to the other side.
   4. Fenestrae (pores) in some capillary endothelial cells increase their permeability to most substances.
E. Secretion by glandular epithelia (Fig. 4-6)
   1. Protein-secreting cells are marked by a well-developed rough endoplasmic reticulum, an extensive Golgi apparatus, and numerous secretory granules (vesicles) in the apical region of the cell.
   2. Steroid hormone-secreting cells are marked by well-developed smooth endoplasmic reticulum and numerous lipid droplets.

Kartagener's syndrome is situs inversus plus immotile cilia syndrome.

Connective Tissue

I. Introduction
- Connective tissue is distributed throughout all the systems and organs of the body.
    A. Functions
        1. Structural support is the primary function of connective tissue.
            - Organs contain a stroma of connective tissue, which supports and nourishes the functional elements, or parenchyma (e.g., secreting cells in glands, myofibers in muscle).
        2. Transport, storage, and protection are specialized functions performed by connective tissue in certain body locations.
    B. Basic components
        1. Cells
        2. The extracellular matrix (ECM) consists of ground substance and fibers.
    C. Classification (Fig. 5-1)
        1. Loose (areolar) connective tissue has a high proportion of cells and ground substance to fibers (Fig. 5-2).
        2. Dense connective tissue has a high proportion of fibers to cells.

II. Cells of Generalized Connective Tissue
    A. Permanent residents are formed locally from undifferentiated mesenchymal cells and remain within the connective tissue.
        1. Fibroblasts synthesize connective tissue fibers and the constituents of the ground substance.

Connective tissue

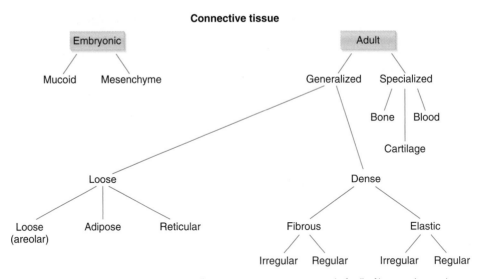

5-1: *Classification of connective tissue. All connective tissues are composed of cells, fibers, and ground substance. They are classified based on the relative amounts and organization of these components.*

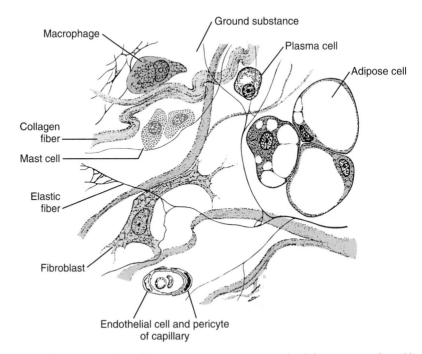

5-2: *Sketch of the cells and fibers of loose connective tissue, as seen with a light microscope. The visible components lie in the optically homogeneous ground substance. (Adapted from Cormack DH: Ham's Histology. Philadelphia: JB Lippincott, 1987, p 170.)*

      a. Active fibroblasts: synthetically active state containing well-developed rough endoplasmic reticulum (RER) and a Golgi complex

      b. Fibrocytes: synthetically inactive state that may revert to the active form during wound healing

  2. Adipose cells store lipid triglycerides in their cytoplasm.

      a. Unilocular (white) adipocytes: one large fat vacuole; the most common form in adults

      b. Multilocular (brown) adipocytes: a large number of lipid droplets; common in embryos and newborn infants

  3. Pericytes are flattened cells that lie adjacent to the capillary endothelium and are enclosed within its basal lamina.

B. Migratory (transient) residents are formed primarily in the bone marrow and migrate from the blood into connective tissue.

  • These cells, which are most numerous during infection and at inflammatory sites, play an important role in the body's defense system (see Chapter 13).

  1. Macrophages, which arise from circulating monocytes, are the most abundant phagocytic cells in connective tissue.

    • Some macrophages are fixed to fibers; others migrate throughout the connective tissue.

  2. Mast cells are filled with membrane-bound granules containing various biologic mediators, including histamine, heparin, and platelet-activating factor.

    • Release of these substances leads to an immediate (type I) hypersensitivity reaction (see Fig. 13-5).

  3. T and B lymphocytes accumulate in large numbers during chronic infection.

  4. Plasma cells originating from B lymphocytes (see Chapter 12), which produce secreted antibodies, are commonly found where microorganisms and toxins can penetrate the epithelial surfaces of the body.

  5. Granulocytes (see Chapter 12)

      a. Neutrophils are highly phagocytic cells found at sites of acute infection.

      b. Eosinophils increase in number during parasitic infection and at sites of allergic reactions.

III. Ground Substance

  • This optically homogeneous material, filling the space between connective tissue cells and fibers, consists of a complex scaffold of macromolecules bathed in tissue fluid.

A. Glycosaminoglycans (GAGs) are unbranched polysaccharides composed of repeating disaccharide subunits.

  1. Common properties of GAGs

      a. All GAGs have regularly spaced, negatively charged groups and exhibit metachromasia (i.e., they stain red with a blue dye).

      b. With the exception of hyaluronic acid, GAGs are covalently attached to core proteins and contain covalently attached sulfate groups.

Hyaluronic acid is a large, abundant, hydrated glycosamino-glycan that impedes the spread of bacteria and tumor cells through the extracellular matrix; it is a joint lubricant.

Invasion of connective tissue by some bacteria (e.g., group A strepto-cocci) and many tumor cells is promoted by hyaluronidase, which is produced by these invaders.

2. Hyaluronic acid
   a. This very large, highly coiled molecule (molecular weight ≈ 106 Da) is synthesized by enzyme complexes embedded in the plasma membrane of fibroblasts.
   b. It can bind many water molecules, forming a viscous hydrated gel that imparts stiffness and resilience to connective tissues.
      • It is the lubricant in synovial fluid.
   c. Hyaluronic acid interacts with itself and with proteoglycans to provide a barrier to the spread of bacteria, tumor cells, and large molecules.
      • It is degraded by hyaluronidase, an enzyme produced by some bacteria and by many tumor cells.
3. Major sulfated GAGs
   a. Chondroitin sulfate (cartilage, bone, blood vessels)
   b. Dermatan sulfate (skin, blood vessels, heart valves)
      • It is present in increased amounts in mitral valve prolapse.
   c. Heparan sulfate (basal laminae, plasma membranes)
      • It imparts a negative charge to the glomerular basement membrane.
   d. Keratan sulfate (cornea, cartilage)
B. Proteoglycans are a diverse group of molecules composed of a core protein from which covalently attached GAG side chains extend.
   • Most proteoglycans are secreted into the extracellular matrix after their synthesis, but some remain attached to the plasma membrane by a transmembrane domain (e.g., syndecans).
   1. Proteoglycan aggregates consist of a central hyaluronic acid molecule to which approximately 100 proteoglycan monomers are bound (Fig. 5-3).

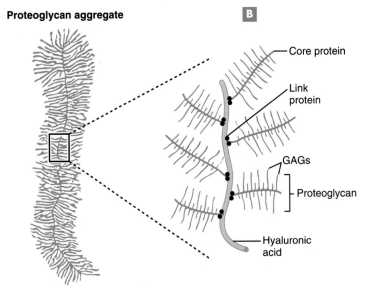

A Proteoglycan aggregate   **B**

Core protein

Link protein

GAGs

Proteoglycan

Hyaluronic acid

5-3: Proteoglycan aggregate. **A,** *Proteoglycans are attached at regular intervals to a central hyaluronic acid molecule. These aggregates may attain a molecular weight of $10^8 D$ and occupy a volume equivalent to that of a bacterium.* **B,** *Each proteoglycan consists of a central core protein and numerous covalently bound glycosaminoglycans (GAGs), as shown in the enlarged view.*

- These large aggregates are particularly abundant in cartilage.
- Aggregates are assembled in the extracellular space from hyaluronic acid and proteoglycan monomers.
  2. Synthesis and turnover of proteoglycans
     a. The core protein is synthesized on the RER of fibroblasts.
     b. GAG side chains are assembled on the core protein, one sugar at a time, in the RER and Golgi complex.
     c. Certain lysosomal enzymes degrade proteoglycans, accounting for their turnover in connective tissue.
        - Mucopolysaccharidoses are characterized by hereditary defects in various lysosomal enzymes (Box 5-1).
  3. Functions of connective tissue proteoglycans
     a. Act as a supporting matrix for cells and fibers
     b. Attract and hold tissue fluid
     c. Permit diffusion of small molecules in solution
     d. Obstruct the movement of large molecules
     e. Bind fibroblast growth factor and other growth factors in the ECM, protecting them from degradation and presenting them to cell-surface receptors
  C. Matrix adhesive (structural) proteins are large glycoproteins that cross-link other ECM components with specific cell-surface proteins.

Hurler's syndrome and other forms of mucopolysaccharidoses result from defective degradation of glycosaminoglycans in lysosomes, leading to their accumulation in various tissues and their excretion in urine.

BOX 5-1

MUCOPOLYSACCHARIDOSES (MPS)

Defects in lysosomal degradation of glycosaminoglycans (GAGs) lead to excretion of GAGs in the urine and their accumulation in many tissues. These defects usually are autosomal recessive and cause various clinical syndromes, which constitute one type of lysosomal storage disease.

Hurler's syndrome (MPS I H): This condition is the prototypical mucopolysaccharidosis and is the most severe of the three allelic forms of MPS I. It causes progressive corneal clouding, severe mental retardation, gargoyle-like facies (low forehead, widely spaced teeth, large tongue), a short neck and trunk, joint contractures, and enlarged liver and spleen. Dermatan sulfate and heparan sulfate are found in the urine. Early death usually occurs as a result of respiratory infection or heart failure.

Hunter's syndrome (MPS II): The severe form is marked by mental retardation, dwarfism, deafness, hernia, clawhand, and valvular heart disease. Dermatan sulfate and heparan sulfate are found in the urine. It is the only X-linked form of MPS. Death typically occurs before age 15 years, usually as a result of heart disease.

Morquio's syndrome (MPS IV): Affected individuals have normal intelligence, dwarfism, hunchback, knock-knees, progressive deafness, and mild corneal clouding. Keratan sulfate is found in the urine.

Fibronectins and laminins bind to other components of the extracellular matrix and to cell-surface proteins, linking cells to the extracellular matrix. They are important in wound healing and tumor invasion.

1. Fibronectins play an important role in cell migration during development and in wound healing.
   a. Specific domains in fibronectins bind the following:
      (1) Collagen and heparan sulfate (ECM components)
      (2) Fibrin (the major component of blood clots)
      (3) Integrins (intrinsic membrane proteins)
   b. Fibroblasts produce connective tissue fibronectins.
   c. Liver cells produce fibronectin that circulates in the blood.
2. Laminins promote the adhesion of epithelial cells to the underlying connective tissue.
   a. All basal laminae contain laminins.
   b. Specific domains in laminins bind the following:
      (1) Type IV collagen and perlecan (a heparan sulfate proteoglycan), both components of the basal laminae
      (2) Integrins in the plasma membrane of epithelial cells

D. Tissue fluid, the fluid part of the ground substance, provides a medium for diffusion of metabolites in the intercellular space.
   • It is constantly being formed from the blood as it passes through arterioles and is resorbed into venules and lymphatic vessels.

IV. Extracellular Fibers
   A. Collagen fibers are inelastic, flexible fibers (1 to 12 μm in diameter) with high tensile strength. They constitute the major fibrous component of connective tissue.
      • A single collagen fiber consists of aggregations of long, thin fibrils (20 to 100 nm in diameter) composed of tropocollagen molecules.
      • Turnover of collagen in adult tissues is much slower than that of most intercellular proteins (e.g., collagen molecules persist for years in bone).
      1. Tropocollagen (Fig. 5-4)
         a. A long, rigid molecule (molecular weight = 300 kDa), tropocollagen is composed of three polypeptide chains (α chains) coiled about one another, forming a triple helix.
         b. The unusual amino acid composition of tropocollagen (30% glycine and 25% proline plus hydroxyproline) contributes to its rigidity and assembly into fibrils.
      2. Collagen fibrils
         a. Triple-helical tropocollagen molecules, which have distinct head and tail regions, are assembled into fibrils that are all oriented in the same direction.
         b. The dark and light periodicity (every 64 to 67 nm, depending on the preparation) of many native collagens reflects the highly organized packing of tropocollagen subunits into fibrils.
      3. Collagen formation: intracellular events (Fig. 5-5)
         a. In RER
            (1) Synthesis of pro-α chains
            (2) Hydroxylation of proline and lysine in pro-α chains, which requires ascorbic acid and the addition of carbohydrate

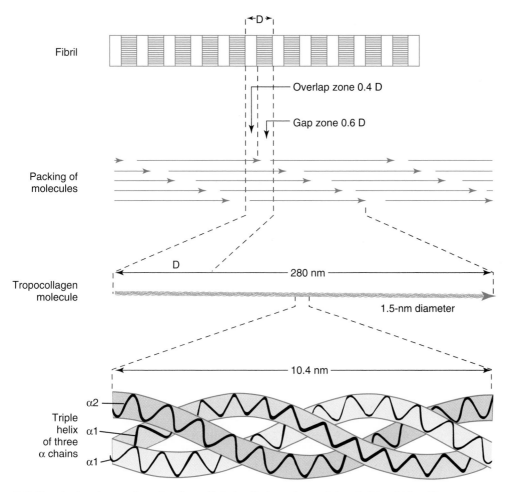

5-4: *Organization of tropocollagen in collagen fibrils that display a characteristic periodicity of 64 nm (D). In these fibrils, tropocollagen molecules are organized in a quarter-staggered array (i.e., the ends of adjacent molecules are displaced approximately one quarter of the length of one molecule). Each tropocollagen molecule is a triple helix of three interwoven α chains, which may be identical or different.*

      (3) Assembly of three-stranded procollagen, which is stabilized by intrachain disulfide bonds in the nonhelical propeptides at both ends

   b. Transfer to the Golgi complex, where oligosaccharide side chains on procollagen are completed

   c. Transfer to the secretory vesicle, which then moves to the cell surface

   d. At the surface of the cell, exocytosis of procollagen and removal of peptides at the amino and carboxyl ends by proteases on the cell surface to yield tropocollagen

  4. Collagen formation: extracellular events

   a. Self-assembly of tropocollagen to form collagen fibrils

   b. Formation of cross-links

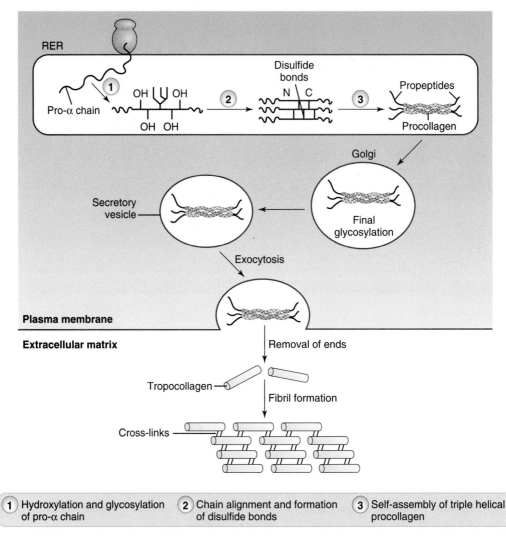

5-5: *Overview of collagen biosynthesis. Synthesis begins in the rough endoplasmic reticulum (RER) and is completed outside the cell, with cleavage of the ends to yield tropocollagen, which assembles into cross-linked fibrils. Side-by-side aggregation of fibrils produces large collagen fibers.*

- Lysyl oxidases deaminate hydroxylysine and lysine to form highly reactive aldehyde groups, which spontaneously form covalent bonds within and between tropocollagen molecules, stabilizing the fibrils.
- Cross-linking increases as collagen ages, so it becomes more insoluble in aqueous solution.
5. Types of collagen
   - Approximately 25 distinct tropocollagen α chains have been identified. Various combinations of α chains in the tropocollagen triple helix give rise to more than 20 biochemically different types of collagen (Table 5-1).

TABLE 5-1:
Properties of Major
Collagen Types

Type	Cells Synthesized	Major Tissues	Function
I	Fibroblast Odontoblast Osteoblast	Bone and dentin; skin; tendons and ligaments; interstitium of internal organs	Resists tension
II	Chondroblast	Cartilage (hyaline and elastic); intervertebral disks; vitreous humor	Resists intermittent pressure
III	Fibroblast	Cardiovascular system; endoneurium; lymph nodes; interstitium of internal organs; lymph nodes	Forms extensive open network that provides structural support in expandable organs Is first collagen in wound healing
IV	Epithelial cell Schwann cell Adipocyte Muscle cell	All basal laminae	Provides support and selective filtration
X	Chondrocyte	Epiphyseal plate	Provides framework for bone formation

   a. Fibrillar (fibrous) collagens account for 80% to 90% of the collagen in the body, including types I, II, and III, which form typical 67-nm banded fibrils.
   b. Reticular fibers, composed of type III collagen with more carbohydrate residues, stain with periodic acid-Schiff and silver salts (unlike other collagens).
B. Elastic fibers can be readily deformed or stretched by a small force, and they reversibly recover their original dimensions.
   • These fibers are prevalent in the extracellular matrix of the skin, blood vessels, and lungs, tissues that must be strong and elastic to function.
   1. Elastin, an amorphous protein composed of tropoelastin subunits, forms the core of elastic fibers.
      a. Elastin has a high proportion of nonpolar, hydrophobic amino acids, making it relatively insoluble.
      b. Joining of tropoelastin subunits into elastin is catalyzed by lysyl oxidases, which form covalent lysine cross-links and two unusual amino acids, desmosine and isodesmosine.
   2. Microfibrils (11 nm in diameter) form a scaffold for elastin, molding it into a fibrous configuration.
      • Several glycoproteins, with the predominant one called *fibrillin,* form microfibrils.
   3. Elastic fiber–producing cells include fibroblasts (generalized connective tissue), smooth muscle cells (large arteries), and chondrocytes (elastic cartilage).

C. Diseases involving defective extracellular fibers
   1. Scurvy results from a severe impairment of collagen synthesis due to prolonged deficiency of vitamin C (ascorbate), which is required for the hydroxylation of proline to hydroxyproline during tropocollagen synthesis.
      • Clinical symptoms include pinpoint hemorrhages in the skin, bleeding gums, and loosened teeth as preexisting normal collagen gradually is lost and is not replaced.
   2. Ehlers-Danlos syndrome is caused by a genetic defect that prevents conversion of procollagen to tropocollagen.
      • This disorder is characterized by fragile skin, weakened blood vessels, rupture of the colon, and hypermobile joints.
   3. Homocystinuria, an autosomal recessive defect in the enzyme cystathionine synthetase, leads to abnormal tropocollagen cross-linking.
      • This disorder is marked by elevated levels of homocystine and methionine in the blood and urine, in addition to musculoskeletal, ocular, and cardiac abnormalities similar to those associated with Marfan syndrome.
      • Increased plasma homocystine predisposes individuals to vessel thrombus.
   4. Marfan syndrome, an autosomal dominant disorder, is caused by a mutation in the fibrillin gene on chromosome 15.
      • Clinical manifestations include abnormally long fingers and toes (arachnodactyly), dislocation of the lens, mitral or tricuspid valve prolapse, and stretching of the ascending aorta, which may lead to a dissecting aortic aneurysm.
   5. Lathyrism is caused by reduced lysyl oxidase activity, usually due to severe copper deficiency or ingestion of an excessive amount of β-amiono-propionitrile (found in some peas).

V. Basement Membrane
   • All epithelia are separated from the subjacent connective tissue by a structurally similar interface, the basement membrane (Table 5-2).

Scurvy and Ehlers-Danlos syndrome (dissecting aortic aneurysm) result from impaired collagen synthesis or surface peptidaic activity.

Homocystinuria is marked by increased plasma homocystine and methionine and by vessel thrombus and marfanoid habitus.

Marfan syndrome is caused by defective formation of elastic fibers. It is marked by arachnodactyly, lens dislocation, dissecting aortic aneurysm, and mitral or tricuspid valve prolapse.

TABLE 5-2:
Terms Referring to Various Epithelia and Subjacent Connective Tissues

Site	Epithelium	Connective Tissue	Epithelium and Connective Tissue
Covering of external body surfaces	Epidermis	Dermis	Skin
Lining of body cavities open to the surface (alimentary, urinary, respiratory tracts)	Epithelium (with or without glands)	Lamina propria	Mucosa
Lining of closed body cavities Coelomic cavity (peritoneal, pericardial, and pleural)	Mesothelium (no glands)	Submesothelium	Serosa
Cardiovascular cavity	Endothelium	Subendothelium	Intima (vessels) Endocardium (heart)

- A basement membrane also surrounds muscle cells, adipose cells, and Schwann cells, and separates epithelial and endothelial cells in kidney glomeruli.
A. Structural elements of the basement membrane
  1. The basal lamina, which ranges in thickness from 40 to 100 nm, is produced by the adjacent epithelium.
     - All basal laminae contain similar components, although their ultrastructural organization may vary in different sites.
     a. The lamina lucida (rara), an electron-lucent zone closest to the epithelium, contains two key proteins:
        (1) Laminin, which binds type IV collagen, herparan sulfate, and cell-surface integrins
        (2) Perlecan, a proteoglycan rich in heparan sulfate
     b. The lamina densa is largely a meshlike network composed of type IV collagen.
  2. The lamina reticularis is produced by the underlying connective tissue.
     - It is rich in collagen and reticular fibers embedded in ground substance.
B. Functions of the basement membrane
  1. Forms a selective barrier to the movement of large molecules and cells
  2. Separates connective tissue from the epithelial cell environment
  3. Provides elastic support
  4. Helps guide the migration of cells during development and regeneration of injured tissue
C. Alport's syndrome
  - This X-linked dominant or autosomal dominant disorder is caused by a mutation in the gene encoding one of the α chains of type IV collagen.
  - The resulting defects in the glomerular basal lamina cause nephritis marked by hematuria and progressive renal failure. Some patients also manifest hearing loss and ocular disorders.

Alport's syndrome is marked by nephritis, hearing loss, and ocular defects. It has autosomal dominant or X-linked dominant transmission.

Nervous Tissue

TARGET TOPICS

- Ultrastructure and classification of neurons
- Functions of neuroglial cells
- Changes associated with nerve injury and recovery
- Generation of action potentials and impulse transmission at the synapses

- Myelination and nodes of Ranvier
- Blood–brain barrier
- Peripheral nerve layers
- Meningitis, degenerative diseases of the central nervous system, Guillain-Barré syndrome, Charcot-Marie-Tooth disease, neurofibromatosis

I. Introduction
   - Nervous tissue is specialized to receive stimuli (irritability) and transmit impulses (conductibility).
   A. Cellular components
      1. Neurons, which conduct impulses, are the fundamental structural and functional unit of the nervous system.
         - They consist of a cell body (perikaryon), which extends into two types of processes, axons and dendrites.
      2. Neuroglial cells, which are nonconducting, support and protect neurons.
   B. Major divisions
      1. The central nervous system (CNS) comprises the brain and spinal cord.
      2. The peripheral nervous system (PNS), consisting of neurons located outside the CNS, transmits impulses to and from the CNS.

II. The Neuron
   A. Formation of neurons
      - Neurons are nonreplicating, postmitotic cells derived from precursor cells that are present only during prenatal development.
      1. Neuroepithelial cells in the embryonic neuroectoderm give rise to neuroblasts, which differentiate into the neurons of the CNS.
      2. Neural crest cells, derived from a specialized region of the neuroectoderm, migrate throughout the body and give rise to the neurons and neuroglial cells of the PNS.

B. Structure of neurons
   1. The cell body contains the nucleus and various cytoplasmic organelles, cytoskeletal elements, and inclusions.
      a. The Golgi complex, located near the nucleus, and mitochondria throughout the cytoplasm
      b. Nissl bodies (or substance), which are composed of rough endoplasmic reticulum (RER) and free ribosomes
      c. Lipofuscin granules, which are the end result of lysosomal activity and increase in number with age
      d. Neurofilaments (intermediate filaments) and neurotubules (microtubules), some of which extend from the cell body into the processes
   2. Neuron processes vary in number, providing the basis for the morphologic classification of neurons (Fig. 6-1).
      a. Axons (nerve fibers) conduct impulses away from the cell body.
         (1) Most axons are long, slender processes that arise from the axon hillock in the cell body and branch at the distal (terminal) end.
         (2) The axonal cytoplasm (axoplasm) lacks ribosomes, RER, and the Golgi apparatus.

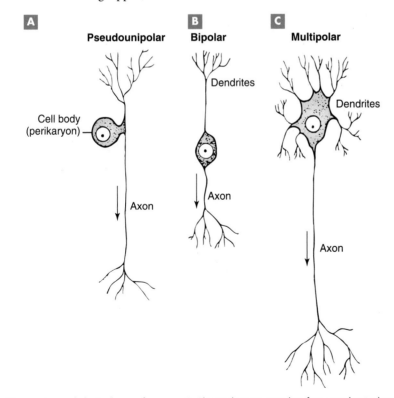

6-1: *Three main morphologic classes of neurons.* **A,** *The single axon extending from pseudounipolar neurons divides into two branches, one functioning as an axon and the other as a dendrite.* **B,** *Bipolar neurons have an axon and a dendrite.* **C,** *Multipolar neurons, which have multiple dendrites and a single axon, are the most abundant. Arrows indicate the direction of impulse conduction.*

(3) The myelin sheath, composed of many layers of modified plasma membrane, covers some axons.
b. Dendrites conduct impulses toward the cell body.
(1) Dendrites usually are relatively short and highly branched.
(2) They contain all the cytoplasmic components found in the cell body except the Golgi apparatus.
C. Axoplasmic transport
• Because the axon terminus lacks components for synthesizing new proteins or degrading old ones, materials must be transported back and forth between the cell body and the terminus.
1. Anterograde transport: Cell body → axon terminal
a. The fast component (50 to 400 mm/day) transports the cytoplasmic proteins and macromolecules that are required for metabolic and synaptic activity.
b. The slow component (1 to 4 mm/day) transports the cytoskeletal components down the axon.
2. Retrograde transport: Axon terminal → cell body
• Used membranous components of the synaptic vesicles move to the cell body, where they are degraded in lysosomes.
D. Functional classification of neurons
1. Sensory neurons transmit impulses from sensory receptors to the CNS.
2. Motor neurons transmit impulses from the CNS to a motor effector organ (muscle or gland).
a. Somatic motor neurons innervate the skeletal muscles.
b. Autonomic motor neurons innervate some glands, cardiac muscle, and involuntary smooth muscles.
• Autonomic neurons are classified into two functional types, which generally have opposite effects on target organs (Table 6-1).
(1) Parasympathetic neurons: cell body of the first-order (presynaptic) neurons in the cranial and sacral regions of the spinal cord; cell body of the second-order (postsynaptic) neurons in or near the organs they innervate
(2) Sympathetic neurons: cell body of the first-order neurons in the thoracic and lumbar regions of the spinal cord; cell body of the second-order neurons in the sympathetic ganglia near the spinal cord

Viruses and toxins can be transported from the periphery to the central nervous system within axons (retrograde transport).

TABLE 6-1:
Selected Effects of Parasympathetic and Sympathetic Stimulation

Target Tissue/Organ	Parasympathetic Effect	Sympathetic Effect
Adrenal medulla	No effect	Stimulates secretion
Bladder	Promotes voiding	No effect
Bronchi	Constricts	Relaxes
Heart pacemaker cells	Decreases heart rate	Increases heart rate
Pupil of eye	Constricts	Dilates
Salivary glands	Stimulates secretion	Inhibits secretion
Stomach, intestines	Promotes motility and gland secretion	Inhibits motility and gland secretion

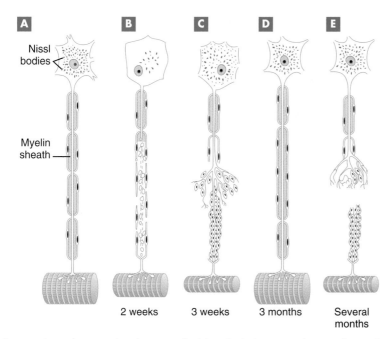

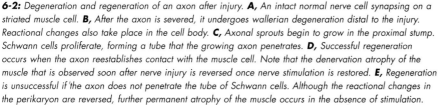

2 weeks   3 weeks   3 months   Several months

6-2: Degeneration and regeneration of an axon after injury. **A,** *An intact normal nerve cell synapsing on a striated muscle cell.* **B,** *After the axon is severed, it undergoes wallerian degeneration distal to the injury. Reactional changes also take place in the cell body.* **C,** *Axonal sprouts begin to grow in the proximal stump. Schwann cells proliferate, forming a tube that the growing axon penetrates.* **D,** *Successful regeneration occurs when the axon reestablishes contact with the muscle cell. Note that the denervation atrophy of the muscle that is observed soon after nerve injury is reversed once nerve stimulation is restored.* **E,** *Regeneration is unsuccessful if the axon does not penetrate the tube of Schwann cells. Although the reactional changes in the perikaryon are reversed, further permanent atrophy of the muscle occurs in the absence of stimulation.*

    3. Interneurons transmit impulses within the CNS and most commonly connect sensory and motor neurons.

  E. Reaction of neurons to injury (Fig. 6-2)

    1. Damage to the cell body generally results in the death of a neuron.

      • Because neurons cannot undergo cell division and no neural precursor cells are present after birth, neurons that are destroyed postnatally cannot be replaced.

    2. Severing or crushing of an axon leads to characteristic changes (see Fig. 6-2A and B).

      a. Wallerian (anterograde) degeneration occurs in the distal portion of the axon (the portion separated from the cell body).

        (1) The axon begins to swell and degenerate, the myelin sheath fragments, and phagocytes remove cellular debris.

        (2) After about 3 weeks, Schwann cells proliferate and form a tube of cells distal to the injury.

      b. Reactional changes occur in the neuron cell body.

        (1) The cell body swells and the nucleus is displaced peripherally.

        (2) Nissl bodies disperse with a concomitant loss in the cytoplasmic basophilia referred to as *chromatolysis.*

    c. Recovery and regeneration of damaged axons (see Fig. 6-2C and D)
- If the lesion in a peripheral neuron is sufficiently distant from the cell body, the nerve may recover.
  (1) Axonal sprouts are produced at the distal end of the axon stump, using materials synthesized in the cell body.
  (2) The axon stump elongates and the sprouts seek the tubes formed by Schwann cells.
  (3) If sprouts penetrate the Schwann cell tube and reestablish contact with an appropriate effector cell, regeneration is likely.

3. Trophic effects of nerve injury
    a. Degeneration of the motor neurons innervating some muscle cells induces muscle atrophy.
- Motor neuron disease is any condition in which progressive degeneration of the motor neurons at the cervical and lumbosacral levels of the spinal cord leads to degeneration atrophy of the limb muscles (e.g., amyotrophic lateral sclerosis, polio).

    b. Degeneration of some neurons is transmitted to neurons with which they synapse, causing transneuronal degeneration.

III. Nerve Impulses
- Nerve impulses represent rapid, transient changes in the membrane potential of neurons, called *action potentials.*

A. Generation of action potentials (Fig. 6-3)

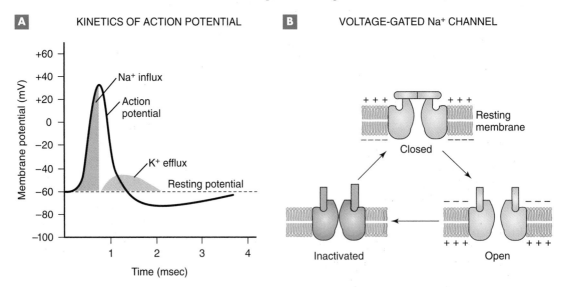

6-3: *Action potential.* **A,** *Time course of an action potential. A sudden massive influx of Na⁺ ions causes a rapid depolarization of the membrane potential from its resting value. Subsequent closing of Na⁺ channels and opening of K⁺ channels leads to efflux of K⁺ ions, briefly hyperpolarizing the membrane potential below its resting value.* **B,** *Schematic diagrams of changes in the conformational states of voltage-gated Na⁺ channels during generation of an action potential. In unstimulated neurons, these channels are closed. Their opening, triggered by a small depolarizing stimulus, leads to rapid depolarization of the membrane potential, as shown in* **A.**

- Action potentials originate at the axon hillock and move as a wave of electrical excitation toward the axon terminal.

B. Synaptic transmission of nerve impulses

- Impulses are transmitted from one neuron (presynaptic) to another neuron (postsynaptic) or from a neuron to an effector cell (muscle or gland cell) at regions of functional apposition, called *synapses.*

1. Chemical synapses (Fig. 6-4A)

   a. Presynaptic axon terminal: a small, knoblike termination (end-foot) of the transmitting neuron, which contains synaptic vesicles filled with a neurotransmitter

   b. Presynaptic membrane: a thickened region in the plasmalemma of the presynaptic axon terminal containing voltage-gated Ca^{2+} channels

      - Arrival of an action potential at an axon terminal → opening of Ca^{2+} channels → influx of Ca^{2+} ions → rise in the cytosolic Ca^{2+} level, which promotes exocytosis of the neurotransmitter into the synaptic cleft

   c. Synaptic cleft: a 20- to 40-nm–wide space separating the presynaptic and postsynaptic membranes across which a neurotransmitter diffuses

   d. Postsynaptic membrane: a thickened region in the plasmalemma of a receiving cell containing neurotransmitter receptors (Box 6-1)

      - At the excitatory synapse: Binding of neurotransmitter to its receptors → opening of Na^+ channels in the postsynaptic membrane → depolarization of the membrane → action potential in the postsynaptic cell

      - At the inhibitory synapse: Neurotransmitter binding → opening of K^+ or Cl^- channels in the postsynaptic membrane → hyperpolarization of the membrane → no action potential in the postsynaptic cell

An action potential is a rapid, transient change in the electrical potential across the plasma membrane involving an influx of Na^+ ions (depolarization) followed by an efflux of K^+ ions (repolarization).

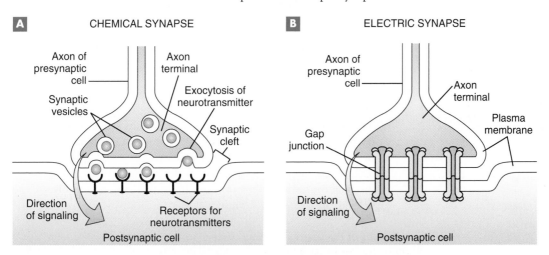

6-4: Synapses. The two types of synapses, chemical **(A)** and electrical **(B)**, differ in structure and in the mechanism of impulse transmission. Impulse transmission is faster at electrical synapses than at chemical synapses, although the latter are much more common. See also Figure 1-7C for the structure of gap junctions. (Adapted from Lodish HA, Berk SL, Zipursky P, Darnell J: Molecular Cell Biology, 4th ed. New York: WH Freeman, 2000, p 914.)

BOX 6-1

EXCITATORY AND INHIBITORY SYNAPSES

Whether a neurotransmitter promotes or inhibits generation of an action potential in postsynaptic cells depends on which receptor it binds to in the postsynaptic membrane. Acetylcholine (ACh) produces an excitatory response in some postsynaptic cells but an inhibitory response in other cells. Most neurotransmitters, however, produce either an excitatory or an inhibitory response. The effects and sites of action of some common neurotransmitters are listed below:

- Excitatory: ACh in skeletal muscle; dopamine, glutamate, and serotonin in the central nervous system (CNS)
- Inhibitory: ACh in heart muscle; γ-aminobutyric acid (GABA), glycine, and met-enkephalin in the CNS
- Excitatory or inhibitory: ACh in the CNS; norepinephrine in the CNS and peripheral nervous system

Important clinical correlations include:

- Decreased serotonin is associated with depression. Tryptophan is a precursor in the biosynthesis of serotonin.
- Increased GABA in the CNS leads to hepatic encephalopathy in patients with chronic liver disease.
- Decreased ACh in the CNS is commonly seen in Alzheimer's disease.
- Tetanus toxin blocks the release of inhibitory neurotransmitters (e.g., glycine), leading to continuous stimulation and contraction of muscles.
- Tyrosine is a precursor in the biosynthesis of dopamine and norepinephrine.

Acetylcholine is a neurotransmitter that is excitatory for skeletal muscle (nicotinic acetylcholine receptor) and inhibitory for heart muscle (muscarinic acetylcholine receptor).

2. Electrical synapse (Fig. 6-4B)
   a. Gap junctions (nexi) directly link the cytoplasm of some presynaptic and postsynaptic cells.
   b. The flow of ions through gap junctions transmits action potentials from presynaptic to postsynaptic cells without the involvement of neurotransmitters.
   c. The speed of impulse transmission at electric synapses is nearly instantaneous, whereas transmission at chemical synapses involves a delay of approximately 0.5 msec.

IV. Components of the Central Nervous System
   A. Two types of tissue are distinguishable in the CNS.
      1. Gray matter consists of the cell bodies of neurons, neuron processes, and neuroglial cells.
      2. White matter contains neuroglial cells and a large number of neuron processes, most of which are myelinated, but it lacks neuron cell bodies.

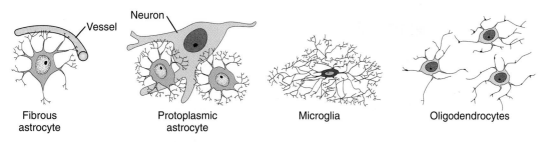

6-5: Neuroglial cells. Both fibrous and protoplasmic astrocytes have end-feet that terminate on vessel walls. Protoplasmic astrocytes, found mainly in the gray matter, also associate closely with neuron cell bodies. Microglia are phagocytes of the central nervous system. Oligodendrocytes myelinate central nervous system neurons.

B. Neuroglial cells of the CNS are approximately 10 times more numerous than neurons (Fig. 6-5).
- Neuroepithelial cells of the embryonic neuroectoderm give rise to all CNS neuroglial cells except microglia, which arise from the embryonic mesoderm.
- Under appropriate conditions, neuroglial cells are capable of cell division.
1. Astrocytes, the largest of the neuroglial cells, have numerous processes with expanded end-feet (pedicles) that terminate on capillaries or on the pia mater.
   a. Fibrous astrocytes: located primarily in the white matter; long, spindly processes with few branches
   b. Protoplasmic astrocytes: located in the gray matter; thick, highly branched processes; closely apposed to neuron cell bodies
   c. Functions of astrocytes
      (1) Regulate the composition of the intercellular environment and the entry of substances into it
      (2) Provide structural support (analogous to fibroblasts)
      (3) Metabolize neurotransmitters
      (4) Mediate the exchange of nutrients and metabolites between the blood and neurons
      (5) Help form noncollagenous scar tissue after injury to the CNS
2. Oligodendrocytes
   a. In white matter, oligodendrocytes are the predominant type of neuroglial cell and produce the myelin sheath around myelinated fibers.
   b. In gray matter, oligodendrocytes are closely associated with neuron cell bodies, functioning as satellite cells along with protoplasmic astrocytes; they also surround the axons of unmyelinated fibers.
3. Microglia are small phagocytic cells that enlarge and become mobile after injury to the CNS.
4. Ependymal cells are ciliated cuboidal cells that line the ventricles of the brain and the central canal of the spinal cord.
   - Within the choroid plexus, ependymal cells are thought to be the principal cell type that secretes cerebrospinal fluid (CSF).

Neuroglial tumors, which arise from astrocytes, oligodendrocytes, and ependymal cells, make up about half of all intracranial tumors.

Microglial cells, the macrophages of the central nervous system, are the reservoir cell for human immunodeficiency virus in patients with acquired immune deficiency syndrome dementia.

BOX 6-2

MENINGITIS

Infection or inflammation of the meninges usually results from pathogens spreading from other, primary sites of infection via the bloodstream. Meningitis often has a sudden onset and is characterized by severe headache, fever, nausea with vomiting, and stiffness in the neck. The diagnosis of meningitis is confirmed by a lumbar puncture (spinal tap) and analysis of the cerebrospinal fluid.

Bacterial meningitis commonly is caused by *Streptococcus pneumoniae* and *Neisseria meningitidis*. This severe, pus-forming infection requires immediate, high-dose antibiotic therapy.

Viral meningitis, caused by coxsackie and mumps viruses, generally is self-limiting and resolves within a few weeks.

Fungal meningitis due to *Candida* or *Cryptococcus* can be serious, especially in immunocompromised patients.

Glioblastoma multiforme, the most malignant type of astrocytoma, is a rapidly growing tumor that usually occurs in the cerebral hemispheres in adults.

C. The meninges are the three membranous layers that cover and protect the brain and spinal cord (Box 6-2).

1. The dura mater (outer meninx) blends with the periosteum of the skull, but is separated from the vertebrae by the epidural space and from the underlying arachnoid by the subdural space.
   - It is composed of dense, fibrous connective tissue.
   - It is lined by a discontinuous mesothelium on its inner surface in the skull and on both surfaces in the spinal column.

2. The arachnoid (middle meninx) is a delicate fibrous layer that extends weblike strands (trabeculae) into the underlying subarachnoid space.
   - It is lined on both surfaces by the mesothelium.
   a. The subarachnoid space lies between the arachnoid and the pia mater and contains blood vessels surrounded by CSF.
   b. The arachnoid villi are specialized projections of the arachnoid that terminate in venous spaces and function to return CSF to the venous system.
      - Meningiomas are derived from arachnoid granulation.

3. The pia mater (inner meninx) is a delicate layer of fibroblasts and collagen fibers directly apposed to the brain and spinal cord.
   a. Perivascular spaces are tunnels covered with pia mater through which blood vessels penetrate the CNS.
      - The pia mater disappears as blood vessels are transformed into capillaries.
   b. The choroid plexus consists of infoldings of the pia mater that project into ventricles of the brain and are covered by a thin layer of specialized ependymal cells (choroid epithelial cells).

      (1) Blood perfuses through the choroid plexus to form CSF, which is
          an exudate of blood.

      (2) Tight junctions between the choroid epithelial cells constitute the
          blood–CSF barrier.

  D. The blood–brain barrier prevents the passage of certain substances from the
     blood to nervous tissue in the CNS.

     • Several properties of CNS capillaries reduce their permeability, contributing
      to the functional blood–brain barrier:

     1. The lack of fenestrations and the paucity of pinocytic vesicles in the
       endothelial cells

     2. The zonulae occludens (tight junctions) between the endothelial cells

     3. Astrocyte pedicles that completely envelop these capillaries

  E. Degenerative diseases of the CNS (Table 6-2)

> Hydrocephalus results from a decrease in the absorption or outflow of cerebrospinal fluid. It typically leads to enlargement of the head and mental retardation.

V. Components of the Peripheral Nervous System

     • The PNS is composed of neuron processes and cell bodies located outside
      the CNS, ganglia that house cell bodies, neuroglial cells, and nerve
      endings.

  A. Neuroglial cells of the PNS

     1. Satellite cells (amphicytes) form a capsule of cells around neuron cell
       bodies located in the peripheral ganglia.

     2. Schwann cells envelop the axons of unmyelinated fibers and elaborate the
       myelin sheath around myelinated fibers.

  B. Myelin sheath

     • In both the CNS and PNS, some axons, but no dendrites, are surrounded
      by a myelin sheath.

     1. Myelin-producing cells

       a. In the CNS, individual oligodendrocytes myelinate portions of several
         axons.

       b. In the PNS, individual Schwann cells myelinate portions of only a
         single axon.

     2. Composition and formation of the myelin sheath (Fig. 6-6)

      • The myelin sheath, which is derived from the plasma membrane of a
       neuroglial cell, is similar in composition to the plasma membrane, but
       has a higher proportion of lipids.

     3. Nodes of Ranvier

       a. These interruptions in the myelin sheath around an axon represent
         gaps between adjacent myelinating cells.

       b. Because Na^+ channels are concentrated at the nodes, impulse
         conduction along myelinated axons involves "jumping" of action
         potentials from one node to the next (saltatory conduction).

  C. Ganglia

     • These encapsulated collections of neuron cell bodies, located outside the
      CNS, also contain satellite cells (amphicytes) and the usual connective
      tissue elements.

     1. Craniospinal ganglia house the cell bodies of sensory neurons, which are
       pseudounipolar or bipolar.

> Alzheimer's disease and Pick's disease are marked by distinct histopathologic changes that cause atrophy of the cerebral cortex, leading to dementia.

> The myelin sheath is formed by Schwann cells in the peripheral nervous system and by oligodendrocytes in the central nervous system.

> Demyelination can result from viral infection of the oligodendrocytes (measles virus), osmotic damage to the Schwann cells (diabetes), or autoantibodies directed against myelin (multiple sclerosis).

TABLE 6-2:
Degenerative Diseases of the Central Nervous System

Disease	Pathogenesis	Clinical Features
Alzheimer's disease	Progressive diffuse atrophy throughout cerebral cortex from degeneration of neurons; senile plaques (extracellular deposits of β-amyloid fibrils); neurofibrillar tangles within neurons	Gradual loss of recent memory (decreased acetyl choline), cognition, and judgment, progressing to dementia Defects in fine motor skills, restlessness, and fearfulness Most common cause of dementia after 65 years of age
Amyotrophic lateral sclerosis	Progressive deterioration of upper and lower motor neurons (corticospinal tract), leading to muscle atrophy	Wasting of muscles, beginning in limbs and progressing proximally Onset usually in middle age; rapid course, leading to severe paralysis, breathing difficulty, and death within 2–5 years
Huntington's chorea	Severe atrophy of caudate nuclei, cerebral cortex, and extrapyramidal system	Rapid, jerky movements (chorea) of head, limbs, and tongue; mental deterioration ending in dementia Autosomal dominant inheritance, with onset at age 25–45 years; death within 15 years
Multiple sclerosis	Patchy autoimmune destruction of myelin throughout central nervous system and peripheral nervous system, resulting in slowed impulse conduction along affected fibers	Numbness in limbs, muscle weakness, incoordination, and visual disturbances Onset in young adulthood, with recurrent attacks of symptoms and remissions
Parkinson's disease	Loss of neurons within substantia nigra (decreased dopamine) and other portions of extrapyramidal system	Mask-like facies, "pill-rolling" involuntary tremor, shuffling gait, slowing of voluntary movement, muscle rigidity
Pick's disease	Progressive atrophy, primarily involving frontal and temporal lobes; globular filamentous inclusions (Pick bodies) within degenerating neurons	Similar to Alzheimer's disease

- Sensory ganglia are associated with most cranial nerves and the dorsal roots of all the spinal nerves (dorsal root ganglia).
  2. Autonomic ganglia house the cell bodies of multipolar motor neurons composing the autonomic nervous system.
     a. Sympathetic ganglia are located beside the vertebral column.
     b. Parasympathetic ganglia are located within or near the target tissue.
  D. Peripheral nerves (Fig. 6-7)

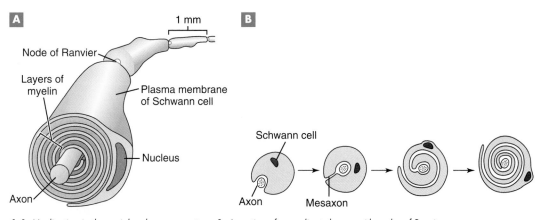

6-6: Myelination in the peripheral nervous system. **A,** A portion of a myelinated axon with nodes of Ranvier between adjacent Schwann cells. **B,** Mechanism of myelination. After a Schwann cell completely surrounds an axon, the region of edge-to-edge contact of the plasma membrane (mesaxon) elongates and wraps around the axon. As consecutive spirals of infolded plasma membrane are formed, the intervening cytoplasm is squeezed out and the cytosolic surfaces fuse (major dense line). The external membrane surfaces are held in close apposition (intraperiod line) by a protein found only in myelinating Schwann cells. In reality, the myelin layers are compacted much more tightly than depicted.

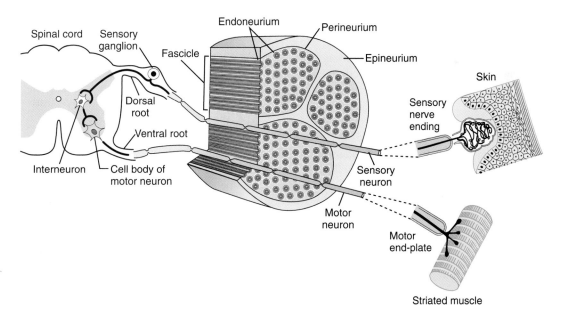

6-7: Schematic depiction of a typical reflex arc, with a cross-sectional view of a mixed peripheral nerve. Note the bundles (fascicles) of fibers in the nerve and the three types of connective tissue layers. Stimulation of sensory nerve endings in the skin triggers an impulse that is transmitted to the spinal cord via the dorsal root ganglion. The sensory impulse is transmitted to a motor neuron (via an interneuron), triggering a motor impulse that passes to a skeletal muscle. The knee-jerk reflex and the heat-induced withdrawal reflex operate in this fashion.

The connective tissue layers of the peripheral nerves:

- The epineurium surrounds an entire nerve and carries blood vessels.
- The perineurium surrounds a fascicle of nerve fibers, forming a permeability barrier.
- The endoneurium surrounds a single nerve fiber, including the myelin sheath, if present.

- A peripheral nerve comprises bundles (fascicles) of nerve fibers (axons) that are surrounded by myelin sheaths or Schwann cells and are invested with three connective tissue elements.
1. Connective tissue elements
   a. Epineurium: a thick, fibrous coat that forms the external covering of a nerve
      - Blood and lymphatic vessels supply the epineurium.
   b. Perineurium: a layer of dense connective tissue around each fascicle of nerve fibers
      - The inner surface is lined with epithelial-like cells joined by zonulae occludens (tight junctions), which provide a permeability barrier.
      - This layer must be rejoined in microsurgery for limb reattachment.
   c. Endoneurium: a thin, reticular layer that surrounds each individual nerve fiber and contains Schwann cells
      - In myelinated fibers, the endoneurium lies outside and encloses the myelin sheath.
2. Functional classification of nerves
   a. Sensory nerves contain axons of sensory neurons (afferent fibers), whose cell bodies are located in craniospinal (dorsal root) ganglia.
   b. Motor nerves contain axons of motor neurons (efferent fibers), whose cell bodies are located in the spinal cord or autonomic ganglia.
   c. Mixed nerves, the most common type, contain both efferent (motor) and afferent (sensory) fibers.
E. Peripheral nerve endings (see Fig. 6-7)
   1. Motor endings are the axonal terminations of motor fibers where they synapse with muscles or glands.
      a. A motor end-plate is the chemical synapse between the axon terminal of a motor fiber and a muscle fiber; it is also called a *neuromuscular junction.*
      b. Neurotransmitter released from motor endings changes the permeability of the effector cell (muscle or gland), causing a wave of depolarization to sweep over the effector cell, bringing about contraction or secretion.
   2. Sensory endings are specialized dendritic terminations that convert various internal or external stimuli into nerve impulses.
      a. Mechanoreceptors respond to stretch, touch, or pressure; they may be free nerve endings or encapsulated corpuscles (see Fig. 8-3).
      b. Chemoreceptors are the free endings of specialized epithelial cells that respond to taste sensations and odors (see Fig. 19-5).
      c. Light receptors are the free endings of photoreceptor cells in the retina (see Fig. 19-2).
      d. Temperature and pain receptors generally are free nerve endings.
F. Diseases of the peripheral nerves
   1. Guillain-Barré syndrome (acute idiopathic polyneuritis): a rapidly progressive ascending motor neuron paralysis that frequently is a sequel to enteric or viral infection

- Clinical manifestations begin with paresthesias of the feet, followed by flaccid paralysis of the legs that moves upward; it is accompanied by a slight fever.

2. Charcot-Marie-Tooth disease (type I): a hereditary (autosomal dominant) disorder marked by loss of innervation to the muscles supplied by the peroneal nerves
   - Clinical onset in children or young adults leads to weakness and atrophy of the calf muscles. Foot deformities (talipes) are common.
   - An inverted champagne bottle appearance results from preservation of the thigh muscles with atrophy of the calf muscles.

3. Neurofibromatosis (type 1): a relatively common autosomal dominant disorder caused by loss of the *NF-1* or *NF-2* tumor-suppressor gene.
   - Clinical features include numerous soft, benign tumors (neurofibromas) over the entire body; café au lait spots on the skin; Lisch nodules (hamartomas of the iris); and multiple types of brain tumors (e.g., acoustic neuromas, meningiomas, optic nerve gliomas).

Muscular Tissue

TARGET TOPICS

- Banding patterns of skeletal muscle in the resting, contracted, and stretched states
- Key structural and functional differences among skeletal, cardiac, and smooth muscle
- Molecular structure of myofibrils and myofilaments

- Sliding filament mechanism of muscle contraction
- Role of T tubules and sarcoplasmic reticulum in contraction
- Muscular dystrophies, Eaton-Lambert syndrome, myasthenia gravis, botulism, and the regenerative capacity of muscle

I. Introduction
- Muscular tissue comprises a population of cells (muscle fibers, myofibers) specialized to perform movement (locomotion) through the processes of contraction and relaxation.

Muscle cell = myofiber = fiber

- All muscles consist of a stroma of connective tissue and a parenchyma of muscle fibers varying in length and diameter.
  A. Classification of muscular tissue
    - Three types vary in their structure, distribution, and functional properties.
    1. Skeletal muscle (muscles of the skeleton)
    2. Cardiac muscle (parenchyma of the heart)
    3. Smooth muscle (muscles associated with blood vessels, viscera, and internal organs)
  B. Basic properties of muscle fibers
    1. Excitability: ability to respond to a stimulus
    2. Conductivity: ability to propagate a limited response
    3. Contractility: ability to shorten
    4. Elasticity and viscosity: ability to relax (return to their original shape) after contraction

II. Structure of Skeletal Muscle
- Skeletal muscle fibers are long, cylindrical cells with numerous, peripherally located nuclei.

A. Development of skeletal myofibers
  1. Prenatal: Embryonic mesodermal cells in somites proliferate, migrate, and fuse into multinucleated myotubes, which differentiate into skeletal muscle fibers.
  2. Postnatal: Growth of muscle before puberty occurs by an increase in the size of muscle fibers (hypertrophy) and in their number (hyperplasia). After puberty, growth occurs by hypertrophy only.
B. Connective tissue stroma of skeletal muscles (Fig. 7-1)
  1. Epimysium envelops an entire muscle.
  2. Perimysium separates small bundles (fascicles) of muscle fibers.
  3. Endomysium envelops each individual muscle fiber.
    a. The external lamina, which is equivalent to the basal lamina in epithelial tissue, lies between the plasma membrane (sarcolemma) and the endomysium.
    b. Satellite cells (pericytes) located within the external lamina function as stem cells that can replace damaged muscle by proliferating, fusing, and differentiating into skeletal muscle fibers.
C. Myofibrils
  • The cytoplasm (sarcoplasm) of a muscle fiber is filled with bundles of myofibrils composed of long myofilaments running parallel to the long axis of the fiber.
  1. Characteristic striations evident in each muscle fiber and myofibril arise from the highly organized pattern of myofilaments (see Fig. 7-1).
    a. A band: a darkly staining region (overlapping thin and thick filaments)
    b. I band: a lightly staining region (thin filaments only)
    c. H band: a lightly staining region that bisects each A band (thick filaments only)
    d. Z line (Z disk): a dense region that bisects each I band
    e. M line: a narrow dark region that bisects each H band
  2. A sarcomere, the regularly repeating unit between successive Z lines, is the smallest unit capable of contraction.
D. Molecular components of myofilaments
  1. Thick (myosin) filaments ($\approx 14\,nm$ thick)
    a. Myosin is a dimeric protein with a long tail and two globular heads at one end.
    b. Tails of hundreds of myosin molecules associate to form a bipolar filament with the heads located at the distal ends and the tails directed toward the central region (Fig. 7-2A).
    c. The heads of the myosin molecules, which project from thick filaments, have actin-binding sites and ATPase activity.
  2. Thin (actin) filaments ($\approx 8\,nm$ thick)
    a. Fibrous F-actin, a double helical filament, is formed by the polymerization of 300 to 400 G-actin monomers (Fig. 7-2B).
      • Each actin monomer possesses a myosin-binding site.
    b. Tropomyosin, a long polymeric protein, runs in the groove of the F-actin helix.

Striations in skeletal muscle:
• A band: dark (thick and thin filaments)
• I band: pale (thin filaments)
• H band: pale, located at the center of an A band (thick filaments)
• Z line: dark, located at the center of an I band
• M line: dark, located at the center of an H band

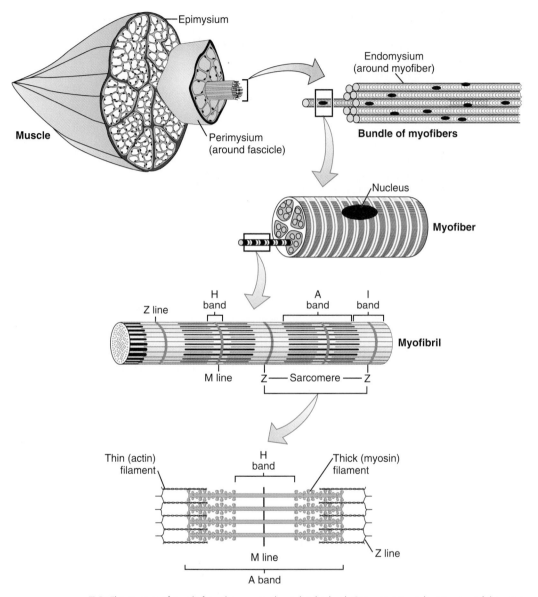

7-1: *The structure of muscle from the gross to the molecular level. Connective tissue layers surround the entire muscle, bundles of myofibers (fascicles), and individual myofibers. The regular array of myofilaments within each myofibril and the alignment of sarcomeres of adjacent myofibrils produce the characteristic banding pattern. In the region where thick and thin myofilaments overlap, each thick filament is surrounded by six thin filaments in a hexagonal array.*

c. Troponin (Tn), a globular protein complex composed of three subunits, attaches to specific sites along the tropomyosin polymer.

(1) Tn-T binds to tropomyosin.

(2) Tn-C binds Ca^{2+}.

(3) Tn-I inhibits the actin–myosin interaction.

An elevated troponin level in blood is seen after acute myocardial infarction.

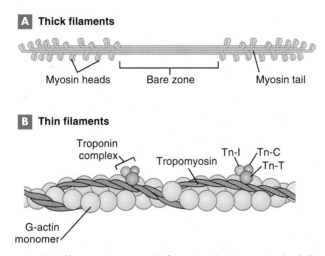

A Thick filaments

Myosin heads   Bare zone   Myosin tail

B Thin filaments

Troponin complex
Tropomyosin
Tn-I   Tn-C
Tn-T

G-actin monomer

7-2: Myofilaments. **A,** Thick filaments are composed of myosin molecules, arranged with their long, coiled tails parallel and their heads projecting from the surface. These filaments are bipolar, with each end covered by heads and the central portion devoid of heads. **B,** Thin filaments are composed primarily of F-actin, resulting from the polymerization of G-actin monomers. In skeletal and cardiac muscle, tropomyosin and the trimeric troponin complex (Tn-T, Tn-I, and Tn-C) that is associated with thin filaments participate in regulating contraction.

E. Proteins that organize myofilaments in skeletal muscle
  1. Titin, a large, fibrous protein, connects the ends of thick filaments to the Z line, centering these filaments in the sarcomere.
  2. α-Actinin attaches thin filaments to the Z line.
  3. A framework of desmin intermediate filaments, which surrounds the Z line and extends into each sarcomere, links myofibrils together laterally and to the sarcolemma.
    • Desmin is an excellent marker for tumors that are derived from skeletal and smooth muscle and that have a nonvascular origin.
  4. Dystrophin is one of the proteins that link the α-actinin–desmin complex to the cytoplasmic side of the sarcolemma.
    • The dystrophin gene, located on the X chromosome, is mutated in patients with Duchenne and Becker muscular dystrophies.
F. Sarcoplasmic membrane system in skeletal muscle (Fig. 7-3)
  1. The sarcoplasmic reticulum (SR), a modified smooth endoplasmic reticulum, constitutes a meshwork of tubules and cisternae surrounding each myofibril.
    • Terminal cisternae: greatly dilated regions of the SR, located at A–I junctions, that store and release Ca^{2+} ions
  2. Transverse (T) tubules are invaginations of the sarcolemma that extend into the sarcoplasm at the level of the A–I junction.
  3. Triads consist of a central T tubule flanked by two terminal cisternae.
G. Types of skeletal muscle fibers
  • Most skeletal muscles contain a mixture of two or three fiber types.
  1. Red fibers have large-diameter myofibrils and are capable of sustained activity over long periods; they are also called *slow-twitch fibers.*

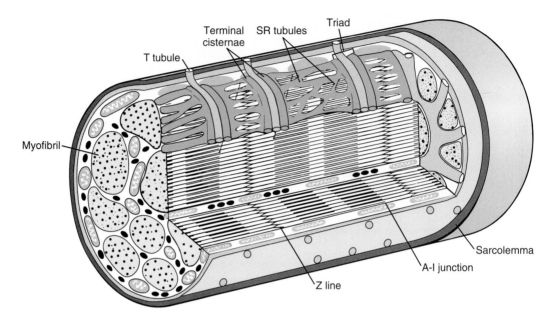

7-3: *Sarcoplasmic reticulum (SR) and transverse (T) tubules in skeletal muscle fibers. Ca²⁺ ions stored in the SR are released to the cytosol via voltage-gated channels in the terminal cisternae. Opening of channels is triggered by depolarization of the sarcolemma, which is conveyed by the T tubules into the sarcoplasm.*

- They have high myoglobin and low glycogen content and many mitochondria.
2. White fibers have small-diameter myofibrils and are capable of fast but brief bursts of activity; they are also called *fast-twitch fibers.*
   - They have low myoglobin and high glycogen content and few mitochondria.
3. Intermediate fibers have characteristics similar to or between those of red and white fibers.

III. Mechanism of Skeletal Muscle Contraction
   A. Sliding filament model
      - When a myofibril contracts, thin filaments move past thick filaments, increasing their overlap.
      - Filament sliding during contraction decreases sarcomere length, but the lengths of myofilaments remain constant (Fig. 7-4).
   B. Contraction cycle (Fig. 7-5)
      - Movement of thick and thin filaments past each other requires adenosine triphosphate (ATP) and involves cyclic interactions between myosin and actin.
      - In the absence of ATP (e.g., after death), myosin cannot dissociate from actin filaments, and muscles remain in a state of rigor mortis.
   C. Regulation of skeletal muscle contraction
      1. Inactive (off) state: In resting muscle, tropomyosin partially covers the myosin-binding sites on thin (actin) filaments, inhibiting the interaction

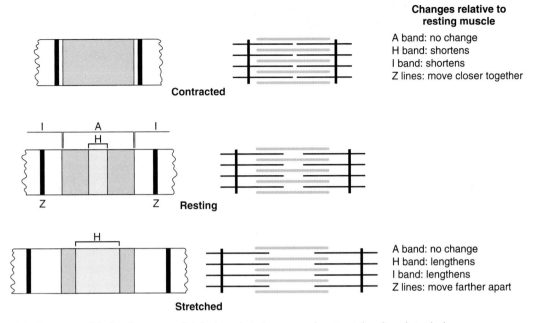

**Changes relative to
resting muscle**

A band: no change
H band: shortens
I band: shortens
Z lines: move closer together

Contracted

Resting

A band: no change
H band: lengthens
I band: lengthens
Z lines: move farther apart

Stretched

7-4: *Comparison of the banding pattern of skeletal muscle in the contracted, resting (relaxed), and stretched states. During contraction and stretching, the overlapping of thick and thin filaments changes, but their lengths remain constant.*

of myosin with actin that occurs during the contraction cycle. In this state, the contraction cycle cannot proceed.

2. Active (on) state: Binding of Ca^{2+} by troponin C (Tn-C) leads to a slight shift in the position of tropomyosin on the thin filament, exposing the myosin-binding sites. In this state, the contraction cycle proceeds if ATP is available.

D. Initiation and cessation of muscle contraction (Fig. 7-6)
 • Contraction of skeletal muscle is triggered by the arrival of a nerve impulse at the motor end-plate or neuromuscular junction.

1. Acetylcholine (ACh) released from motor nerve endings binds to receptors in the sarcolemma of the muscle fiber.

2. A wave of depolarization (action potential) sweeps over the sarcolemma and T tubules and is relayed across the gap between the T tubules and the terminal cisternae.

3. Opening of voltage-gated Ca^{2+} channels in the SR terminal cisternae releases stored Ca^{2+} into the cytosol.

4. An increase in cytosolic Ca^{2+} switches actin thin filaments from the off to the on state, permitting myofibrils to contract. The contraction cycle will continue as long as the cytosolic Ca^{2+} level remains high enough.

5. The Ca^{2+} ATPase in the SR membrane pumps Ca^{2+} back into the SR, reducing the cytosolic Ca^{2+} level.
 • When cytosolic Ca^{2+} is reduced enough, the thin filaments return to their off state and fiber relaxes.

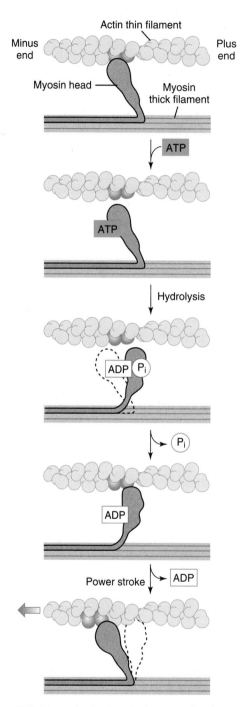

In the absence of a bound nucleotide, the myosin head is tightly bound to the actin filament in a "rigor" state.

Binding of ATP causes a slight conformational change in myosin that weakens its interaction with actin, leading to dissociation.

Hydrolysis of ATP causes a conformational change that displaces the myosin head a short distance along the actin filament. ADP and P_i remain bound to myosin.

Release of P_i permits strong binding of myosin to a new site on the actin filament and generates force for the power stroke.

As ADP is released, myosin returns to its original conformation, causing the actin filament to move. At the end of the power stoke, myosin is ready to begin the cycle again.

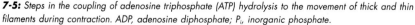

7-5: Steps in the coupling of adenosine triphosphate (ATP) hydrolysis to the movement of thick and thin filaments during contraction. ADP, adenosine diphosphate; P_i, inorganic phosphate.

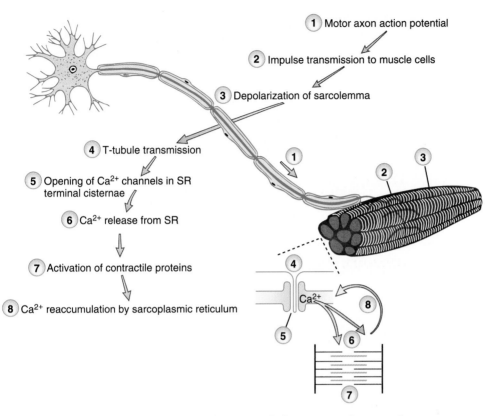

① Motor axon action potential

② Impulse transmission to muscle cells

③ Depolarization of sarcolemma

④ T-tubule transmission

⑤ Opening of Ca²⁺ channels in SR terminal cisternae

⑥ Ca²⁺ release from SR

⑦ Activation of contractile proteins

⑧ Ca²⁺ reaccumulation by sarcoplasmic reticulum

Ca²⁺

7-6: *Summary of events leading to the contraction of skeletal muscle fibers. SR, sarcoplasmic reticulum. (Adapted from Ross RB, Reith EJ: Histology: A Text and Atlas, 4th ed. New York: Harper & Row, 1985, p 204.)*

IV. Disorders of Skeletal Muscle
- The two major classes of muscle disorders, myopathy and neuropathy, generally lead to muscle atrophy marked by a decrease in the cross-sectional area of muscle fibers and in the number of myofibrils.
  A. Myopathies: Innervation to the muscle fibers remains intact.
    - Proximal, symmetrical muscle weakness commonly occurs in myopathies.
    1. Muscular dystrophies are hereditary diseases in which muscle fibers exhibit shrinkage and enlargement, centrally located nuclei, and eventual necrosis (Table 7-1).
      - Ring fibers, formed by wrapping one dystrophic fiber around another, are a distinctive feature of myotonic muscular dystrophy.
    2. Aging, malnutrition, and immobilization can lead to muscle atrophy with retention of innervation.
  B. Neuropathies: Innervation to the muscle fibers is lost.
    - Distal, asymmetrical muscle weakness commonly occurs in diseases caused by degeneration of the motor neurons (e.g., amyotrophic lateral sclerosis, Guillain-Barré syndrome, and Charcot-Marie-Tooth disease; see Chapter 6).

Duchenne muscular dystrophy is X-linked. It is caused by an absence of dystrophin and is the most severe form of muscular dystrophy, with fairly rapid progression.

Becker muscular dystrophy is X-linked. It is caused by defective dystrophin. It is similar to Duchenne muscular dystrophy, but with later onset and slower progression.

Eaton-Lambert syndrome is caused by autoantibodies that block the release of acetylcholine from the motor end-plate. It causes weakening of the limb muscles, but the ocular muscles usually are spared.

TABLE 7-1: Muscular Dystrophies

Type	Inheritance	Onset/Progression	Signs and Symptoms
Duchenne muscular dystrophy (DMD)	X-linked (dystrophin gene mutated)	Early onset Usually fatal by maturity	Progressive weakness of pelvic and limb girdles Early Gowers' sign Extensive pseudohypertrophy of calf muscles (replacement of lost fibers by connective tissue and fat) Swaying gait, with legs kept wide apart Cardiac involvement
Becker muscular dystrophy	X-linked (dystrophin gene mutated)	Late onset Slow progression	Similar to DMD, but less severe
Limb-girdle muscular dystrophy	Autosomal recessive	Variable onset (10–30 years of age) Usually slow progression	Weakness and wasting of proximal muscles of upper and lower limbs
Myotonic muscular dystrophy	Autosomal dominant	Childhood onset common but may be later Slow progression	Sustained muscle contraction (myotonia), especially in face and neck, followed by muscle atrophy Distinctive ring fibers Cataracts, gonadal atrophy, frontal balding, cardiac defects

Myasthenia gravis is caused by autoantibodies that block acetylcholine receptors in muscle. It causes weakening of muscles, especially those of the eye, face, and throat.

Botulinum toxin inhibits the release of acetylcholine at motoneuron endings. Bungarotoxin and other neurotoxins in certain snake venoms bind to and inactivate acetylcholine receptors at neuromuscular junctions.

C. Disorders in which impulse transmission at the neuromuscular junction is disrupted
1. Eaton-Lambert syndrome is an autoimmune disease in which autoantibodies to voltage-gated Ca^{2+} channels in motoneuron endings inhibit the release of ACh.
   • Muscle weakness affects the limbs but usually does not involve the ocular or bulbar muscles. It is often associated with oat cell (small cell) carcinoma of the lung.
2. Myasthenia gravis is an autoimmune disease in which autoantibodies to ACh receptors in muscle cells block the binding of ACh.
   • Gradual weakening (atrophy) of skeletal muscles, especially the most active ones, occurs. Ptosis, diplopia, dysphagia, and dysarthria are often present.
3. Botulism is a type of food poisoning in which an endotoxin produced by *Clostridium botulinum* inhibits the release of ACh at motoneuron endings.
   • Visual disorders, muscle weakness, difficulty swallowing, and sometimes nausea and vomiting may occur. The condition is fatal if untreated, usually due to respiratory failure.

4. Certain snake venoms (e.g., bungarotoxin) bind to and inactivate ACh receptors at the neuromuscular junctions, leading to paralysis.

V. Cardiac Muscle (Table 7-2)
- Cardiac muscle is striated because of the organization of thick and thin filaments, as in skeletal muscle.
  A. Major structural features that characterize cardiac muscle
   1. Cell shape and size: branched cells that are shorter than skeletal muscle cells
   2. Nucleus: single, centrally located

TABLE 7-2:
Comparison of Types of Muscular Tissues

Property	Skeletal Muscle	Cardiac Muscle	Smooth Muscle
Structural Properties			
Location	Muscles of skeleton	Heart	Vessels, organs, and viscera
Cell size/shape	Long; cylindrical	Short; branched	Variable size; spindle shape
Nuclei	Many; peripherally located	Single; centrally located	Single; centrally located
Striations	Yes	Yes	No
Z lines	Yes	Yes	Cytoplasmic dense bodies replace Z lines
T tubules and sarcoplasmic reticulum (SR)	Triads at A-I junction	Diads at Z line	Caveolae replace T tubules; sparse SR
Cell junctions	None	Intercalated disk (adherens, occludens, and nexi)	Nexi (gap junctions)
Connective tissue	Epimysium Perimysium Endomysium	Endomysium	Reticular fibers
Association of fibers	Bundles (fascicles)	Sheets	Sheets (primarily)
Functional Properties			
Mode of contraction	Voluntary; all or none	Involuntary; rhythmic all or none	Involuntary; slow, sustained
Stimuli inducing contraction	Neural (somatic efferent)	Intrinsic (pacemaker) modified by autonomic efferent; spread via nexi	Intrinsic (stretching), neural (autonomic efferent), and hormonal; spread via nexi
Mitosis	No	No	Yes
Regeneration	Limited (differentiation of satellite cells)	None	High

3. Sarcoplasmic membrane system
   a. T tubules: located at the Z line instead of at the A–I junction because they are found in skeletal muscle
   b. Terminal cisternae: relatively small and discontinuous
   c. Diads: one terminal cisterna associated with a T tubule at each Z line
4. Intercalated disks
   - These complex steplike junctions connect adjacent cardiac fibers end-to-end.
   a. Transverse parts, which run at right angles to the long axis of cardiac fibers, contain adherens and occludens components.
      - Thin filaments of adjacent cells attach to the transverse parts.
   b. The lateral part, which runs parallel to the long axis of cardiac fibers, contains numerous large gap junctions (nexi).
      - Action potentials spread rapidly from one fiber to another via these gap junctions, synchronizing contraction of the individual cardiac muscle fibers.

B. Contraction of cardiac muscle
   - The mechanism of contraction is the same as that in skeletal muscle.
   - Certain specialized cardiac myofibers contract through intrinsically generated impulses, which are passed to neighboring cells via gap junctions, resulting in the rhythmic heartbeat (see Chapter 11).

C. Absence of cardiac muscle regeneration
   - Cardiac myofibers are postmitotic cells incapable of cell division and are not associated with any stem cells, such as the pericytes in skeletal muscle.
   - Injured cardiac muscle generally is replaced by fibrous connective (scar) tissue.

VI. Smooth Muscle (see Table 7-2)
   - Smooth muscle lacks striations because the thin and thick filaments are not organized in the highly ordered arrays found in skeletal and cardiac muscle.

A. Major structural features that characterize smooth muscle
   1. Cell shape and size: fusiform (spindle-shaped); considerable variation in size, depending on location
   2. Nucleus: single, centrally located
   3. Sarcoplasmic membrane system: very sparse and lacking T tubules
   4. Caveolae: depressions in the sarcolemma that may function in regulating the cytosolic Ca^{2+} level
   5. Dense bodies: regions in the sarcoplasm that may be analogous to Z lines
      a. Thin (actin) filaments are anchored to sites on the sarcolemma and to dense bodies.
      b. Intermediate filaments extend from one dense body to another.
   6. Gap junctions (nexi): abundant in the sarcolemma of smooth muscle fibers, enabling rapid transmission of action potentials to adjacent fibers, which are not separately innervated

B. Contraction of smooth muscle
   1. Sliding of thin filaments relative to thick filaments results in shortening and thickening of smooth muscle fibers.

In adults, smooth muscle cells undergo mitosis, but skeletal and cardiac muscle cells do not.

2. An increase in the cytosolic Ca^{2+} level triggers contraction (as in skeletal muscle), but the mechanism by which it does so differs from that in skeletal muscle.
3. The rate of ATP hydrolysis by myosin is slower than in skeletal muscle, so contraction is relatively slow and sustained.
4. Initiation of smooth muscle contraction is triggered by various stimuli.
   a. Nerve impulses in vascular smooth muscle (usually)
   b. Stretching of muscle in visceral smooth muscle
   c. Oxytocin in the uterus during the terminal stages of pregnancy
   d. Epinephrine in smooth muscle elsewhere in the body

C. Regeneration of smooth muscle
   • Because smooth muscle cells actively divide, damaged fibers are regenerated.

Regeneration of muscle:
- High in smooth muscle because cells actively divide
- Limited in skeletal muscle because of the differentiation of satellite cells
- None in cardiac muscle, which lacks any stem cells. Injured fibers are replaced by scar tissue.

Integumentary System

I. Introduction
- The integumentary system consists of the skin and its appendages (hair follicles, nails, sweat glands, and sebaceous glands).

The skin is the largest organ of the body, accounting for 8% to 16% of adult body weight.

  A. Major components of the skin
1. Epidermis: the superficial layer of stratified squamous keratinized epithelium; primarily of ectodermal origin
2. Dermis (corium): the dense, fibrous, irregular connective tissue layer beneath the epidermis; mesodermal origin
3. Hypodermis: the layer of loose connective tissue that underlies the dermis and corresponds to the superficial fascia of gross anatomy
   - The hypodermis, which is not actually part of the skin, binds the skin to the subjacent tissue.
   - It may contain fat cells, which can form a thick layer (panniculus adiposus) in obese individuals or in certain regions of the body.

  B. Functions of the skin
1. Protective barrier
   a. Prevents desiccation (loss of fluids)
   b. Inhibits entry of foreign substances and microorganisms
   c. Disperses light (keratinized layers) and absorbs ultraviolet (UV) radiation (melanin)
   d. Undergoes wound healing

2. Thermoregulation
   a. Body temperature is regulated by control of sweat gland activity and blood flow through the dermal capillary network.
   b. The number of sweat glands is decreased in the elderly, predisposing them to heat stroke.
3. Regulation of blood pressure
   a. Opening of the dermal capillary network lowers blood pressure.
   b. Closing of the dermal capillary network raises blood pressure.
4. Excretion of metabolic waste products
5. Sensory reception (touch, pressure, temperature, and pain)
6. Synthesis of provitamin D
   • Photolysis of 7-dehydrocholesterol in the skin by UV radiation produces cholecalciferol (provitamin D), which is converted to active vitamin D in the liver (25-hydroxylation) and kidneys (1-α-hydroxylation).

II. Epidermis
   A. Epidermal strata (Fig. 8-1)
      • Keratinocytes, the predominant cell type of the epidermis, form a stratified squamous keratinized epithelium containing five strata in the following order, from deepest to most superficial:
      1. Stratum basale: a single, mitotically active layer of cuboidal to columnar keratinocytes
         a. Hemidesmosomes attach keratinocytes to the adjacent basement membrane.
         b. Low–molecular-weight keratins are produced by keratinocytes in the basal layer.
         c. Basal cells give rise to additional nondifferentiating stem cells, which remain in this layer, and to differentiating keratinocytes, which move into the stratum spinosum.

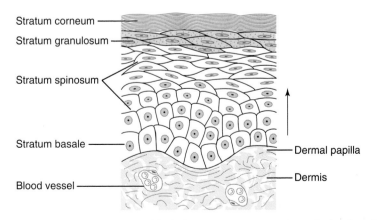

8-1: *Strata of thin skin, which covers most of the body. Keratinocytes arise in the stratum basale and move toward the surface as they differentiate (arrow), a process that normally takes 15 to 30 days. The connective tissue dermis contains blood vessels and nerve endings. The stratum lucidum, a thin layer just below the stratum corneum, is evident only in thick skin (the palms and soles).*

The layers of the epidermis from the base to the surface are the stratum basale, stratum spinosum, stratum granulosum, stratum lucidum (thick skin only), and stratum corneum.

The absence of tyrosinase in the melanocytes is responsible for albinism.

2. Stratum spinosum: several layers of polyhedral-shaped keratinocytes (prickle cells) that proliferate and differentiate
   a. High–molecular-weight keratins are produced and assembled into intermediate filaments (tonofibrils) that terminate in numerous desmosomes.
   b. Lamellar bodies (membrane-coated granules) containing lipid, carbohydrate, and hydrolytic enzymes become evident.
   c. Stratum germinativum = stratum basale + stratum spinosum.
3. Stratum granulosum: three to five layers of flattened keratinocytes that cannot divide
   a. Disulfide bonds begin to cross-link keratin filaments, which associate with numerous keratohyalin granules.
   b. Glycolipid and sterols secreted from the lamellar bodies into the intercellular space form an impermeable, waterproof barrier.
   c. Lysosomal activity degrades organelles as cells move toward the next stratum.
4. Stratum lucidum: a clear, homogeneous layer composed of flat keratinocytes that lack nuclei and organelles
   a. This layer is well defined only in thick skin (palm of the hand and sole of the foot).
   b. Cytoplasm consists almost entirely of keratin filaments.
5. Stratum corneum: 5 to 50 layers of flattened, keratinized (cornified) dead cells
   a. Cells of this superficial layer, called squames, are filled with cross-linked keratin filaments embedded in a globular amorphous matrix.
   b. Squames are continuously shed from the surface and replaced by differentiating cells from the basal layer.
      • Cytomorphosis of keratinocytes in the stratum basale to squames in the stratum corneum takes 15 to 30 days.

Melanocytes synthesize melanin, which is seen in pigmented melanophores and chromatophores.

B. Nonkeratinocytes in the epidermis
   1. Melanocytes synthesize a dark brown pigment (melanin) that absorbs UV radiation, thereby protecting DNA in the dividing cells of the skin from UV-induced damage.
      • An elevated corticotropin level increases melanin synthesis.
      a. Location: in the stratum basale, the papillary layer of the dermis, and the hair follicles
      b. Origin: derived from embryonic neural crest cells that migrate into the skin of a 12- to 24-week embryo
      c. Melanin formation and release
         (1) Synthesis occurs in the melanosomes, membrane-bounded granules that contain tyrosinase and other enzymes involved in the conversion of tyrosine to melanin.
         (2) Processes containing melanin-filled melanosomes are transferred via cytocrine secretion from melanocytes to the cytoplasm of keratinocytes (melanophores) in the stratum basale and stratum spinosum.

(3) Chromatophores are pigmented cells in the dermis that take up melanin by phagocytosis.
2. Langerhans cells have long dendritic processes that radiate throughout the epidermis.
   a. Location: primarily in the stratum spinosum
   b. Origin: derived from precursor cells in the bone marrow
   c. Function: involved in the immune response as antigen-presenting cells (see Chapter 13)
3. Merkel cells contain small, dense-cored granules filled with catecholamines (similar to granules in the cells of the adrenal medulla).
   a. Location: in the stratum basale near the well-vascularized, highly innervated dermis; present only in thick skin
   b. Function: may act as sensory mechanoreceptors or as diffuse neuroendocrine cells

C. Thickness of the epidermis
   • Skin is classified as thin or thick based on the relative thickness of the viable epidermis (stratum germinativum) and the stratum corneum.
   1. Thin skin covers most of the body (see Fig. 8-1).
      a. Epidermis: 50 to 70 μm thick
      b. Viable strata thicker than the stratum corneum
      c. Appendages: present
      d. Stratum lucidum: absent
   2. Thick skin lines the palms of the hands and the soles of the feet.
      a. Epidermis: 400 to 1500 μm thick
      b. Stratum corneum thicker than the viable epidermis
      c. Appendages: not present
      d. Stratum lucidum: present

D. Skin color
   • Skin thickness, vascular supply, and the presence of pigments determine the color of skin.
   1. Black or brown color is due to melanin.
      • Although blacks and whites have the same number of melanocytes, these cells are larger and transfer more melanin to the keratinocytes in blacks.
   2. Yellow color is due to carotene in the stratum corneum and in the adipose cells of the dermis.
   3. Red color is due to oxyhemoglobin in the blood.

E. Disorders involving the epidermis
   1. Epidermal neoplasms (Box 8-1)
      • Skin tumors arise from cells that are actively mitotic, including keratinocytes in the viable epidermis and melanocytes.
   2. Psoriasis: chronic skin disease marked by dry, scaly plaques and papules, most commonly on the scalp, knees, elbows, and trunk
      • Psoriatic lesions result from increased proliferation of keratinocytes in the stratum germinativum, faulty keratinization, and a reduction in transit time from the basal layer to the skin surface.

Langerhans cells in the epidermis function as antigen-presenting cells.

BOX 8-1

EPIDERMAL TUMORS

Basal cell carcinoma: the most common form of malignant skin tumor, arising from keratinocytes in the stratum basale. It usually occurs as small, pearly nodules with a central crater that may erode, crust, and bleed. It is locally invasive and aggressive, but rarely metastatic, and is most common on the faces of adults, especially on sun-exposed areas.

Squamous cell (epidermoid) carcinoma: a slow-growing malignant tumor that often originates in sun-damaged areas of the skin and also develops from the squamous epithelium in the lung and other sites. Actinic (solar) keratosis is a precursor lesion for squamous cell skin cancer. Tumor cells resemble prickle cells of the stratum spinosum and are characterized by "keratin pearls." Skin lesions commonly are firm, red, painless small bumps, which initially are localized and superficial but may later invade and metastasize.

Malignant melanoma: any malignant neoplasm arising from melanocytes. The most common type (superficial spreading melanoma) often occurs on the lower leg or back and presents as flat, pigmented skin patches that develop over several months or years. Malignant melanomas are deeply invasive and may metastasize throughout the body.

Verruca plana: a generally benign epidermal tumor caused by papillomavirus infection of keratinocytes. Small, slightly raised, tan or flesh-colored lesions (warts) often occur in large numbers on the face, neck, back of the hands, wrists, and knees.

Seborrheic keratosis: a benign skin tumor arising from basal cells and usually occurring in middle age. Lesions often develop rapidly in crops, presenting as yellow or brown raised soft plaques. A rapid increase in size and number of these lesions, known as Leser-Trélat sign, may indicate internal malignancy, especially of the gastrointestinal tract.

Ichthyosis vulgaris is an autosomal dominant disease that causes hyperkeratosis and absence of the stratum granulosum. It is the most common inherited disease affecting keratinization.

3. Ichthyosis vulgaris: the most common inherited disorder (autosomal dominant) of keratinization, with onset in childhood
   • Dry scales are present on the trunk and extremities; histologic features include hyperkeratosis and absence of the stratum granulosum.
4. Pemphigus vulgaris: a chronic autoimmune disease marked by flaccid, fragile bullae that rupture, leaving painful denuded regions
   • Autoantibodies to the adherens junctions between keratinocytes mediate this disease, the most common form of pemphigus.

III. Dermis
   • The dermis, composed of dense, fibrous, irregular connective tissue, varies in density, thickness, and elasticity in different body locations.

A. Dermal layers
  • Both layers of the dermis contain an elastic fiber network that is continuous throughout the bundles of collagen (primarily type I).
  1. Papillary layer: moderately dense connective tissue arranged in fine, interlacing bands of thin collagenous bundles
    • Irregular contour that sends projections (dermal papillae) into the adjacent basal layer of the epidermis
  2. Reticular layer: dense connective tissue arranged in thick, interlacing collagenous bands
    • Continuous with the hypodermis
B. Cells and other structural components of the dermis
  • Similar elements are also found in the underlying hypodermis.
  1. Fibroblasts
  2. Adipocytes
  3. Smooth muscle fibers
  4. Nerves and nerve endings
  5. Blood vessels
  6. Extensions of epidermal derivatives (hair follicles, sweat glands, and sebaceous glands)
C. Variation in the thickness of the dermis
  1. On the back, the dermis is very thick.
  2. On the abdomen, the dermis is very thin.
D. Disorders involving the dermis
  1. Keloids: abnormal scar tissue that is elevated, firm, and rounded, with irregular margins
    • These lesions result from abnormal wound healing or skin injury involving excessive formation of type III collagen in the dermis.
  2. Elastosis: loss of skin elasticity (wrinkles) accompanied by an increase in stainable elastin in the dermis
    • This condition commonly occurs with aging and can result from excessive exposure to sunlight.

IV. Appendages of the Skin
  • The skin's appendages are derived from the epidermal layer, but hair follicles and glands extend into the dermis and sometimes the hypodermis.
A. Hair and hair follicles (Fig. 8-2)
  1. Structure
    a. Hair shafts are located in multilayered follicles.
      • The ducts of the sebaceous glands and apocrine sweat glands empty into hair follicles.
    b. A dermal sheath surrounds each follicle and extends a protrusion (hair papilla) through the follicular layers and into the base of the shaft (hair bulb).
    c. The arrector pili muscle (smooth muscle) originates on the dermal sheath of the hair follicle and inserts into the papillary layer of the dermis.
      • Contraction elevates the hair (piloerection) and depresses the skin where the muscle attaches to the dermis, causing "goose bumps."

Basal cell carcinoma is derived from the stratum basale. It is rarely metastatic. Small lesions have a central crater, and it commonly occurs on the face.

Squamous cell carcinoma is a slow-growing lesion that is rarely metastic. It causes firm, painless bumps, with keratin pearls visible in the cells.

Malignant melanoma is derived from the melanocytes. It is deeply invasive and metastatic and causes flat, pigmented skin lesions on the lower leg and back.

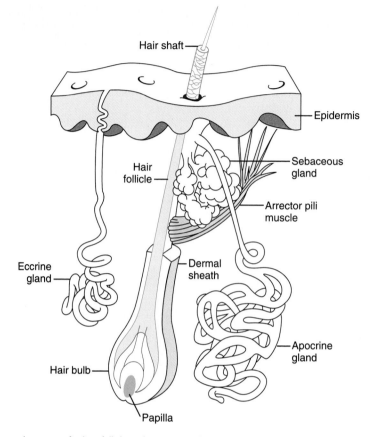

8-2: *General structure of a hair follicle and its associated structures. Both the hair shaft and the follicle are epidermal derivatives and contain several histologically distinguishable cell layers. Sebaceous glands and apocrine sweat glands empty into hair follicles, whereas eccrine sweat glands empty into pores on the skin surface.*

 2. Hair growth
  a. A hair shaft grows from the hair bulb, which is composed of a germinal layer of mitotically active basal cells and a keratogenous zone where hair cells become keratinized.
  b. Sex hormones influence hair growth in both males and females.
  c. Usually, hair growth is asynchronous.
  d. When hair growth is synchronous (e.g., postpartum, while taking oral contraceptives), massive hair loss occurs.
 B. Glands in the skin (see Fig. 8-2)
  • Prominent features of the sebaceous, eccrine sweat, and apocrine sweat glands are summarized in Table 8-1.
 1. Sebum: oily secretion of the sebaceous glands of the skin
  a. A mixture of sebum and sweat is mildly bactericidal and protects the skin against drying.
  b. Androgen receptors in the sebaceous glands function in controlling sebum production.

Androgen receptors in the sebaceous glands function in the androgen-mediated control of sebum production.

TABLE 8-1:
Glands of the Skin

	TYPE OF GLAND		
Property	**Sebaceous**	**Eccrine Sweat**	**Apocrine Sweat**
Location within skin	Dermis	Dermis	Dermis and hypodermis
Body distribution	Throughout body, except for palms and soles	Throughout body	Axilla, mons pubis, areola of nipple, perianal region
General structure	Branched acinar gland with short duct	Simple tubular gland	Large, complex gland
Myoepithelial cells	Absent	Present	Present
Type of secretion	Thick, lipid-containing substance (sebum)	Clear, watery secretion	Viscous substance rich in protein and cellular debris
Secretion mechanism	Holocrine	Merocrine	Mixed
Duct opening	Hair follicle (usually)	Surface of skin (sweat pore)	Hair follicle
Period of activity	Inactive until puberty	Active throughout life	Inactive until puberty
Other features	Excess androgen-mediated secretion can plug hair follicles, predisposing to acne	Secretion stimulated by high temperature and stress	Activity linked to menstrual cycle in female

2. Seborrhea: any of several skin diseases marked by very oily skin resulting from overproduction of sebum
3. Acne vulgaris: a chronic inflammatory disease of the pilosebaceous apparatus
   a. Pathogenic features include abnormal keratinization of the follicular epithelium, increased sebum production (androgen-controlled), and lipase production by *Propionibacterium acnes,* leading to release of fatty acid and an inflammatory reaction.
   b. Lesions take various forms, including blackheads (comedones), pink papules, and pus-filled cysts, primarily on the face, chest, and upper back.
C. Nails
   • Nails are hard, keratinized plates resting on a bed of epidermis at the distal end of each digit.
   1. The proximal root is embedded in a deep fold of epidermis.
      a. Eponychium (cuticle): stratum corneum of the nail fold, which overlies the proximal root
      b. Nail matrix: a region of epidermal cells covered by the eponychium where nail synthesis occurs
      c. Lunula: extension of the nail matrix beyond the eponychium, visible as a whitish crescent

2. The distal (free) edge is underlain by the hyponychium, a thickened stratum corneum.
3. Abnormal nails are associated with some diseases.
   - Nails should appear pinkish due to the blood vessels in the underlying dermis.
   a. A pale or bluish nail bed may indicate cardiovascular problems or poor oxygenation of the circulating blood (cyanosis).
   b. Split nails are associated with nutritional deficiencies.
   c. Clubbing (thickening) at the nail base may indicate lung cancer.
   d. Spoon-shaped nails (koilonychia) are associated with iron deficiency anemia.

V. Vasculature and Innervation of the Skin
   A. Blood supply to the skin
      - The epidermis lacks blood vessels; however, the dermis, hypodermis, and all skin appendages have an extensive network of small vessels.
      1. Arterial plexuses
         a. The rete cutaneum (reticular plexus) is located at the dermis–hypodermis border.
         b. The rete subpapillare (papillary plexus) is located at the border of the papillary and reticular layers of the dermis.
            - Arterioles from this plexus give rise to a single capillary loop around each dermal papilla.
      2. Venous plexuses
         a. At the middle of the dermis
         b. Between the papillary and reticular layers of the dermis
         c. At the dermis–hypodermis border
      3. Arteriovenous anastomoses (arteriovenous shunts)
         a. Direct connections between the arterioles and the venules, which occur in deeper parts of the skin, are important in thermoregulation.
         b. Blood flow through the arteriovenous shunts is regulated by autonomic nerve fibers and certain hormones.
      4. Kaposi's sarcoma
         a. Clinically, Kaposi's sarcoma is characterized by bluish-red cutaneous nodules, usually first appearing on the legs, toes, or feet, that slowly enlarge and spread to more proximal sites.
            - In patients with AIDS, Kaposi's sarcoma is associated with herpes infection (HHV8).
         b. Histologically, the lesions exhibit vascular proliferation with slitlike channels composed of malignant spindle-shaped cells, probably of endothelial origin.
   B. Nerves of the skin
      1. Motor nerves: postganglionic fibers from the sympathetic ganglia of the paravertebral chain
         - The autonomic nerve supply functions primarily in thermoregulation by regulating blood flow to the skin, secretion by sweat glands, and piloerection.

Sympathetic innervation of the skin functions largely in thermoregulation by controlling blood flow, secretion of sweat glands, and piloerection.

Kaposi's sarcoma is a spindle cell carcinoma of vascular origin that commonly arises in the skin and presents as bluish-red nodules. It is the most common cancer found in patients with AIDS, and it is associated with HHV8 infection. The lesions are aggressive and often metastasize.

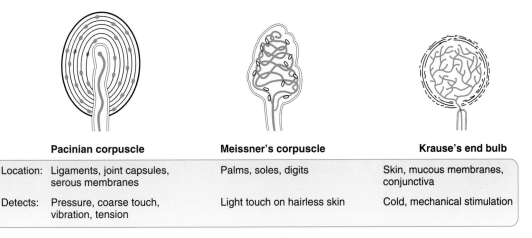

Pacinian corpuscle	Meissner's corpuscle	Krause's end bulb
Location: Ligaments, joint capsules, serous membranes	Palms, soles, digits	Skin, mucous membranes, conjunctiva
Detects: Pressure, coarse touch, vibration, tension	Light touch on hairless skin	Cold, mechanical stimulation

8-3: *Encapsulated mechanoreceptors. Their relative size is pacinian corpuscle > Meissner's corpuscle > Krause's end bulb (not to scale).*

2. Sensory nerve endings: most dense on the hands and feet, on the face (especially around the mouth), and in the anogenital region
   a. Free nerve endings, located at the epidermal opening and in the root sheath of the hair follicles, function as mechanoreceptors.
   b. Encapsulated sensory receptors, located in the skin and associated mucous membranes, are summarized in Figure 8-3.

Cartilage, Bone, and Joints

I. Cartilage
- A specialized avascular connective tissue, cartilage functions primarily to support soft tissues and in the development and growth of long bones.
  A. Structure of cartilage
    1. Cartilage cells, which arise from stellate mesenchymal cells, synthesize and secrete extracellular matrix components.
       - Eventually these cells become roundish and completely surrounded by matrix except for the small spaces, or lacunae, in which they reside.
       a. Chondroblasts: a less mature form that actively produces the matrix
       b. Chondrocytes: a more mature form that is less active in matrix synthesis
    2. The matrix of cartilage consists of fibers, ground substance, and water.
       a. The fibrous component contains collagen types I and II, elastic fibers, and reticular fibers, depending on cartilage type.
       b. Ground substance contains hyaluronic acid and chondroitin sulfate and keratan sulfate proteoglycans, primarily in the form of aggregates (see Fig. 5-3).

       c. Bound water provides an avenue for the diffusion of nutrients and oxygen to chondrocytes and confers a gel-like property to the cartilage matrix.

    3. Perichondrium, the vascularized connective tissue investment surrounding most cartilage, comprises two layers.

       a. The outer fibrous layer of the fibroblasts

       b. The inner chondrogenic layer

B. Types of cartilage (Table 9-1)

C. Growth of cartilage

    1. Interstitial growth results from mitosis of pre-existing chondrocytes and chondroblasts in the lacunae.

       a. Isogenous (isogenic) groups of two or four daughter cells trapped in lacunae are formed by interstitial growth.

       b. Cartilaginous fetal bones elongate by interstitial growth.

    2. Appositional growth results from differentiation of mesenchymal cells in the chondrogenic layer of the perichondrium.

       a. This growth process involves the formation of new chondrocytes and additional matrix at the periphery.

       b. Cartilaginous fetal bones increase in width by appositional growth.

D. Calcification of cartilage

    1. When chondrocytes hypertrophy, they release alkaline phosphatase, which leads to precipitation of calcium phosphate in the matrix.

    2. The calcified matrix compromises the nutrient supply so that cartilage cells die.

    3. During endochondral ossification, large spicules of calcified cartilage function as scaffolding for bone formation.

TABLE 9-1:
Properties of Cartilage Types

Cartilage Type	Primary Fibers	Major Body Locations	Other Properties
Hyaline (most abundant)	Type II collagen	Articular surfaces at diarthrotic joints Ventral ends of ribs (costal cartilages) Tracheal rings Larynx	Functions as temporary skeleton during fetal growth Matrix has smooth, glassy appearance on light microscopy
Elastic	Type II collagen Elastic fibers	Pinna of external ear Wall of external auditory canal Epiglottis Larynx (cuneiform and corniculate cartilages)	Found in flexible, semirigid structures Has yellowish color when unstained Matrix shows elastic fibers on light microscopy
Fibrocartilage (least abundant)	Type I collagen	Pubic symphysis Intervertebral disks	Located where support and tensile strength needed Lacks perichondrium

TABLE 9-2:
Comparison of Cartilage and Bone

Property	Cartilage	Bone
Ground substance	Proteoglycan aggregates Hyaluronic acid No mineral component	Proteoglycans Osteonectin and osteocalcin Hydroxyapatite crystals and small amounts of other minerals
Collagen fibers	Type I (fibrocartilage) Type II (hyaline and elastic cartilage)	Type I
Blood supply	Lacking (nutrients diffuse through ground substance)	Present
Nerve supply	Lacking	Present
Mitotic activity	Chondroblasts: Yes Chondrocytes: Yes	Osteoprogenitor cells: Yes Osteoblasts: Maybe Osteocytes: No
Regenerative ability	Low	High
Communicating gap junctions	None	Between osteocytes

II. Bone (Table 9-2)
- A specialized vascular connective tissue, bone contains several cell types embedded in or on a mineralized matrix.
   A. The bone matrix is a roughly 1:1 mixture of inorganic and organic components.
      1. Hydroxyapatite crystals, $Ca_{10}(PO_4)_6(OH)_3$, constitute the bulk of the inorganic part of the bone matrix.
      2. Osteoid, the organic part of the matrix, is composed of type I collagen fibers; proteoglycans; osteonectin, which anchors mineral salts to collagen; and osteocalcin, a calcium-binding protein.
         a. It is eosinophilic if unmineralized.
         b. It is basophilic after mineralization.
   B. Covering tissues
      1. Periosteum: a vascularized connective tissue that covers most external surfaces of bone
         a. An outer fibrous layer and an inner osteogenic layer compose the periosteum.
         b. Sharpey's fibers, which are collagen fibers present in the periosteum, sweep into bone, anchoring the periosteum to it.
      2. Endosteum: a thin cell layer that lines the internal surfaces of bone and has osteogenic capability
   C. Bone cells
      1. Osteoblasts are bone-forming cells that arise from stellate mesenchymal cells and retain their stellate morphology.
         a. These cells produce osteoid (unmineralized bone matrix) and have a basophilic cytoplasm containing well-developed rough endoplasmic reticulum and a Golgi apparatus typical of protein-synthesizing cells.

Four major cell types in bone:
- Osteoblasts = bone-forming cells.
- Osteocytes = relatively inactive osteoblasts in the lacunae.
- Osteoclasts = bone-resorbing cells.
- Osteoprogenitor cells = undifferentiated mesenchymal cells that give rise to osteoblasts.

b. Separate receptors for vitamin D and parathyroid hormone are present on the surface of osteoblasts.

2. Osteocytes (mature bone cells) are osteoblasts that have been trapped within the matrix they produce.

a. Cells retain their stellate shape and are housed within matrix-bound lacunae.

b. Tunnels (canaliculi) form around cytoplasmic processes as matrix is deposited.

- Tissue fluid in the small space between the matrix of the canaliculi and the osteocyte plasmalemma supplies nutrients and metabolites to the osteocytes.

c. Adjacent osteocytes communicate with each other via gap junctions between their cytoplasmic processes.

d. Osteocytes are relatively inactive in osteoid production but are capable of osteocytic osteolysis, the removal of some calcium from newly mineralized matrix.

e. Because osteocytes do not undergo cell division, there is no interstitial growth of bone (in contrast to cartilage).

3. Osteoclasts are bone-resorbing cells located at sites of active bone resorption.

- They often are located in depressions, called *Howship's lacunae*, in the bone being resorbed.

a. Morphology of osteoclasts

(1) Multinucleated giant cells formed by the fusion of several monocytes

(2) Ruffled border on the resorptive surface adjacent to the eroding bone

(3) Many mitochondria, vesicles, and lysosomes; well-developed rough endoplasmic reticulum and Golgi apparatus

b. Resorptive activity of osteoclasts

(1) Collagenase and other enzymes (e.g., lysosomal hydrolases) secreted by osteoclasts digest the osteoid, releasing previously stored minerals in the bone matrix.

(2) Parathyroid hormone increases osteoclastic activity by inducing the release of osteoclast-activating factor (interleukin-1) from osteoblasts, leading to an increase in blood Ca^{2+}.

(3) Calcitonin and estrogen decrease osteoclastic activity, the latter by inhibiting osteoclast-activating factor.

4. Osteoprogenitor (osteogenic) cells are undifferentiated mesenchymal cells located in the inner layer of the periosteum (osteogenic layer) and in the endosteum.

a. The proliferation and differentiation of these cells generates osteoblasts.

b. Although relatively inactive in adults, osteoprogenitor cells begin to proliferate under certain conditions (e.g., after a fracture).

D. Types of bone (Fig. 9-1A)

1. Cancellous (spongy) bone consists of endosteum-covered spicules of bone and has a honeycomb appearance.

Vitamin D and parathyroid hormone promote bone growth by stimulating the proliferation and differentiation of osteoprogenitor cells into osteoblasts.

Osteoporosis is caused by increased osteoclastic activity (postmenopausal form) or decreased osteoblastic activity (senile form), leading to a decrease in bone mass.

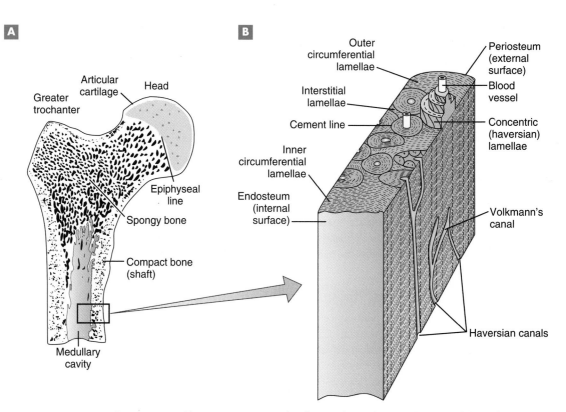

9-1: *Two views of bone structure. **A,** Spicules of spongy bone adjacent to the marrow-filled shaft of a long bone are surrounded by compact bone containing numerous haversian systems (osteons). **B,** An enlarged section through the shaft of a long bone shows the lamellar organization of compact bone.*

Metastases to bone are much more common than primary tumors arising in bone. Osteolytic metastases cause increased bone resorption; osteoblastic metastases cause increased bone density.

- • After birth, cancellous bone is found adjacent to the epiphyseal plates and to cavities filled with bone marrow.
- 2. Compact bone, which has no spicules, forms the shaft of typical long bones surrounding the medullary cavity.
  - • The matrix of compact bone is deposited in lamellae (rows), leaving cells trapped in the lacunae.
  - a. The outer circumferential lamellae are produced by the periosteum.
  - b. The inner circumferential lamellae are produced by the endosteum.
  - c. Haversian lamellae are circular lamellae located between the inner and the outer circumferential lamellae.
  - d. Interstitial lamellae are derived from incompletely resorbed haversian lamellae produced during remodeling of bone.
- E. Haversian system (osteon) in compact bone
  - 1. Osteon structure (Fig. 9-1B)
    - a. Groups of concentric (haversian) lamellae surround a central vascular channel, forming a long cylindrical structure that runs parallel to the long axis of the bone.
    - b. The cement line, a thin zone that lacks canaliculi, defines the periphery of an osteon.

2. The formation of osteons occurs continually as a consequence of bone remodeling.
    a. Resorption tunnels created by osteoclasts are "filled in" by osteoblasts, forming new osteons.
    b. Osteon formation proceeds from the outside toward the center, with the oldest lamellae at the outer edge and the youngest lamellae adjacent to the haversian canal.
3. Volkmann's canals are vascular canals that branch from the haversian canals at various angles and interconnect osteons.
F. Bone disorders unrelated to vitamin deficiencies (Box 9-1)

III. Histogenesis of Bone
A. Intramembranous ossification
    • This process of bone formation involves differentiation of mesenchyme directly into bone without formation of an intervening cartilaginous model.
    • The flat bones of the skull and subperiosteal lamellar bone are formed by intramembranous ossification.
    1. Steps in intramembranous ossification
        a. Stellate mesenchymal cells differentiate into osteoblasts, forming spicules of aggregated cells.
        b. Osteoblasts begin producing osteoid, which eventually traps some osteoblasts as osteocytes in the interior of spicules.
        c. Mineralization of the developing spicule occurs gradually.
            (1) Basophilic core = mineralized, older osteoid
            (2) Thin, eosinophilic peripheral zone = nonmineralized, younger osteoid
        d. Spicules anastomose with each other, producing immature (woven) bone, which has the following characteristics:
            (1) Absence of lamellae
            (2) Loosely packed, randomly arranged collagen fibers, which impart a woven appearance
            (3) High cell density (greater than that of mature bone)
        e. Anastomosing spicules eventually enclose mesenchymal areas, which contain blood vessels and nerves.
        f. Appositional deposition of the osteoid is greatest on the side of the spicule nearest the vessels and nerves, thereby forming an immature osteon.
    2. Remodeling of immature bone yields mature (compact) bone.
B. Endochondral ossification
    • This process of bone formation begins with differentiation of the mesenchyme into a hyaline cartilage model, which is reworked into adult (compact) bone.
    • The long bones of the limbs, as well as the vertebral column, shoulder and pelvic girdles, and ribs, are formed by endochondral ossification.
    1. Formation of the diaphyseal (primary) center of ossification (Fig. 9-2, steps 1 to 4)

BOX 9-1

BONE DISORDERS

Osteogenesis imperfecta: a group of diseases caused by mutation in a gene encoding one of the α chains of type I collagen, leading to a disturbance in the amount and quality of bone collagen. It is marked by fragile bones that are prone to fracture, lax joints, and discolored teeth. Characteristic blue sclerae result from thinning of the sclerae and increased visibility of the underlying choroidal veins. The most common and mildest form (type I) exhibits autosomal dominant transmission.

Osteopetrosis: a hereditary disease characterized by abnormally dense bone usually due to decreased resorption by dysfunctional osteoclasts. The most severe form (autosomal recessive), occurring in infancy and childhood, leads to obliteration of marrow cavity and lack of bone remodeling. Bone fractures, anemia, and cranial nerve palsies (bone entrapment) are common complications. Bone marrow transplants have been helpful.

Osteoporosis: a metabolic disorder characterized by decreased bone mass caused by an imbalance between bone formation (decreased) and bone resorption (increased). All forms are associated with increased risk of fracture after minor trauma and may cause pain (especially in the lower back), loss of body height (compression vertebral fractures), and deformities.

- Postmenopausal osteoporosis, occurring in women 3 to 20 years after menopause, results from excessive bone resorption by osteoclasts. A lowered estrogen level in postmenopausal women is a risk factor because estrogen inhibits osteoclast-activating factor.
- Senile osteoporosis, occurring in both men and women older than age 70 years, results from decreased bone formation by osteoblasts.
- Immobilization, endocrine disorders (e.g., hyperparathyroidism), and other diseases also can cause osteoporosis.

Paget's disease of bone (osteitis deformans): a chronic, often asymptomatic bone disorder that occurs primarily in individuals older than 40 years. Repeated episodes of increased osteoclastic activity, followed by excessive attempts at repair (osteoblastic activity), result in weakened, thickened bones, called *mosaic bone*. Bowing of long bones, spinal curvature (kyphosis), bone pain, and multiple fractures are common manifestations.

Osteosarcoma (osteogenic sarcoma): the second most common malignant tumor of bone origin, mainly affects young males. It generally involves the metaphysis of the distal femur or proximal tibia and often spreads to the lungs. Tumors are highly variable and are classified based on their major histologic component.

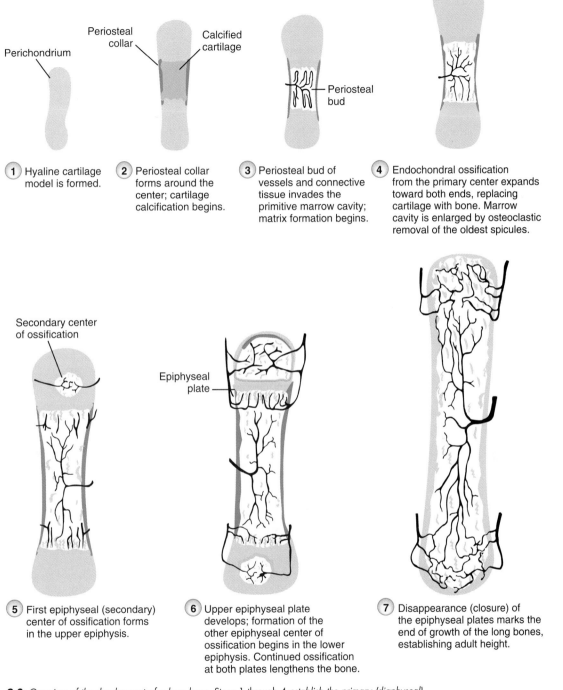

1 Hyaline cartilage model is formed.

2 Periosteal collar forms around the center; cartilage calcification begins.

3 Periosteal bud of vessels and connective tissue invades the primitive marrow cavity; matrix formation begins.

4 Endochondral ossification from the primary center expands toward both ends, replacing cartilage with bone. Marrow cavity is enlarged by osteoclastic removal of the oldest spicules.

5 First epiphyseal (secondary) center of ossification forms in the upper epiphysis.

6 Upper epiphyseal plate develops; formation of the other epiphyseal center of ossification begins in the lower epiphysis. Continued ossification at both plates lengthens the bone.

7 Disappearance (closure) of the epiphyseal plates marks the end of growth of the long bones, establishing adult height.

Labels: Perichondrium; Periosteal collar; Calcified cartilage; Periosteal bud; Secondary center of ossification; Epiphyseal plate

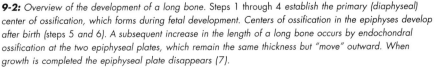

9-2: *Overview of the development of a long bone. Steps 1 through 4 establish the primary (diaphyseal) center of ossification, which forms during fetal development. Centers of ossification in the epiphyses develop after birth (steps 5 and 6). A subsequent increase in the length of a long bone occurs by endochondral ossification at the two epiphyseal plates, which remain the same thickness but "move" outward. When growth is completed the epiphyseal plate disappears (7).*

a. The hyaline cartilage model, formed from fetal mesenchyme, contains chondroblasts and chondrocytes and is surrounded by perichondrium, except at the ends.

b. Interstitial growth increases the length of the model, and appositional growth from the perichondrium increases its width.

c. Vascularization of the perichondrium induces differentiation of osteoblasts from regional mesenchyme, thereby transforming the outer layer into the periosteum.

d. The periosteal collar of bone is produced by intramembranous ossification of the periosteum around the center of the model.

e. Hypertrophy and death of the chondrocytes at the center of the cartilage model leaves spicules of calcified cartilage and empty lacunae that form a primitive marrow cavity.

f. Enlargement of the marrow cavity occurs by the addition of bone on the outside of the diaphyseal collar and removal of bone from its endosteal surface.

g. The periosteal bud, containing blood vessels, osteoprogenitor cells, and mesenchymal cells, extends from the diaphyseal periosteum into the center of the degenerating cartilage model.

h. The osteoprogenitor cells of the periosteal bud attach to "naked" spicules of calcified (basophilic) cartilage and become osteoblasts, establishing the primary center of ossification.

i. Osteoblasts begin elaborating the matrix, the oldest of which soon becomes mineralized, forming a spicule.
   • Spicules have a center of calcified cartilage surrounded by a mineralized bone matrix. The surface of the matrix is covered by a thin zone of unmineralized (eosinophilic) matrix directly underneath the layer of osteoblasts.

j. Bone formation proceeds toward both epiphyseal ends by repetition of steps *b* through *i* (discussed earlier).

k. The marrow cavity is enlarged by osteoclastic removal of the oldest spicules of endochondral ossification.

2. Formation of epiphyseal (secondary) centers of ossification (Fig. 9-2, steps 5 to 7)

a. After birth, a secondary center of ossification develops in each epiphysis by the same endochondral process used in the formation of the diaphyseal center.

b. The epiphyseal and diaphyseal centers of ossification are separated by epiphyseal plates composed of hyaline cartilage.

c. The continual addition of new hyaline cartilage at the epiphyseal ends of the long bones and its replacement by bone at the diaphyseal ends "move" the epiphyseal plates outward, leading to lengthening of the long bones.

d. The epiphysis is enlarged by interstitial growth of the hyaline cartilage in the articular region and its ossification.

e. The epiphyseal surface remains covered by the hyaline (articular) cartilage and has no periosteum.

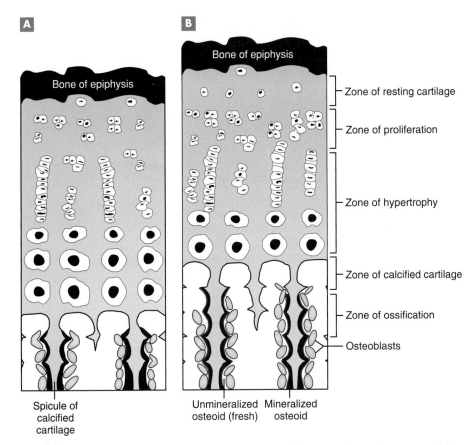

9-3: *Endochondral ossification at an epiphyseal plate of a growing long bone. The two diagrams are of the same regions, but **A** shows an earlier stage in the process, and **B** shows a later stage. The formation of new cartilage at the epiphyseal end of the plate and its ossification at the diaphyseal end lead to lengthening of the bone shaft. In the zone of ossification, osteoblasts attached to spicules of calcified cartilage secrete osteoid onto the spicule surface. In time, the osteoid is mineralized (dark band), starting with the oldest, which is closest to the cartilage spicule. At the diaphyseal end of the mineralized spicules (not shown), osteoclasts remove the calcified cartilage–mineralized matrix complex, thereby enlarging the diaphyseal marrow cavity.*

C. Epiphyseal plates
- Pituitary growth hormone stimulates overall growth, especially bone formation at the epiphyseal plates.
1. Zones in the epiphyseal plates can be distinguished histologically and occur as follows, from the epiphyseal to the diaphyseal side (Fig. 9-3):
   a. Zone of resting cartilage: small, randomly arranged chondrocytes
   b. Zone of proliferation: interstitial growth of chondrocytes, giving rise to rows of isogenous cell groups
   c. Zone of hypertrophy: enlarged chondrocytes that release alkaline phosphatase
   d. Zone of calcified cartilage: dying or dead chondrocytes and calcified cartilage spicules (intensely basophilic)

e. Zone of ossification: continuous secretion of osteoid (eosinophilic) by osteoblasts attached to spicules of calcified cartilage and subsequent mineralization of older osteoid (basophilic), producing the tricolored appearance of spicules

2. Closure of the epiphyses refers to the change within the epiphyseal plates that makes them nonfunctional.
   a. Depending on the bone, closure occurs in young adults at 20 to 30 years of age.
   b. Epiphyseal closure marks the end of growth in the length of long bones.
   c. The epiphyseal line in "older" long bones marks the site of the former epiphyseal plate.

D. Effect of vitamin and hormonal abnormalities on bone formation
   1. Vitamin C deficiency impairs collagen synthesis by osteoblasts, although the osteoid that is produced is mineralized.
      • Results in thin spicules of mineralized bone, as seen in scurvy (see Chapter 5)
   2. Vitamin D deficiency causes poor intestinal absorption of calcium and phosphorus, leading to poor mineralization of osteoid (soft bone).
      • Results in thick spicules of bone containing excessive amounts of eosinophilic, unmineralized osteoid
      a. Rickets in children is due to poor mineralization before closure of the epiphyseal plates.
         • Clinical features include short stature, flaring of the ribs, bowlegs, knock-knees, craniotabes (soft skull), and rachitic rosary (nodular swellings where the ribs join the cartilage).
      b. Osteomalacia in adults is due to poor mineralization after closure of the epiphyseal plates.
         • Clinical features include thickened osteoid seams, bone pain, muscle weakness, and fatigue.
   3. Excess vitamin A causes premature epiphyseal closure, resulting in short stature.
   4. Excess growth hormone stimulates liver-derived somatomedin, leading to excessive bone formation.
      a. Before epiphyseal closure → pituitary gigantism (elongated long bones)
      b. After epiphyseal closure → acromegaly (thickened long bones)
   5. Deficiency of growth hormone before epiphyseal closure causes pituitary dwarfism.

E. Remodeling of bone
   1. Continual bone remodeling results from the combined activity of osteoclasts (bone resorption) and osteoclasts (bone formation).
   2. Immature bone is remodeled more rapidly than mature bone.
   3. A typical adult bone turns over completely in approximately 7 to 10 years, so that a new skeleton is formed roughly each decade.
   4. Bone density is promoted by weight-lifting and walking and reduced by lack of gravity in space.

Bone formation by osteoblasts requires vitamin C for synthesis of collagen fibers and vitamin D for intestinal absorption of the Ca^{2+} and phosphorus used in mineralization of osteoid.

Serum alkaline phosphatase (released by enlarged chondrocytes) is three to five times higher in children than in adults because of the rapid bone growth in children.

Growth hormone deficiency before epiphyseal closure causes pituitary dwarfism.

Growth hormone excess before epiphyseal closure causes pituitary gigantism marked by elongated long bones. Growth hormone excess after epiphyseal closure causes acromegaly marked by thickened long bones.

F. Broken bones and their repair
   1. Initial events after a fracture
      a. Thrombus formation
      b. Arrival of neutrophils and macrophages, which remove debris
      c. Hypoxia of the bone matrix distal to a fracture caused by blood vessel damage
      d. Death of osteocytes in osteons
   2. Development of a bony callus on the internal and external surfaces at a fracture site
      a. Differentiation of osteoprogenitor cells in the endosteum and periosteum into chondroblasts and chondrocytes
      b. The formation of a cartilaginous bridge, or callus, across the break on the periosteal side (external callus) and endosteal side (internal callus)
      c. Endochondral ossification of a callus to produce cancellous bone
   3. Remodeling of a bony callus into mature compact bone across the fracture site
      a. Forces of stress (weight bearing) cause remodeling of the original architecture.
      b. Bone develops the structure that is most suited to resist the forces acting on it (Wolff's law).

IV. Joints
   A. Synarthroses
      • These immovable joints are classified based on the type of tissue connecting the bones.
      1. Syndesmoses: bone joined to bone by dense, fibrous connective tissue (e.g., sutures of the skull during childhood)
      2. Synchondroses: bone joined to bone by cartilage (e.g., epiphyseal plate, which is temporary, and the union between the ribs and sternum)
      3. Synostoses: bone joined to bone by bone (e.g., sutures of the skull in an adult)
   B. Amphiarthroses
      • These slightly movable joints are composed of fibrocartilage (e.g., pubic symphysis and intervertebral disks).
   C. Diarthroses
      • These freely movable joints, which generally unite long bones, are also known as *synovial joints.*
      1. The synovial fluid-filled cavity separates two bones.
      2. The hyaline (articular) cartilage covers the opposing bone surfaces, which lack perichondrium.
         • Parallel collagen fibers lie close to the joint cavity. Deeper fibers run in arches or arcades.
         • Small pieces of cartilage ("joint mice") broken off during joint function may be present in the synovial fluid.
      3. The joint capsule connects the ends of adjacent bones.
         a. The inner capsular layer contains nonepithelial cells that secrete hyaluronic acid, the joint lubricant.

- This layer, also called the *synovial membrane,* functions in the formation of a blood dialysate that enters the joint cavity and, together with hyaluronic acid, forms synovial fluid.
        b. The outer capsular layer supports the synovial membrane.
- The fibrous type withstands pressure.
- The areolar type allows sliding.
- The adipose type provides a cushion.
    4. Menisci are cushions of fibrocartilage that are present in some synovial joints (e.g., knee).
D. Joint disorders
    1. Osteoarthritis: a noninflammatory, degenerative disease that commonly affects the joints of the hand, cervical and lumbar spine, hip, and knee
- Pathologic changes include degeneration of the articular cartilage, thickening and polishing of subchondral bone (eburnation), and formation of bony spurs (osteophytes) that often extend into the joint.
    2. Rheumatoid arthritis: chronic inflammatory arthritis caused by autoimmune mechanisms and involving systemic effects
- Inflammation and proliferation of the synovial membrane lead to the formation of a rheumatoid pannus, the characteristic joint lesion. Muscle atrophy and ankylosis occur at later stages.
    3. Ankylosing spondylitis: a chronic degenerative inflammatory disease that primarily affects males younger than age 30 years and initially involves the spine
- Marked by synovitis without pannus formation and inflammation of ligaments at their insertion into bone; may progress to ankylosis of the spinal column
- Often associated with inflammatory intestinal diseases

Osteoarthritis is the most common noninflammatory joint disease. It causes degeneration of the articular cartilage with osteophyte formation at the joint margins.

Rheumatoid arthritis is a disease of autoimmune origin. It causes synovitis with pannus formation, muscle atrophy, and ankylosis (late).

The majority of patients with ankylosing spondylitis are HLA-B27–positive.

Respiratory System

TARGET TOPICS

- Histologic features characterizing the different portions of the respiratory tract
- Cell types composing the respiratory epithelium
- Pathway of gaseous exchange (air–blood interface)

- Cell types in the alveoli
- Lung cancer, chronic bronchitis, asthma, respiratory distress syndrome, emphysema, pneumoconiosis (coal miner's lung, silicosis, asbestosis), heart-failure cells

I. Introduction
   - The structures throughout the respiratory system possess characteristic lining epithelia, supporting tissues, and glands (Table 10-1).
   A. The conducting portion comprises a series of progressively smaller passageways that convey inspired air to small conducting bronchioles within the lungs.
      - No gaseous exchange occurs in these airways, which constitute the dead air space of pulmonary physiology.
   B. The respiratory portion, located entirely within the lungs, comprises structures where gaseous exchange occurs between blood and air.

II. Respiratory Epithelium
   - The pseudostratified ciliated columnar epithelium, commonly known as the *respiratory epithelium,* lines all or part of the larger conducting structures.
   A. Cell types composing the respiratory epithelium
      1. Goblet cells secrete mucus, which traps inhaled particles (bacteria, pollen, dust).
      2. Ciliated columnar cells beat their cilia toward the oropharynx, thereby moving mucus upward so it can be swallowed or expectorated.
      3. Nonciliated columnar cells have microvilli on their apical surface but no cilia.
      4. Basal cells are undifferentiated stem cells whose progeny can differentiate into goblet cells or columnar cells (ciliated and nonciliated).

TABLE 10-1:

Histology of the Components of the Respiratory System

Structure	Epithelium*	Cilia	Goblet Cells	Supporting Tissue	Other Features
Conducting Portion					
Nasal cavity					
Respiratory	Respiratory	Yes	Yes	Bone, hyaline cartilage	Nasal sinuses; glands
Olfactory	Olfactory	No	No	Bone	Olfactory bipolar neurons; Bowman's glands
Nasopharynx	Respiratory, oral	Yes	Yes	Muscle	Pharyngeal tonsil; glands
Larynx	Respiratory, oral	Yes	Yes	Hyaline and elastic cartilages	Epiglottis and vocal cords; glands
Trachea and primary bronchi	Respiratory	Yes	Yes	C-rings (hyaline cartilages); smooth muscle (trachealis)	Glands
Intrapulmonary bronchi	Respiratory	Yes	Yes	Hyaline cartilage blocks; smooth muscle	Glands
Conducting bronchioles	Respiratory to simple cuboidal	Some	In larger ones	Smooth muscle	Clara cells
Respiratory Portion					
Respiratory bronchioles	Simple cuboidal	Some	None	Smooth muscle	Clara cells; some alveoli
Alveoli and alveolar ducts	Pneumocytes (type I and II)	None	None	Elastic and reticular fibers in interalveolar septa	Surfactant covering surface; alveolar macrophages

*Respiratory epithelium, pseudostratified ciliated columnar epithelium containing five cell types; oral epithelium, nonkeratinized stratified squamous epithelium.

    5. Small granule cells are neuroendocrine cells that synthesize and release catecholamines.

  B. The lamina propria beneath the respiratory epithelium
- Formed of loose, areolar connective tissue that contains glands (seromucous, mucous) and diffuse lymphatic tissue, including plasma cells, lymphocytes, and macrophages

III. Conducting Portion
- During its passage through the conducting portion, inspired air is warmed, moistened, and somewhat cleaned.
- The structures of the conducting portion are arranged in the following order: nasal cavity → nasopharynx and oropharynx → larynx → trachea → bronchi → bronchioles → terminal bronchioles

A. Nasal cavity and nasopharynx
   1. Portions of the nasopharynx that experience "wear and tear" (e.g., uvula) are covered by nonkeratinized stratified squamous epithelium, or oral epithelium, rather than respiratory epithelium.
   2. The watery secretion of the glands in the lamina propria moistens inspired air.
   3. The many blood vessels in the lamina propria help to warm inspired air.
   4. Olfactory mucosa is present on the superior aspect of each nasal cavity (see Chapter 19).
B. Larynx
   • Several hyaline and elastic cartilages help support the thin walls of the larynx and function in phonation.
   1. The epiglottis, the anterior superior extension of the larynx, is shared by the respiratory and digestive systems.
      • During swallowing, the epiglottis folds on itself, closing the airway.
      a. Elastic cartilage forms the core of the epiglottis and is surrounded by a lamina propria.
      b. The digestive part, which constitutes the anterior aspect, tip, and upper part of the posterior aspect, is covered by oral epithelium.
      c. The respiratory part, which constitutes the lower part of the posterior aspect, is covered by respiratory epithelium.
   2. The vocal apparatus, distal to the epiglottis, consists of two pairs of folds of the laryngeal mucosa, spanning the laryngeal space.
      a. The false vocal cords (vestibular folds) are the superior pair of folds, which play no role in phonation.
         • Covered by respiratory epithelium and containing seromucous glands in the lamina propria
      b. The true vocal cords (folds) are the inferior pair of folds, which produce sound as air passes over them.
         • Covered by oral epithelium and lacking seromucous glands in the lamina propria
         (1) Vocal ligament: a mass of elastic tissue forming the core of each vocal cord
         (2) Vocalis muscle: a small skeletal muscle deep to the vocal ligament
C. Trachea
   1. The surface of the mucosa is covered by respiratory epithelium, with an underlying lamina propria; a prominent basement membrane separates these.
   2. The submucosa, containing many seromucous glands, is separated from the mucosa by a layer of elastic fibers.
   3. C-shaped hyaline cartilages (C-rings) lie deep to the submucosa.
      • These supporting cartilages are covered by a perichondrium, which is surrounded by an adventitia of loose connective tissue shared with the esophagus.
      a. The open end of each C-ring faces posteriorly, toward the esophagus.
      b. Smooth muscle (trachealis) bridges the open end of each cartilage.

4. Extrapulmonary (primary) bronchi, which arise by division of the trachea outside the lungs, are histologically similar to the trachea.

D. Intrapulmonary bronchi
- Within the lungs, the bronchi divide many times.
1. The hyaline cartilages are variably shaped and eventually break up into small pieces in the walls of the intrapulmonary bronchi.
2. The respiratory epithelium and other histologic layers of the wall progressively diminish in thickness.

E. Conducting bronchioles
1. Characteristic features
   a. Absence of cartilages (i.e., loss of rigid support)
   b. Abundant smooth muscle in the walls
      - Contraction and relaxation of smooth muscle determines the diameter of the bronchioles.
      - Epinephrine relaxes this muscle.
   c. Transition of the epithelium as the bronchioles become smaller:
      - Respiratory epithelium → ciliated columnar → ciliated cuboidal → nonciliated cuboidal
   d. Absence of seromucous glands
   e. Mucus-producing goblet cells only in the larger bronchioles

2. Terminal bronchioles
   - Constitute the smallest (diameter <0.5 mm), most distal part of the conducting tree and terminate in the first component of the respiratory division
   a. Some ciliated cuboidal cells but no goblet cells are present, ensuring that all mucus production occurs upstream of the cilia.
   b. Parallel branching converts turbulent airflow to laminar airflow.

3. Clara cells
   a. Prevalence: As the number of ciliated cells decreases in the conducting bronchioles, the number of Clara cells increases.
   b. Morphology: These cells have a rounded, dome-shaped apical surface (with short, blunt microvilli, but no cilia); the cytoplasmic ultrastructure is typical of secretory cells.
   c. Function
      (1) Secretion of a surface-active lipoprotein that prevents the collapse of terminal bronchioles, especially during exhalation
      (2) Metabolism of airborne toxins by cytochrome P-450 enzymes

F. Diseases involving the bronchi and bronchioles
1. Bronchogenic carcinoma (a squamous cell carcinoma)
   - Cigarette smoke, which is ciliotoxic and stimulates excess production of mucus, is the most common causative agent.
   a. Carcinogenesis involves progressive changes in the respiratory epithelium of the bronchi, as illustrated in Figure 10-1.
   b. Cessation of smoking can lead to reversal of dysplastic changes but not anaplastic changes.

> Terminal bronchioles are the primary site for "small airway" diseases, such as asthma.

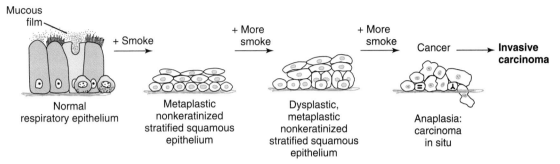

10-1: *Changes in the respiratory epithelium caused by smoking. Normal respiratory epithelium first undergoes metaplasia (replacement of one adult cell type by another adult cell type) to normal-appearing nonkeratinized stratified squamous epithelium. These metaplastic cells then undergo atypical changes in their size, shape, and organization (dysplasia). Further dysplastic changes lead to complete cytologic disorganization of the epithelium (anaplasia), initially producing a carcinoma in situ (confined to the epithelium above the basement membrane) and then an invasive carcinoma (extending through the basement membrane into adjacent tissues).*

  (1) Reversal results from differentiation of the remaining basal cells into goblet cells and ciliated and nonciliated columnar cells, thereby restoring the normal respiratory epithelium.
  (2) The risk of carcinoma slowly returns to almost normal with no exposure to smoke.
 2. Chronic bronchitis results from irritation of the bronchi, commonly by cigarette smoke, leading to excess production of mucus and narrowing of the airway, primarily the terminal bronchioles.
    • Defined clinically as a sputum-producing cough for at least 3 months per year for 2 successive years
 3. Asthma is marked by recurrent bronchospasms in which widespread constriction of smooth muscle in the bronchi and bronchioles decreases their diameter, leading to expiratory wheezing.
    a. Asthma attacks often are associated with immediate (type I) hypersensitivity reactions during which vasoconstrictive mediators are released (see Fig. 13-5).
    b. Common treatment for mild asthma is β_2-agonists (e.g., albuterol), which relax the bronchiolar smooth muscle and decrease its tonus, thus enlarging the air passages.

β_2-Agonists used to treat asthma (e.g., albuterol) reduce bronchospasm and enlarge the airways by relaxing bronchiolar smooth muscle.

IV. Respiratory Portion
  A. Pulmonary lobules
    • Distal to the terminal bronchioles, the lung is composed of lobules, each containing a central respiratory bronchiole that gives way to alveolar ducts whose distal end terminates in one or more alveolar sacs.
    1. Deoxygenated blood is carried into each lobule by a branch of the pulmonary artery that accompanies the respiratory bronchiole and terminates in the dense capillary networks in the walls of the alveoli.
    2. Oxygenated blood is drained from the periphery of each lobule by pulmonary veins contained in the delicate connective tissue septa arising from the visceral pleura.

Lobar pneumonia results from the spread of microorganisms throughout the lung via the pores of Kohn, which connect adjacent alveoli.

Atelectasis is proximal plugging of the terminal bronchioles with mucus. In this condition, air in the alveoli is resorbed through the pores of Kohn.

Type II pneumocytes secrete pulmonary surfactant, which reduces the surface tension of pulmonary fluids, thereby contributing to the elasticity of the alveoli and the patency of the small airways on expiration.

Deficiency of pulmonary surfactant causes respiratory distress syndrome, which is most common in premature infants or those with diabetic mothers.

B. Alveoli

- These saclike evaginations in the walls of the respiratory bronchioles, alveolar ducts, and alveolar sacs are the sites of gaseous exchange.
- Alveoli are the smallest (200 to 300 μm in diameter) and most abundant (300 million per lung) air-containing structures in the respiratory tract.

1. Interalveolar septa: connective tissue partitions separating adjacent alveoli and containing pulmonary capillaries
2. Pores of Kohn: holes in the interalveolar septa through which adjacent alveoli normally share air (thus equalizing the pressure)
3. Alveolar walls: lined by an epithelium composed of two types of pneumocytes
   a. Type I pneumocytes have an extremely thin cytoplasm and cover approximately 95% of the alveolar surface.
      - Tight junctions connect adjacent type I cells.
      - The basal lamina of these cells may be fused with the basal lamina of nearby capillary endothelial cells.
   b. Type II pneumocytes (great alveolar cells) are somewhat rounded cells that bulge into the alveolar lumen, covering approximately 5% of the alveolar surface.
      - These cells, the primary repair cells of the alveoli, can divide and replace damaged type I pneumocytes, which normally do not divide.
4. Pulmonary surfactant: a phospholipid–protein mixture secreted by type II pneumocytes that spreads over the alveolar walls
   a. A reduction in surface tension due to surfactant permits the alveoli to expand easily during inspiration without collapsing during expiration.
   b. Respiratory distress syndrome of the newborn is caused by a deficiency in the amount and quality of pulmonary surfactant.
      - This disorder is most common in premature infants (surfactant production normally begins late in gestation) and in infants with diabetic mothers (insulin inhibits surfactant production).
      - Labored breathing is evident shortly after birth, followed by cyanosis of the skin and mucous membranes. If the newborn survives for 3 to 5 days, the disease usually resolves.
5. Pulmonary emphysema: an abnormal increase in the residual volume of the lungs (hyperinflation) accompanied by a decrease in vital capacity and an increase in total lung capacity
   a. A decrease in the normal elasticity of the alveolar walls eventually causes distention of the alveoli, rupture of their walls, and obliteration of the alveolar capillaries.
      - Decreased elasticity can result from cigarette smoke or from a hereditary condition that reduces the activity of α_1-antitrypsin, which normally protects the lungs' elastic fibers from degradation by elastase released from neutrophils.
   b. In advanced cases, chronic hypoxemia (low arterial Po_2) causes pulmonary artery hypertension, which makes the right side of the heart work excessively, resulting in cor pulmonale associated with right ventricular hypertrophy.

C. Gaseous exchange
1. Mechanism: Oxygen diffuses from the alveolar airspace across the air–blood interface into the red blood cells, where it binds to heme groups in hemoglobin, releasing bound carbon dioxide, which diffuses back to the alveolar airspace.
2. Respiratory membrane (air–blood interface): Approximately 0.2 μm thick at its thinnest points and comprises the following components in the air-to-blood direction (Fig. 10-2):
   - Surfactant → type I pneumocyte → basal lamina of a type I pneumocyte → basal lamina of a capillary endothelial cell → endothelial cell → blood plasma → plasmalemma of a red blood cell
D. Alveolar macrophages (dust cells)
   - These phagocytic cells, derived from monocytes that migrate out of the capillaries in the interalveolar septa, wander over the alveolar surface, ingesting bacteria and other inhaled particles.
   1. Pneumoconiosis: accumulation of nondegradable particulate matter in phagocytic cells in the lungs
      a. Anthracosis (coal miner's lung, black lung) caused by deposition of inert carbon particles
         - Pulmonary fibrosis and emphysema eventually develop.
      b. Silicosis resulting from deposition of silica dust
         - Acute exposure can lead to pulmonary edema and alveolar damage.
         - Prolonged exposure is marked by the development of fibrous nodules that may enlarge, causing massive fibrosis of the lungs.
      c. Asbestosis resulting from deposition of asbestos fibers
         - Interstitial fibrosis of the lungs occurs to varying degrees. It is often associated with benign pleural plaques, pleural mesothelioma, and bronchogenic carcinoma (the most common cancer).

> Pneumoconiosis is any disease caused by the accumulation of airborne, nondegradable particles in the lungs, including anthracosis (coal miner's lung, black lung), asbestosis, and silicosis.

> Emphysema, caused by decreased elasticity of the alveolar walls, can lead to cor pulmonale (right-sided ventricular hypertrophy) with pulmonary hypertension.

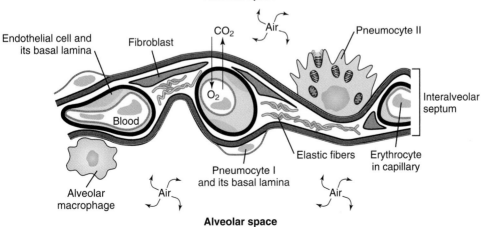

10-2: Interalveolar system. The thin cytoplasm and underlying basal lamina of type I pneumocytes extend over most of the alveolar surface, which is covered with a layer of surfactant secreted by type II pneumocytes. Gas exchange is most efficient where the membrane is thinnest.

BOX 10-1

FORMATION OF HEART-FAILURE CELLS

Left-sided heart failure causes sluggish blood flow in the lungs resulting from a backup of blood from the failed left side of the heart into the pulmonary veins and capillaries. As pulmonary capillary pressure increases, blood, plasma, and red blood cells (RBCs) escape into the interalveolar septa. Excess tissue fluid and extravascular RBCs eventually move into the alveolar air spaces, causing pulmonary edema. As alveolar macrophages ingest and digest the RBCs, the macrophages become filled with hemosiderin, a brownish breakdown product derived from hemoglobin. Accumulation of these heart-failure cells leads to brown induration of the lung and to rusty-colored sputum.

     2. Heart-failure cells: hemosiderin-containing macrophages found in the pulmonary alveoli and sputum in left-sided heart failure (Box 10-1)

V. Visceral and Parietal Pleurae
  A. Serous membranes, consisting of a surface mesothelium and the underlying lamina propria, enclose the pleural cavity.
    • Visceral pleura invests the lungs; parietal pleura lines the thoracic cavity.
    • Sliding of these pleurae over each other, facilitated by a small amount of serous secretion lying between them, permits movement of the lungs within the thoracic cavity.
  B. Mesothelioma, resulting from malignant transformation of the mesothelium, can be triggered by exposure to asbestos.
    • It is most commonly seen in shipyard workers and individuals who have worked as roofers for more than 20 years.

Cardiovascular System

TARGET TOPICS

- Histologic features distinguishing different types of arteries, veins, and lymphatic vessels
- Properties of continuous, fenestrated, and sinusoidal capillaries
- Formation of tissue fluid and lymph

- Cardiac tunics and their relationship to the pericardium
- Pathway of impulse conduction in the heart
- Arteriosclerosis, edema, tumor angiogenesis, ischemic heart disease, and valvular stenosis

I. Blood Vessels
  A. Vascular tunics
    - The walls of all blood vessels, except the capillaries, consist of three layers (Fig. 11-1).
    - The composition and thickness of the vascular tunics vary in different types of vessels.
    1. Tunica intima (inner layer)
      a. Endothelium and basal lamina
        - von Willebrand's factor VIII, a platelet adhesion factor produced in the endothelial cells, is an immunochemical marker for endothelium.
      b. Subendothelial connective tissue
      c. Internal elastic membrane
    2. Tunica media (middle layer)
      a. Circular smooth muscle and some fibroblasts
      b. Collagen and elastic fibers
    3. Tunica adventitia (outer layer)
      a. Loose, areolar connective tissue
      b. Irregular fibroelastic connective tissue containing adipocytes (outer aspect)
      c. Small vessels (vasa vasorum) and nerves
  B. Arterial vessels
    - As arteries extend outward from the heart, they become progressively smaller and the composition of their tunics changes (Table 11-1).

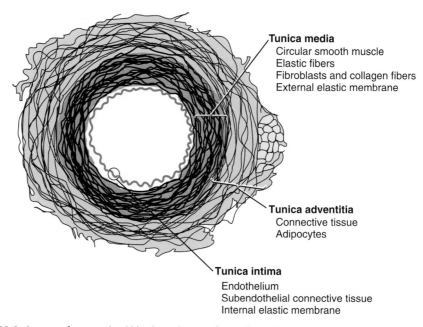

Tunica media
  Circular smooth muscle
  Elastic fibers
  Fibroblasts and collagen fibers
  External elastic membrane

Tunica adventitia
  Connective tissue
  Adipocytes

Tunica intima
  Endothelium
  Subendothelial connective tissue
  Internal elastic membrane

11-1: *Structure of a generalized blood vessel. Except for capillaries, blood vessels contain three well-defined tunics. Some arteries possess an external elastic membrane between the media and the adventitia. See Table 11-1 for variations among different-sized arteries.*

TABLE 11-1:
Selected Characteristics of Arterial Tunics

Tunica Components	Elastic Arteries	Muscular Arteries	Arterioles
Intima			
Endothelium	Yes	Yes	Yes
Basal lamina	Yes	Yes	Yes
Subendothelial layer	Yes	Yes	In some
Internal elastic membrane	Incomplete	Thick, complete	Few elastic fibers
Media			
Smooth muscle (circular)	Interspersed between elastic membranes	Many layers	1–3 layers
Fenestrated elastic laminae	Many	None	None
Fibroblasts and collagen	Yes	Yes	Yes
External elastic membrane	No	Yes	No
Adventitia			
Loose connective tissue	Yes	Yes	No
Adipose connective tissue	Abundant	Some	Little
Vasa vasorum	Yes	In some	No
Nerve fibers	Yes	Yes	Yes

1. Elastic (conducting) arteries include the aorta, the pulmonary trunk, and their large branches.
   a. During systole, elastic arteries stretch as they receive blood.
   b. During diastole, their passive elastic recoil plays a major role in maintaining diastolic blood pressure.
2. Muscular (distributing) arteries include all other named arteries of the gross anatomy.
   a. The transition from the elastic to the muscular type of artery occurs gradually.
   b. Smooth muscle in the tunica media contracts and relaxes in response to hormonal and autonomic stimulation (e.g., facial blush).
   c. The diameter of the lumen and the thickness of the tunica media decrease as muscular arteries get farther from the heart.
3. Arterioles are small arteries that have only one to three smooth muscle layers in their tunica media.
   a. They give rise to metarterioles, the smallest arteries, which possess a discontinuous layer of smooth muscle cells.
   b. Maintenance of mean arterial pressure depends primarily on proper tonus of the smooth muscle in the arterioles (peripheral resistance arterioles).
      (1) Vasodilation: decreased tonus that leads to decreased diastolic blood pressure, which can result in shock
      (2) Vasoconstriction: increased tonus that leads to increased diastolic blood pressure
4. *Arteriosclerosis* refers to any condition marked by thickening and hardening of the arterial walls.
   a. Atherosclerosis: deposition of fibrous fatty plaques (atheromas) in the tunica intima of the arteries, weakening the wall of elastic arteries and reducing the luminal diameter of muscular arteries
      • Subsequent exposure of subendothelial collagen fibers to blood may cause platelet aggregation and thrombus formation (see Chapter 12).
   b. Medial calcific sclerosis (Mönckeberg's arteriosclerosis): calcium deposition in the tunica media of the large and medium-sized arteries (e.g., uterine arteries)
   c. Hyperplastic arteriolosclerosis: hyperplasia of the smooth muscle cells in the arterioles, leading to an onionskin appearance; occurs in malignant hypertension
   d. Hyaline arteriolosclerosis: deposition of hyaline material in the wall of the arterioles, with consequent narrowing of the lumina; occurs in diabetes mellitus and hypertension

C. Capillaries
   • Capillaries, which branch from the metarterioles, consist of a single endothelial layer rolled into a tube that is surrounded by a basement membrane and occasional pericytes.
1. The capillary bed is an intricate network of capillaries interposed between the arterioles and the venules (Fig. 11-2).
   a. Precapillary sphincters control blood flow into the capillaries.

In atherosclerosis of the muscular arteries, the luminal diameter of the arteries is reduced by deposition of fibrous fatty plaques in the tunica intima.

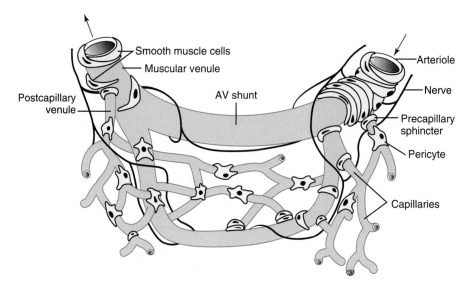

11-2: *Simplified view of a capillary bed. Arrows indicate the direction of blood flow. Capillary walls are designed for the transport of gases, nutrients, and waste products between the blood and tissue spaces. AV shunt, arteriovenous anastomosis.*

      b. The lumen of the capillaries (7 to 9 μm in diameter) is just sufficient to permit the passage of red blood cells one at a time.

      c. Arteriovenous anastomoses (AV shunts) provide direct connections between arterioles and venules. They are numerous in the lips, ears, toes, nose, and fingertips.

        (1) A closed AV shunt directs blood into the capillary bed.

        (2) An open AV shunt permits blood to bypass the capillary bed.

  2. Pericytes are undifferentiated mesenchymal cells that wrap around the capillaries and are encased within the basal lamina (see Fig. 11-2).

      a. The presence of actin and myosin in pericytes suggests that they may be contractile and may help to move blood through the capillaries.

      b. Normally, pericytes are quiescent, but they can be activated (e.g., during wound healing) to differentiate into fibroblasts and other cell types.

  3. The classification of capillaries is based on differences in the structure of their endothelial cells (Fig. 11-3).

      a. Continuous capillaries

        • Transendothelial transport of larger molecules is mediated by pinocytic vesicles. Maculae occludens between adjacent cells permit the passage of water and small hydrophilic molecules.

      b. Fenestrated capillaries (e.g., glomerular capillaries)

        • Transendothelial transport occurs primarily through pores (fenestrae) in the endothelial cells.

      c. Sinusoidal capillaries (e.g., splenic sinusoids)

        • Transendothelial transport occurs primarily through large paracellular gaps.

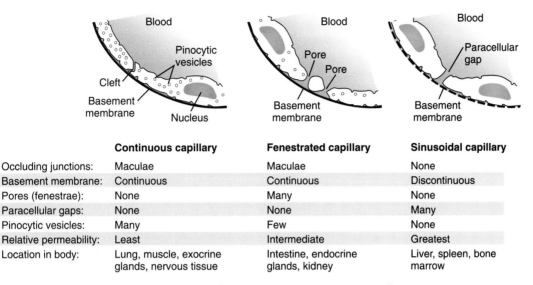

	Continuous capillary	Fenestrated capillary	Sinusoidal capillary
Occluding junctions:	Maculae	Maculae	None
Basement membrane:	Continuous	Continuous	Discontinuous
Pores (fenestrae):	None	Many	None
Paracellular gaps:	None	None	Many
Pinocytic vesicles:	Many	Few	None
Relative permeability:	Least	Intermediate	Greatest
Location in body:	Lung, muscle, exocrine glands, nervous tissue	Intestine, endocrine glands, kidney	Liver, spleen, bone marrow

11-3: Comparison of endothelial cells in three types of capillaries. In contrast to continuous capillaries in most tissues (shown here), those in nervous tissue have few pinocytic vesicles, have zonulae occludens (tight junctions), and have a thick basement membrane, all of which reduce their permeability (blood–brain barrier). Except in renal glomeruli, a thin diaphragm bridges the pores in fenestrated capillaries.

    4. The portal system consists of two capillary beds connected by one or more veins.
      a. Liver portal system: intestinal capillary beds → portal vein → liver sinusoids → central vein → hepatic vein
      b. Hypophyseal portal system: capillary beds in the median eminence → hypophyseal portal veins → capillary beds in the pars distalis
  D. Venous vessels
    • Veins have larger lumens, thinner walls, and a lower hydrostatic pressure than comparable arteries.
    1. Valves, or paired folds of the tunica intima, are present in many veins that work against gravity.
      • These valves prevent backward blood flow and pooling of blood in the extremities, especially the lower ones.
    2. A layer of longitudinal smooth muscle is found in the walls of the largest veins (e.g., inferior vena cava).
      • This extra muscle layer, located in the inner aspect of the tunica adventitia (not in the tunica media), makes the adventitia the thickest of the three tunics in these veins.
  E. Interstitial fluid
    • The formation and recovery of interstitial (tissue) fluid occurs primarily in the capillary beds (Fig. 11-4).
    1. Forces driving fluid movement in and out of vessels
      a. Osmotic pressure, created by a high concentration of albumin in the blood, draws fluid into the capillaries from the surrounding interstitium.

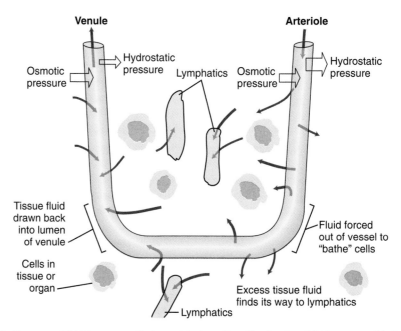

11-4: *Movement of fluid between capillaries and the interstitium. The direction of fluid movement (black arrows) at any point within a capillary loop depends on the difference between the hydrostatic pressure, which decreases from the arterial to the venous side, and the osmotic pressure, which is constant. Fluid forced out at the arterial end of a capillary loop forms the interstitial, or tissue, fluid. This fluid is returned at the venous end or enters blind-ended lymphatic vessels, forming the lymph.*

Transudate, a protein- and cell-poor fluid, is produced in edema resulting from increased hydrostatic pressure or decreased osmotic pressure.

      b. Hydrostatic pressure, created by blood flow against the capillary walls, forces fluid out of the capillaries and into the surrounding interstitium.

  2. Arterial side: Hydrostatic pressure > osmotic pressure.
- Net effect: Fluid, but not formed elements (a transudate), is forced out of the blood, forming interstitial fluid.

  3. Venous side: Osmotic pressure > hydrostatic pressure.
- Net effect: Most, but not all, interstitial fluid returns to the blood.
- Blind-ending lymphatic capillaries take up interstitial fluid that is not returned to the venous blood, forming the lymph.

F. Causes of edema (excess interstitial fluid in a body region)

  1. Increased venous hydrostatic pressure
- Left-sided heart failure → pulmonary edema
- Pregnant uterus pressing on the common iliac veins → pitting edema of the lower extremities
- Right-sided heart failure → pitting edema of the lower extremities

  2. Obstruction of lymphatic drainage
- Axillary node removal (surgical) or radiation → lymphedema of the ipsilateral superior extremity
- Parasitic infection of the lymphatic vessels → elephantiasis

3. Increased permeability of the endothelium
   • Acute inflammation with a histamine-enhanced increase in venule permeability → accumulation of protein- and cell-rich fluid (exudate) in the interstitial space
4. Reduction in the osmotic pressure of the blood due to decreased concentration of macromolecules in the blood
   • Hepatic cirrhosis, nephrotic syndrome, and malnutrition → increased loss of fluid on the arterial side of the capillary bed and decreased return on the venous side → abdominal ascites and pitting edema of the lower extremities

G. Tumor angiogenesis (neoangiogenesis)
   1. Tumor angiogenesis factor, produced by tumor cells, stimulates nearby endothelial cells to proliferate, migrate into the neoplasm, and form new blood vessels supplying it.
      • Growth of a tumor to a large size requires a direct blood supply to provide nutrients to cells throughout the mass.
   2. Inhibitors of neoangiogenesis may be useful in treating tumors.
      • Monoclonal antibody to tumor angiogenesis factor and two natural proteins, endostatin and angiostatin, prevent neoangiogenesis, so that neoplasms must rely on the diffusion of local nutrients only and thus remain small.

II. Lymphatic Vessels
   • The system of lymphatic vessels drains most tissues except the nervous system and bone marrow.
   A. Lymphatic capillaries begin as blind-ending endothelial tubes near the blood capillaries.
      1. Unique structural features of lymphatic capillaries
         a. A single layer of highly attenuated endothelial cells
         b. Absent or intermittent basal lamina
         c. Anchoring filaments that extend from the exterior surface of the endothelium into the surrounding connective tissue
            • These filaments prevent the very thin-walled lymphatic capillaries from collapsing.
      2. Absorption by lymphatic capillaries
         a. Excess tissue fluid and macromolecules in the interstitium are absorbed relatively easily by lymphatic capillaries.
         b. Lipids from a fatty meal are taken up by lymphatic vessels, called *lacteals*, in the intestinal villi (see Fig. 14-4).
   B. Larger lymphatic vessels possess valves and are generally similar in structure to the small veins, but have larger lumens and thinner walls.
      • Lymph is filtered in the lymph nodes, which are interspersed along the lymphatic tree (see Fig. 13-7).
   C. The right lymphatic duct and thoracic duct, the large trunks resulting from the convergence of the lymphatic vessels, have three tunics, similar to blood vessels.

Exudate, a protein- and cell-rich fluid, is produced in edema resulting from increased endothelial permeability (e.g., pus formed in acute inflammation).

In cirrhosis of the liver and nephrotic syndrome, blood albumin levels decrease, reducing osmotic pressure of the blood and promoting edema.

Because of their thin, weak walls, lymphatic capillaries are easily invaded by cancer cells, leading to lymphatic spread of cancer.

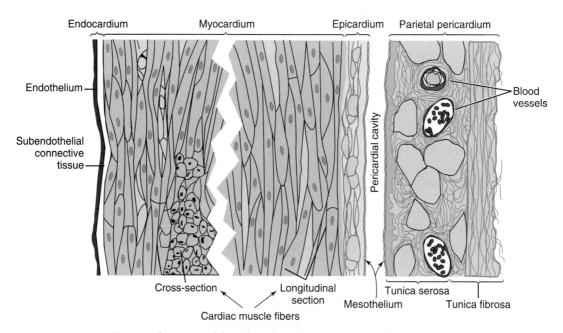

11-5: *Cardiac tunics and their relationship to the pericardium. The three tunics are homologous to those of blood vessels: endocardium = tunica intima; myocardium = tunica media; and epicardium = tunica adventitia. The pericardium is composed of two layers: the outer parietal pericardium and the epicardium, or visceral pericardium, which is in contact with the heart and roots of the great vessels. The parietal pericardium has two regions: a serosa facing the pericardial cavity and, peripheral to that, a fibrosa.*

Cardiac tunics (inside → outside):

- Endocardium (endothelium + subendothelial connective tissue), no adipose cells
- Myocardium (cardiac muscle)
- Epicardium (fibroelastic connective tissue + mesothelium) with adipose cells

Damaged cardiac muscle does not regenerate because these cells cannot divide. Lost cells are replaced by scar tissue, with hypertrophy of the adjacent cardiomyocytes.

III. Heart
 A. Cardiac tunics: three layers composing the wall of the heart; homologous to those of the blood vessels (Fig. 11-5)
  1. The endocardium (inner layer), comprising an endothelium and a thin subendothelial connective tissue layer, is continuous with the tunica intima of major blood vessels entering and leaving the heart.
   - Between the endocardium and the myocardium is a thin connective tissue layer, the subendocardium, which contains the nerves and components of the impulse-conducting system.
  2. The myocardium, the parenchyma of the heart, consists of cardiac muscle cells and is thickest in the ventricles.
   a. Cardiac myocytes are incapable of cell division.
    (1) Cardiac muscle cells that are lost, as in myocardial infarction, are replaced by scar tissue (healed myocardial infarction), which stains blue with trichrome stain.
    (2) Adjacent parenchymal cells assume the extra workload, leading to their hypertrophy.
   b. Atrial natriuretic peptide (ANP) is produced by myofibers in the left and right atria and is stored in neuroendocrine granules.
    (1) Increased blood volume in the atria stretches the myofibers, causing the release of ANP.

(2) ANP increases the secretion of sodium and water by the distal convoluted tubules in the kidney, leading to a decrease in blood volume.

3. The epicardium (outer layer) is equivalent to the visceral layer of the pericardial sac.
   a. Simple squamous epithelium (mesothelium) covers the external surface facing the pericardial cavity.
   b. The underlying fibroelastic connective tissue contains adipocytes, nerves, and coronary vessels.

B. Cardiac skeleton: the dense, collagenous connective tissue from which the myocardial fibers originate and into which they insert

C. Heart valves: endocardial folds with a core of dense connective tissue (dermatan sulfate) that is continuous with the cardiac skeleton

D. Impulse-conducting system
   - The heartbeat is initiated and regulated by several structures composed of cells that are specialized for conduction rather than contraction.
   1. The sinoatrial (SA) node, located in the wall of the superior vena cava at its junction with the right atrium, normally functions as the heart's pacemaker.
      - Small cardiomyocytes in the SA node spontaneously generate impulses that are transmitted to ordinary atrial myofibers, causing atrial contraction.
   2. The atrioventricular (AV) node, located in the wall of the right atrium near the tricuspid valve, receives impulses from the SA node by way of the atrial myocytes.
      - The AV node is histologically similar to the SA node and can act as the pacemaker if the SA node becomes nonfunctional.
   3. The AV bundle (bundle of His) is a band of small special myocytes that radiate from the AV node into the interventricular septum.
      - After dividing into two branches, the bundles enter the subendocardium and continue as Purkinje fibers on either side of the septum.
   4. Purkinje fibers are large, specialized cardiac muscle cells that carry impulses to ordinary cardiac myocytes first in the papillary muscle of each ventricle and at the apex of the heart, then the rest of of the myocardium causing ventricular contraction in such a manner that the heart empties from apex to base. Early contraction of the papillary muscles increases tension on the chorda tendineae, thus prevents prolapse of the AV valve cusps.
      - These cells contain a few peripherally displaced myofibrils and possess perinuclear masses of glycogen.

> Cardiac impulse conduction: Sinoatrial node (pacemaker) → atrioventricular node → bundle of His → Purkinje fibers → papillary muscles

E. Cardiovascular disorders
   - Numerous acquired or congenital defects in the heart muscle, the heart valves, or the impulse-conducting system can compromise heart function.
   1. Ischemic heart disease results from interruption in the coronary artery blood supply to the heart muscle.
      a. Angina pectoris: myocardial pain, often radiating to the arms, in the absence of ischemic necrosis of cardiac muscle

Rheumatic fever is the most common cause of mitral valve stenosis, which may be accompanied by aortic valve stenosis.

      b. Acute myocardial infarction: severe pain, often with pallor, perspiration, nausea, and shortness of breath, associated with ischemic necrosis of cardiac muscle

2. Arrhythmias include any changes in the normal pattern of the heartbeat.
   - Heart block commonly involves impairment of impulse conduction in the AV node or bundle of His.

3. Valvular stenosis involves narrowing of any of the heart valves.
   a. The most important long-term sequela of untreated rheumatic fever in childhood is scarring and reduced elasticity of the mitral valve (most common) and the aortic valve.
   b. Elderly individuals often have isolated aortic stenosis resulting from calcific degeneration. Severe left ventricular hypertrophy develops; dizziness and syncope on exertion are common symptoms.

Blood Cells and Their Formation

I. Introduction
- Blood is a specialized connective tissue of mesodermal origin.
A. Constituents of blood
1. The formed elements, the erythrocytes, leukocytes, and platelets, constitute approximately 45% of blood volume.
2. Plasma, the fluid matrix in which the formed elements are suspended, constitutes approximately 55% of blood volume.
a. Major plasma proteins include albumin, fibrinogen, and the globulins. Gamma globulins function as antibodies (see Chapter 13).
b. Serum is the supernatant remaining after blood has clotted.
B. Turnover of blood cells
1. The life span of almost all blood cells is relatively short, and millions are formed each day to replenish the supply.
2. Hematopoiesis, the formation of new blood cells, occurs primarily in the red bone marrow.

II. Blood Cells
A. Numeric measures of blood cells
- Table 12-1 summarizes the size, number, and life span of the blood's formed elements.
1. Hematocrit: the volume of formed elements determined by centrifugation of whole blood

Normal hematocrit (volume of formed elements in centrifuged blood) is 45. Lower values indicate disorders such as anemia or chronic hemorrhage.

TABLE 12-1:
Number, Size, and Life Span of Peripheral Blood Cells

Cell Type	No./mm³	Differential Count (%)	Diameter in Smear (μm)	Life Span
Erythrocytes	$4.5–5.5 \times 10^6$		7–8	120 days
Platelets	$1.5–4 \times 10^5$		2–5	7–12 days
Leukocytes:	$5–9 \times 10^3$			
Neutrophils		50–70	10–12	Hours to days
Eosinophils		1–3	10–12	8–12 days
Basophils		0.5–1	10–12	? (quite long)
Lymphocytes		20–40	7–12	Months to years
Monocytes		1–6	9–12	Months

Deviations from normal blood counts are indicated by suffixes. Above-normal counts are indicated by *-cytosis* or *-philia* (e.g., monocytosis, eosinophilia). Below-normal counts are indicated by *-penia* (e.g., neutropenia).

Hemoglobin A (HbA) is a major normal hemoglobin in adults (two α-globin and two β-globin chains). HbA₂ is a minor normal hemoglobin in adults (two α-globin and two δ-globin chains). HbF is a normal hemoglobin in fetuses (two α-globin and two λ-globin chains). HbS is an abnormal hemoglobin associated with sickle cell anemia.

Iron deficiency anemia is microcytic-hypochromic anemia caused by decreased hemoglobin synthesis.

- Because red blood cells (RBCs) are much more numerous than other formed elements, the hematocrit is determined largely by the number of RBCs.
2. Blood count: the number of each type of blood cell per cubic millimeter of blood
3. Differential count: the number of each type of white blood cell (WBC) expressed as a percentage of the total WBC count
B. Erythrocytes (RBCs)
 1. Morphology: small, highly deformable biconcave disks that lack a nucleus (anucleate) and most cytoplasmic organelles
 2. Hemoglobin: iron-containing protein in RBCs that carries oxygen and carbon dioxide
 3. Effect of tonicity on RBCs
  - The interior of RBCs has a tonicity equivalent to that of 0.9% saline.
  a. In isotonic medium (0.9% saline), RBCs retain their normal size and shape.
  b. In hypertonic medium (>0.9% saline), water leaves the cells, so RBCs shrink and become wrinkled (crenation).
  c. In hypotonic medium (<0.9% saline), water enters the cells, so RBCs swell and burst (hemolysis).
 4. Erythrocyte cytoskeleton
  - An extensive cortical microfilament network maintains the shape of RBCs. This network is linked to the plasma membrane by spectrin and other proteins (see Chapter 2).
 5. Anemia: any condition characterized by a low count of normal RBCs or a decreased amount of hemoglobin in the peripheral blood (Table 12-2)
C. Platelets (thrombocytes)
 1. Morphology: anucleate, disk-shaped fragments of megakaryocyte cytoplasm
  a. Granulomere: a central, densely staining region marked by granules of various sizes
   (1) Alpha (α) granules (largest) contain platelet-derived growth factor, thromboplastin, von Willebrand's factor VIII, fibrinogen, and factor V.

TABLE 12-2:
Selected Anemias

Disease	Cause	Red Blood Cell (RBC) Morphology	Other Clinical Features
Iron deficiency anemia	Impaired hemoglobin (Hb) production resulting from low iron intake, chronic blood loss, or increased demand for iron (e.g., in pregnancy)	Small RBCs, with large area of central pallor (microcytic-hypochromic anemia)	Pallor Brittle nails, oral lesions Gastroesophagal symptoms
Pernicious anemia	Impaired production of RBCs resulting from vitamin B_{12} deficiency because of inadequate synthesis of intrinsic factor	Large, abnormal RBC precursors in bone marrow and blood (megaloblastic anemia)	Weakness; bilateral tingling and numbness in hands and feet Red, painful tongue Subacute degeneration of posterior and lateral spinal column
Sickle cell anemia	Production of abnormal HbS resulting from mutation in β chain; autosomal recessive (heterozygotes usually asymptomatic)	Fragile, mis-shapen RBCs (sickle cells) with decreased survival time (hemolytic anemia)	Joint pain; attacks of abdominal pain Increased bilirubin levels Ulcerations of lower extremities Increased risk of *Salmonella* osteomyelitis
Hereditary spherocytosis	Mutation in spectrin causing defect in RBC membrane; usually autosomal dominant	Fragile, round, hyperchromic RBCs sensitive to lysis	Jaundice Splenomegaly
β-Thalassemia	Various mutations in Hb β chain; autosomal recessive (heterozygotes asymptomatic or show mild disease)	Small, pale, short-lived RBCs (microcytic, hypochromic, hemolytic anemia)	Splenomegaly Bone deformities

(2) Delta (δ) granules (mid-size) contain serotonin, histamine, and adenosine diphosphate.

(3) Lambda (λ) granules (smallest) contain lysosomal enzymes.

b. Hyalomere: a peripheral, light-staining region filled with microtubules and microfilaments

- A system of canaliculi that open to the surface aids in delivering the granule contents to the outside.

Pernicious anemia is megaloblastic anemia caused by decreased production of red blood cells. Impaired absorption of vitamin B_{12} is usually due to reduced synthesis of intrinsic factor.

Aspirin and other nonsteroidal anti-inflammatory drugs reduce the synthesis of thromboxane A_2 in platelets by inhibiting cyclooxygenase. As a result, the formation of platelet thrombi is curtailed.

When individuals who are taking aspirin cut themselves shaving, cessation of bleeding takes much longer than normal due to the absence of platelet thrombi to stop blood flow.

Anticoagulants (e.g., warfarin, heparin), which inhibit the coagulation system, block the formation of venous thrombi.

Aspirin in low doses reduces the incidence of acute myocardial infarction and stroke by decreasing the development of platelet thrombi in arteries.

2. Role of platelets in hemostasis and disease
   a. Injury of small vessels (e.g., capillaries, venules) is followed by adherence of platelets to the injured endothelium and their aggregation to form platelet plugs bound together by fibrin strands (thrombi).
      (1) von Willebrand's factor VIII, which is produced by both megakaryocytes and endothelial cells, mediates platelet adhesion.
      (2) Adenosine diphosphate, which promotes platelet aggregation, is released from platelet delta (δ) granules after adhesion occurs.
      (3) Thromboxane A_2, a potent aggregating and vasoconstricting agent, is synthesized by platelets after the initial release reaction.
   b. Arterial thrombi usually develop over areas of turbulence (e.g., atherosclerotic plaques) in both muscular and elastic arteries.
      • Arterial thrombi are primarily composed of platelets held together by fibrin strands.
      (1) In muscular arteries (e.g., coronary arteries), thrombi may lead to vessel occlusion and infarction (e.g., coronary thrombosis → acute myocardial infarction).
      (2) In elastic arteries (e.g., aorta, bifurcation of the carotid arteries), thrombi contribute to the formation of fibrofatty plaques, the primary lesion of atherosclerosis, and also may occlude the vessel, leading to infarction (e.g., a thrombus overlying an atheromatous plaque at the bifurcation of the carotid arteries → brain infarction or stroke).
   c. Venous thrombi most commonly develop in the deep veins of the calf.
      (1) Stasis of blood causes activation of the clotting system, leading to the formation of fibrin clots on top of the platelet thrombus.
      (2) Red blood cells and platelets are trapped in the clots, and eventually the vessel lumen is occluded.
3. von Willebrand's disease (vascular hemophilia) is caused by a genetic defect that results in reduced synthesis of von Willebrand's factor (vWF) by endothelial cells and platelets.
   • Sudden nosebleeds and bleeding from the gums occur in severe cases.
D. Leukocytes (WBCs)
   • All WBCs are nucleated and contain the usual cytoplasmic organelles as well as nonspecific azurophilic granules.
   • They commonly migrate from the blood through spaces between capillary endothelial cells, entering areas of connective tissue.
   1. Granulocytes
      • Three types of WBCs, the granulocytes, possess characteristic nuclear shapes and cell type–specific granules containing degradative enzymes or inflammatory mediators (Table 12-3).
      a. Neutrophils, the premier cells for phagocytosing and killing bacteria, commonly are found at sites of acute inflammation.
         (1) Mature neutrophils are also called *polymorphonuclear leukocytes* (PMNs).
         (2) Bands (stabs) are immature neutrophils with a nonlobed, bean-shaped nucleus; normally, they constitute 1–3% of peripheral WBCs.

TABLE 12-3:
Selected Properties
of Granulocytes

Property	Neutrophil	Eosinophil	Basophil
Nuclear shape	3 to 5 lobes	Bilobed	Irregular
Azurophilic granules	Many	Few	Few
Color of specific granules (Giemsa or Wright stain)	Dusty rose	Red/orange	Dark blue to black
Size of specific granules	Small	Large	Large
Phagocytic activity	High (bacteria)	Moderate (antigen–antibody complexes)	None
Other	H_2O_2 formed during phagocytosis	Specific granules are lysosomes with a crystalline core of major basic protein	Degranulation induced by allergens releases histamine

      b. Eosinophils participate in allergic reactions and in the response to invasive parasitic infections.

      c. Basophils contribute to immediate hypersensitivity reactions (see Fig. 13-5).

  2. Lymphocytes (B and T cells)

      a. Have a large, round nucleus surrounded by a thin rim of cytoplasm containing few organelles and azurophilic granules

      b. Possess antigen-binding receptors in their plasma membrane and are responsible for specific immune responses (see Chapter 13)

  3. Monocytes

      a. Have a characteristic kidney-shaped nucleus, with a clumpy, stringy chromatin pattern

      b. Migrate into tissues and give rise to macrophages, which are phagocytic and present antigens to T cells

  4. Leukocytic disorders

      a. Lazy leukocyte syndrome is due to a genetic defect in the contractile actin microfilaments of PMNs that severely impairs their mobility.

        • Clinically, this disorder is marked by a severe decrease in the number of circulating PMNs as well as by recurrent low-grade infections (e.g., sinusitis, stomatitis, and otitis media).

      b. Leukocyte-adhesion deficiency results from a defect in several integrins that are normally expressed on the surface of leukocytes.

        • Defective leukocytes have reduced ability to migrate into tissues and adhere to target cells.

        • Affected individuals have recurrent bacterial infections and impaired wound healing. In newborns, the umbilical cord fails to separate.

III. Inflammation

    • A localized protective response to tissue infection or injury, inflammation is aseptic if no bacteria are involved and septic if bacteria are involved.

    • Various inflammatory mediators are released from leukocytes in connective tissue near the site of infection or injury.

A. Classic signs of acute inflammation
- Histamine released from mast cells causes vasodilation and increased permeability.
    1. Dilation of vessels, with subsequent increased blood flow to the affected area, causes rubor (redness) and calor (heat).
    2. Increased vessel permeability leads to tumor (swelling, or edema) resulting from excess tissue fluid and to dolor (pain) resulting from pressure on the nerve endings and the presence of bradykinin and prostaglandin E_2.

B. Stages in the inflammatory response
    1. Acute phase: PMNs migrate from the bloodstream into the damaged area.
        a. Adherence of circulating PMNs to the endothelium (margination) is mediated by cell-adhesion molecules in the plasma membranes of the interacting cells.
        b. Diapedesis involves movement of the adhered PMNs from the endothelial cells into the surrounding connective tissue.
        c. Chemotactic factors that "attract" neutrophils also play a role in neutrophil adherence and transendothelial migration.
    2. Subacute phase: Lymphocytes, monocytes, and plasma cells enter the affected tissue, mixing with PMNs.
    3. Chronic phase: Macrophages predominate, with lymphocytes and plasma cells also present; few PMNs are present.

C. Changes in the band count during acute infection
    1. Shift to the left: Severe infection results in the release of immature PMNs (bands, or stabs) from the bone marrow, leading to an increase in the band, or stab, count.
    2. Shift to the right: As inflammation subsides, the band, or stab, count decreases toward normal.

IV. Hematopoietic Sites
A. Prenatal sites of blood formation
    1. Yolk sac of the embryo
        a. Blood islands, or angiogenic cell clusters, in the wall of the yolk sac give rise to nucleated erythrocytes from about 2 to 8 weeks' gestation.
        b. No leukocytes form during this stage.
    2. Liver and spleen
        a. The formation of erythrocytes and leukocytes occurs primarily in the fetal liver and spleen from 8 to 28 weeks' gestation.
        b. Hematopoiesis in the liver and spleen normally ceases at about the time of birth.
    3. Red bone marrow
        - Starting at 6 months' gestation, the red bone marrow exhibits hematopoietic activity and soon becomes the major site of hematopoiesis.
B. Postnatal sites of blood formation
    1. Before puberty: Hematopoiesis occurs in the skull, ribs, sternum, vertebrae, clavicles, pelvis, and long bones.

Four cardinal signs of inflammation are rubor (redness), calor (heat), tumor (edema), and dolor (pain).

A higher than normal band, or stab, count (left shift) indicates infection.

2. After puberty: Hematopoiesis occurs in the same sites, except for the long bones.
3. Extramedullary hematopoiesis: Formation of blood cells occurs in the liver and spleen after birth in certain disease states.
C. Histology of the red bone marrow
   1. The stroma contains fibroblasts (which produce collagen and reticular fibers), reticular cells, fat cells, and endothelial cells.
      • Hematopoietic growth factors are synthesized and secreted by stromal cells.
   2. The parenchyma contains hematopoietic cells of different lineages in various stages of differentiation.
   3. Hematopoietic cords are bands of parenchyma and stroma lying between sinusoids that connect arterial and venous vessels within the red bone marrow.
      • Mature blood cells produced in the parenchyma of the cords gain access to the circulation by passing through sinusoid walls.
D. Distribution of hematopoietic cells within the bone marrow parenchyma
   1. Total number of cells
      a. 60% in granulocytopoiesis (formation of neutrophils, basophils, and eosinophils)
      b. 30% in erythrocytopoiesis (formation of erythrocytes)
      c. 10% in thrombocytopoiesis, monocytopoiesis, and lymphocytopoiesis (formation of platelets, monocytes, and lymphocytes, respectively)
   2. Myeloid-to-erythroid (M/E) ratio: ratio of the total volume (or number) of cells undergoing granulocytopoiesis to the total volume (or number) of cells undergoing erythrocytopoiesis in the red bone marrow
      a. The normal M/E ratio is 3:1 (range, 2:1 to 4:1).
      b. A high M/E ratio (e.g., 8:1) indicates decreased erythrocytopoiesis or increased granulocytopoiesis (as in chronic myelogenous leukemia).
      c. A low M/E ratio (e.g., 1:5) indicates increased erythrocytopoiesis (as in polycythemia) or decreased granulocytopoiesis.

> The iliac crest is the primary site for bone marrow biopsy; the secondary site is the sternum.

V. Stages in Hematopoiesis
   • The formation of each type of blood cell progresses through distinct cell kinetic "compartments" during which the degree of developmental potentiality decreases and the extent of differentiation increases.
A. Stem cell compartment
   • This compartment comprises vegetative intermitotics (VIMs), which are self-sustaining and self-renewing cells. The various stem cell populations are cytologically indistinguishable.
   • Hematopoietic stem cells are referred to as *colony-forming units* (CFUs) because they give rise to self-renewing colonies in the spleen of irradiated mice injected with bone marrow.
   1. Totipotent stem cells (CFUs) are capable of giving rise to all types of blood cells.
   2. Pluripotent stem cells arise from daughter cells of totipotent stem cells that become committed to either the myeloid or the lymphoid pathway.

    a. Lymphoid stem cells (CFU-Lys) give rise to lymphocytes.

    b. Myeloid stem cells (CFU-GEMMegs, or CFU-Ss) give rise to all the other blood cell lines.

  3. Unipotent and multipotent stem cells arising from myeloid stem cells are committed to one of three lineages (Fig. 12-1):

    a. Erythrocyte line (CFU-E)

    b. Megakaryocyte–platelet line (CFU-Meg)

    c. Granulocyte–monocyte line (CFU-GM)

      • CFU-GMs subsequently give rise to CFU-Gs, which are committed to the granulocyte line, and CFU-Ms, which are committed to the monocyte line.

B. Differentiating or multiplicative compartment

  • Each lineage of committed stem cells gives rise to differentiating intermitotics (DIMs), or precursor cells, which undergo continuous cell division and cytodifferentiation in this compartment.

  • The first histologically distinct precursors of mature blood cells arise at this stage.

  • All the daughter cells eventually differentiate into highly specialized, postmitotic cells; thus, this compartment must be replenished by an influx from the stem cell compartment.

C. Functional compartment

  • Mature blood cells in each lineage and their immediate precursors compose this compartment. The mature cells enter the bloodstream or are held in reserve until they are needed.

  • These fixed postmitotic cells (FPMs) function, age, and in time die (see Table 12-1). They are replaced by cell influx from the differentiating compartment.

D. Time course of hematopoiesis

  1. Stem cell → granulocytes: approximately 12 days

  2. Stem cell → erythrocytes: approximately 7 days

E. Hematopoietic growth factors (see Fig. 12-1)

  • Three general classes of growth factors—colony-stimulating factors (CSFs), interleukins, and erythropoietin—are responsible for directing cells into different hematopoietic pathways and promoting proliferation and cytodifferentiation within lineages.

  1. Granulocyte–monocyte colony-stimulating factor (GM-CSF) stimulates granulocytopoiesis and monocytopoiesis.

    • Treatment with GM-CSF ameliorates neutropenia associated with myelosuppressive chemotherapy or radiation therapy.

  2. Granulocyte colony-stimulating factor (G-CSF) directs CFU-Gs to differentiate along the neutrophilic pathway.

    • Treatment with G-CSF, which produces a dose-dependent neutrophilia, shortens the duration of neutropenia after myelosuppressive chemotherapy or radiation therapy.

  3. Monocyte colony-stimulating factor (M-CSF) commits CFU-GMs to the monocytic pathway, thereby increasing monocytopoiesis.

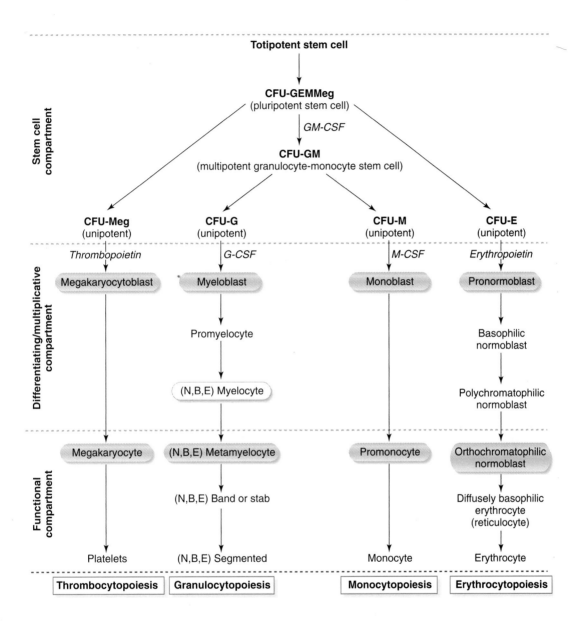

12-1: *Flow chart of hematopoiesis showing the named stages of cytodifferentiation, the key stimulating factors (shown in italics), and the cell kinetic compartments. The first histologically distinct cells in the two non–stem cell compartments are indicated by shading. The three granulocyte lineages—neutrophilic (N), basophilic (B), and eosinophilic (E)—become distinguishable from each other at the myelocyte stage. Totipotent stem cells also give rise to lymphoid stem cells, whose differentiation into lymphocytes is not shown. CFU, colony-forming unit (stem cell); CSF, colony-stimulating factor; E, erythrocyte; G, granulocyte; M, monocyte; Meg, megakaryocyte.*

F. Clinical uses of hematopoietic stem cells
- Patients with cancer who receive aggressive chemotherapy or radiation often require a bone marrow transplant to restore their hematopoietic stem cells, which are destroyed by such treatments.
- Separation of stem cells from harvested bone marrow greatly reduces the volume of marrow that must be infused into a patient.

VI. Histology of Blood Cell Precursors
- Each of the hematopoietic stem cells committed to a particular lineage proceeds through a series of histologically distinct precursors as it undergoes cytodifferentiation.

A. Granulocytopoiesis: CFU-G → neutrophil, basophil, and eosinophil

> Granulocytopoiesis: CFU-Gs → myeloblasts → promyelocytes → myelocytes → metamyelocytes → bands → mature stages

1. Granulocyte precursors (see Fig. 12-1)
   a. G-CSF stimulates CFU-Gs to proliferate and differentiate into the first histologically recognizable granulocyte precursor, the myeloblast, a relatively large cell that is similar in all three granulocyte lineages.
   b. The three lineages—neutrophilic (N), basophilic (B), and eosinophilic (E)—are first distinguishable with the appearance of lineage-specific cytoplasmic granules at the myelocyte stage (N, B, E).
   c. Maturation of each lineage, yielding segmented neutrophils (PMNs), basophils, and eosinophils, is completed within the bone marrow.
2. Common cytologic changes during granulocytopoiesis
   a. The number of both nonspecific and specific granules increases.
   b. The entire cell and the nucleoli decrease in size.
   c. Lobation of the nucleus increases.
   d. Cell deformability increases.
   e. Cell motility increases.
   f. Adhesiveness increases.
   g. Phagocytic capability increases.

B. Erythrocytopoiesis: CFU-E → erythrocyte
1. Erythropoietin, produced in the kidney, stimulates CFU-Es to proliferate and differentiate into the first histologically recognizable erythrocyte precursor, the pronormoblast (proerythroblast).
   - A decrease in the O_2 saturation of the blood stimulates erythropoietin production.
2. A diffusely basophilic erythrocyte, or reticulocyte, the final stage of erythrocytopoiesis within the bone marrow, represents an immature, anucleated RBC.
   a. After entering the bloodstream, reticulocytes lose their remaining ribosomes and mitochondria, becoming mature RBCs.
   b. Reticulocytes normally constitute 1% to 3% of circulating RBCs.
   c. Excessive loss of mature RBCs (e.g., during chronic hemorrhage) causes the release of more reticulocytes from the bone marrow, and their percentage in the blood increases.
3. Secondary polycythemia: any abnormal increase in the total RBC mass resulting from tissue hypoxia, which stimulates the release of erythropoietin from the kidney

      a. Tetralogy of Fallot, a congenital heart defect, is accompanied by hypoxia because not enough blood is routed to the lungs to be oxygenated. Children with this defect commonly are polycythemic.

      b. Cigarette smoke contains carbon monoxide, which binds to hemoglobin much more tightly than oxygen, producing hypoxia. Thus, smokers tend to be polycythemic.

    4. Polycythemia vera: a neoplastic disease involving the stem cells (myeloproliferative disease) marked by an increased RBC mass with low erythropoietin levels

      • Clinical manifestations include headache, dizziness, ruddy face, thrombotic episodes, and hepatosplenomegaly.

C. Thrombocytopoiesis: CFU-Meg → platelets

    1. A megakarycytoblast, the first differentiating precursor in this pathway, undergoes deoxyribonucleic acid replication but not cytokinesis, a process called *endoreduplication.*

    2. A megakaryocyte, a giant, polyploid cell with a huge, multilobed nucleus, is generated by repeated endoreduplication.

      a. The ploidy level varies among postmitotic megakaryocytes, with most cells being $8n$, $16n$, or $32n$ (lower n = younger cell).

      b. Filopods (thin pseudopodia) are extended through the walls of marrow sinusoids into the lumen.

        • Also known as *proplatelets,* filopods "shatter," releasing platelets directly into the circulation.

D. Monocytopoiesis: CFU-M → monocyte

    1. A monoblast, the first differentiating precursor, gives rise to a promonocyte, which matures into a monocyte.

    2. Monocytes enter the bloodstream, circulate for 1 or 2 days, and then migrate into connective tissue areas and body cavities. where they function as tissue macrophages.

E. Lymphocytopoiesis: CFU-Lys → pre-B and pre-T cells → mature B and T cells

    1. Pre-B cells develop into mature, antigen-recognizing B cells in the bone marrow.

    2. Pre-T cells migrate from the bone marrow to the thymus, where they develop into mature, antigen-recognizing T cells.

    3. Proliferation and differentiation of mature B and T cells

      a. Unlike the other types of blood cells, lymphocytes released from the bone marrow and thymus are not fixed postmitotics incapable of cell division.

      b. After encountering a specific antigen, appropriate B and T cells proliferate (clonal expansion) and differentiate into effector cells and memory cells that function in specific immune responses (see Chapter 13).

F. Leukemias: abnormal proliferation and development of leukocytes and their precursors in the bone marrow

    • Common symptoms include fatigue, pallor, dyspnea on exertion, hepatosplenomegaly, and generalized lymphadenopathy.

Thrombocytopoiesis: CFU-Megs → megakaryoblasts → megakaryocytes → platelets

All forms of leukemia are characterized by abnormal proliferation of one or more types of immature blood cells within the bone marrow.

Acute myelogenous leukemia is the most common type of leukemia in people between the ages of 15 and 59 years.

Leukemic cells in chronic myelogenous leukemia have a short chromosome 22 (Philadelphia chromosome) and a long chromosome 9 with the *bcr-abl* oncogene.

Acute lymphoblastic leukemia is the most common cancer of any type affecting children.

Chronic lymphocytic leukemia is the most common of all the leukemias. It is found most commonly in patients older than 60 years of age.

1. Acute myelogenous leukemia (AML) is marked by the accumulation of blast cells containing Auer rods (red refractile bodies) in the bone marrow.
   • It most commonly occurs in individuals 15 to 59 years of age.
2. Chronic myelogenous leukemia (CML) is associated with Philadelphia chromosome resulting from a translocation between chromosomes 9 and 22.
   • Clinical features include leukocytosis and massive splenomegaly. Progression to acute leukemia is typical.
   • Adults 35 to 55 years of age are most commonly affected.
3. Acute lymphoblastic leukemia (ALL) is characterized by the proliferation of blast cells with lymphocyte differentiation markers. It is classified into three types (L1 to L3), based on the morphology of the blast cells.
   • ALL primarily affects children.
4. Chronic lymphocytic leukemia (CLL) usually involves B cells, with many broken cells (smudge cells) seen in a peripheral blood smear.
   • Complications include hypogammaglobulinemia and autoimmune hemolytic anemia.
   • Adults older than 60 years of age are most commonly affected.

Immune System

I. Introduction
   A. General components of the immune system
      1. Lymphoid tissues and organs
      2. B and T lymphocytes (B and T cells), which have specific antigen-binding receptors in the plasma membrane
      3. Phagocytic cells and antigen-presenting cells (Table 13-1)
   B. General functions of the immune system
      1. Recognition and destruction of non-self substances (antigens)
         - Antigens may be soluble or may present on the surface of microorganisms and cells.
      2. Removal of defective, worn-out self-cells and cell products
      3. Functional branches
         a. The antibody-mediated (humoral) response primarily involves B cells (B lymphocytes).
         b. The cell-mediated response involves T cells (T lymphocytes).
   C. Clonal expansion of B and T lymphocytes (Fig. 13-1)
      1. "Virgin," or immunocompetent, lymphocytes are activated by exposure of an appropriate antigen to blastlike cells.
      2. The proliferation and differentiation of blastlike cells generates large numbers of two types of cells:

The immune system has two major cellular components:

- B cells, which are involved in antibody-mediated immunity
- T cells, which are involved in cell-mediated immunity

TABLE 13-1:
Cells of the
Immune System

Cell Type	Primary Functions in Host Defense
Lymphocytes	
T cells	Destruction of cells bearing intracellular (endogenous) antigens (cytotoxic T cells)
	Secretion of cytokines that regulate intensity and duration of immune responses (T_H cells)
B cells	Clearance of extracellular (exogenous) antigens by secreted antibodies
	Processing and presentation of exogenous antigens to T_H cells
Natural killer cells	Antigen-specific and nonspecific cytotoxicity for tumor cells and virus-infected cells
Granulocytes	
Neutrophils	Release of inflammatory mediators
	Nonspecific phagocytosis and killing of bacteria
Eosinophils	Defense against parasitic organisms
Basophils	Release of mediators in certain allergic reactions
Other	
Mast cells	Release of mediators in certain allergic reactions
Macrophages	Nonspecific phagocytosis of exogenous antigens, dead host cells, cellular debris, and bacteria
	Processing and presentation of antigens to T_H cells
Dendritic cells (various types)	Processing and presentation of exogenous antigen to T_H cells

a. Effector cells, which have various functions in clearing antigen from the host
b. Memory cells, which have no effector function but can react more quickly than virgin lymphocytes to a second exposure to the same antigen

D. Immunologic tolerance
1. Self-tolerance: During the fetal and early neonatal periods, a host normally develops tolerance to its own self-antigens but not to the foreign antigens of others.
2. Tolerance to foreign antigens: Introduction of a foreign antigen before the end of the tolerance-generating period will induce tolerance to that antigen.

E. Autoimmune diseases
• A breakdown in the mechanisms ensuring natural tolerance to self-antigens leads to numerous clinical manifestations, depending on the self-antigens recognized and the nature of the response; for example:
1. Hashimoto's disease: Autoantibodies to thyroid proteins block iodine uptake and cause an inflammatory response against thyroid tissue.
   • Hypothyroidism eventually develops.
2. Insulin-dependent diabetes mellitus (type 1): A delayed hypersensitivity reaction causes destruction of insulin-producing (beta) cells in the pancreas.

An individual is naturally tolerant of his or her own self-antigens, but not of foreign (non-self) antigens.

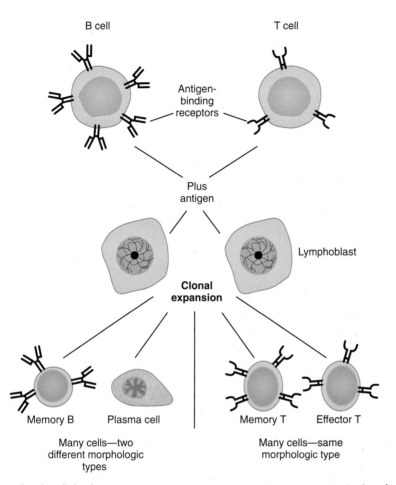

B cell

T cell

Antigen-binding receptors

Plus antigen

Lymphoblast

Clonal expansion

Memory B   Plasma cell

Memory T   Effector T

Many cells—two different morphologic types

Many cells—same morphologic type

13-1: *T-cell and B-cell clonal expansion in response to exposure to an appropriate antigen. Binding of an appropriate antigen to cell-surface receptors on virgin T and B cells activates them to lymphoblasts. These divide mitotically (clonal expansion), producing many daughter cells, which differentiate into effector cells or memory cells with the same antigen specificity as the activated lymphocyte from which they arose.*

- Insulitis with a subsequent decrease in insulin production occurs as a result.
3. Systemic lupus erythematosus: Autoantibodies against erythrocytes, platelets, and other self-antigens (e.g., anti–double-stranded deoxyribonucleic acid, anti-Sm) trigger tissue-destroying inflammatory reactions.
   - Vasculitis, erythematous rash, arthritis, neutropenia, and hemolytic anemia are common manifestations.
4. Goodpasture's syndrome: Autoantibodies to the capillary basement membranes in the kidneys and lungs mediate tissue destruction.
   - Lung hemorrhage, nephritis with proteinuria, and renal failure may result.

5. Other autoimmune diseases include Graves' disease (see Chapter 1), myasthenia gravis (see Chapter 7), and pemphigus vulgaris (see Chapter 8).

II. Cell-Mediated Immunologic Response
- Intracellular pathogens, virus-infected cells, foreign grafts, and autologous neoplasms bearing tumor-specific antigens trigger cell-mediated responses.
- A. Antigen recognition by T cells occurs only when antigen is present on the membrane of a cell in association with a major histocompatibility complex (MHC) molecule.
  1. MHC molecules are membrane proteins that have binding sites for antigenic peptides in their extracellular domain.
     a. Class I MHC molecules are found on the surface of most somatic cells.
     b. Class II MHC molecules are found on the surface of antigen-presenting cells only.
  2. Antigen-presenting cells internalize exogenous antigens (produced outside the cell) and degrade them into smaller peptides, which associate with class II MHC molecules on the cell surface (Fig. 13-2).

An immune response is triggered by antigen exposure followed by clonal expansion of activated antigen-specific B or T cells.

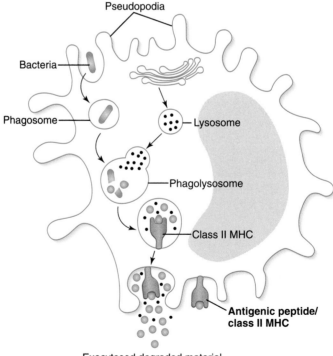

13-2: *Phagocytosis, processing, and presentation of an antigen by macrophages. Phagocytosed material is degraded by lysosomal enzymes, and most of the products are exocytosed. However, antigenic peptides that interact with class II major histocompatibility complex (MHC) molecules form complexes that move to the cell surface for presentation to T$_H$ cells.*

- Dendritic cells, macrophages, Langerhans cells (in the dermis), and B cells, as well as glial cells and vascular endothelial cells, function as antigen-presenting cells.

3. Target cells degrade endogenous antigens (produced within the cell) into smaller peptides, which associate with class I MHC molecules on the cell surface.
   - Common target cells are virus-infected cells, defective self-cells, tumor cells, and foreign graft cells.

B. Effector T cells are divided into two major types, which have different functions and express different CD (cluster of differentiation) antigens on their surface.

1. Activated T helper (T_H) cells
   - Arise by clonal expansion and differentiation of T_H cells, which express CD4 and recognize antigen–class II MHC complexes (Fig. 13-3A)
   - Produce and release cytokines, which are small, soluble protein factors that regulate the intensity and duration of immune responses (Table 13-2)
     a. T_H1 cells promote the formation of cytotoxic T lymphocytes (T_C) and the activation of macrophages.
     b. T_H2 cells help B cells respond to antigenic stimulation.

2. Cytotoxic T lymphocytes
   - Arise by clonal expansion and differentiation of T_C cells, which express CD8 and recognize antigen–class I MHC complexes (Fig. 13-3B)
   - Cause lysis of target cells by a perforin-mediated process

C. Natural killer cells belong to the population of peripheral lymphocytes (null cells) that do not express antigen-specific receptors and other surface markers that are characteristic of B and T cells.
   - Exhibit both nonspecific (antigen-independent) cytotoxicity and specific cytotoxicity, which depends on the presence of antibody on target cells (e.g., tumor cells and virus-infected cells)
   - Perform a surveillance function by attacking tumor cells that arise regularly

D. Macrophages, which express class II MHC molecules but no antigen-specific receptors on their membrane, are derived from monocytes in the blood that migrate into tissues and differentiate.

1. Types of macrophages
   - Fixed macrophages are attached to reticular fibers, whereas free macrophages are motile and wander throughout the stroma of different organs.
     a. Kupffer cells in the liver
     b. Alveolar macrophages in the lung
     c. Histiocytes in connective tissue
     d. Microglial cells in the brain

2. Functions of macrophages
   a. Phagocytosis and degradation of aged, defective, and dead self-cells
   b. Nonspecific processing and presentation of non–self-antigens in the context of class II MHC molecules (see Fig. 13-2)

B and T cells express antigen-binding receptors on their surface; natural killer cells, a third type of lymphocyte, do not.

T helper cells are CD4+ and class II major histocompatibility complex–restricted. T_c cells are CD8+ and class I major histocompatibility complex–restricted.

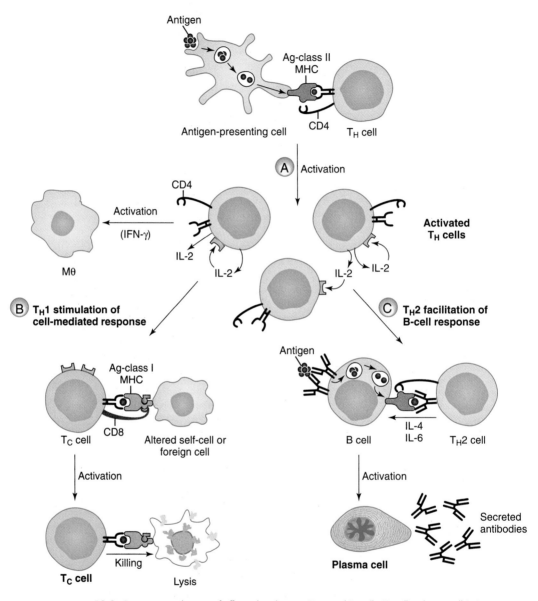

13-3: *Generation and action of effector lymphocytes (activated T_H cells, T_C cells, plasma cells). An antigen (Ag)-presenting cell activates T_H cells (A). Cytokines secreted by the T_H1 and T_H2 subsets of activated T_H cells preferentially promote cell-mediated responses (B) and antibody-mediated responses (C). IFN, interferon; IL, interleukin; Mθ, macrophage.*

      c. Secretion of complement proteins and various cytokines that promote inflammation, elimination of pathogens and tumor cells, and hematopoiesis

   E. Transplantation-associated immune responses

      1. Graft rejection is caused primarily by the host's cell-mediated response to antigens expressed on the cells of a grafted tissue or organ.

Cytokine	Secreted by	Major Biologic Functions
Interleukin (IL)-1	Macrophages, other antigen-presenting cells	Promotes activation of T_H cells
IL-2	T_H1 cells	Promotes proliferation of T_H and T_C cells Enhances activity of NK cells
IL-4	T_H2 cells, mast cells	Promotes clonal expansion of B cells Enhances synthesis of IgG and IgE by plasma cells
IL-6	T_H2 cells, macrophages	Promotes terminal differentiation into plasma cells
Interferon-γ	T_H1 cells, NK cells	Enhances activity of macrophage's Inhibits response of T_H2 cells

TABLE 13-2:
Properties of Selected Cytokines

IFN, interferon; Ig, immunoglobulin; IL, interleukin; NK, natural killer; T_H, T helper.

- The intensity of rejection reactions depends on the type of graft:
  a. Autografts (from self to self) and isografts (between genetically identical individuals) usually are accepted.
  b. Allografts (between individuals of the same species) and xenografts (between individuals of different species) are rejected unless the immune response is suppressed.
     (1) Immunosuppressive drugs (e.g., cyclosporine) that selectively suppress the function of T_H cells and natural killer cells reduce graft rejection but significantly increase the risk of cancer (e.g., squamous cell cancer of the skin).
     (2) Natural suppression of maternal cell-mediated immunity during pregnancy helps prevent rejection of allogeneic fetal tissue.
  2. Graft-versus-host disease occurs when donor T_H cells in a graft recognize the recipient's cells as non-self and mount a cell-mediated response, leading to destruction of the recipient's tissue.
     - Graft-versus-host disease is most likely to occur when a graft containing immunocompetent donor T_H cells is transplanted into a recipient with a compromised immune system.

Donor T_c cells in transplanted tissue may mediate an immune response against the recipient's cells, causing graft-versus-host disease.

III. Antibody-Mediated (Humoral) Immunologic Response
  - Soluble antigens (e.g., foreign proteins) and antigenic substances on the surface of extracellular pathogens trigger humoral responses.
  - Clonal expansion and differentiation of B cells requires direct B cell–T_H cell interaction and cytokines released from activated T_H cells (see Fig. 13-3A and C).
  A. Plasma cells are the only type of effector B lymphocyte.
     - Plasma cells, which arise from antigen-stimulated B cells (primarily within lymph nodules), are terminally differentiated cells and cannot divide. They have the following characteristic properties:
     1. Production and secretion of immunoglobulins, the active agents of humoral immunity
     2. Absence of antigen-binding receptors on their surface (unlike effector T cells)

Plasma cells, which secrete circulating antibody, arise by differentiation of antigen-stimulated B cells.

3. Short life span (approximately 2 to 3 weeks)
4. Abundant rough endoplasmic reticulum and a well-developed Golgi apparatus, typical of protein-secreting cells
5. Eccentric nucleus with a clock face chromatin pattern
B. Immunoglobulins function as antibodies (i.e., they interact specifically with antigens).
   1. Secreted (soluble) and membrane-bound antibodies
      a. Immunoglobulins secreted by plasma cells bind to antigens, forming antigen–antibody complexes that are cleared from the body by various mechanisms that may involve complement proteins.
      b. Immunoglobulins expressed on the surface of mature virgin B cells function as antigen-binding receptors.
   2. Antibody structure and specificity
      a. Monomeric immunoglobulins have a Y-shaped structure consisting of two identical heavy (H) chains and two identical light (L) chains (Fig. 13-4A).
      b. Antigen-binding sites, located at the outer ends of the "arms" of the molecule, exhibit variable amino acid sequences.

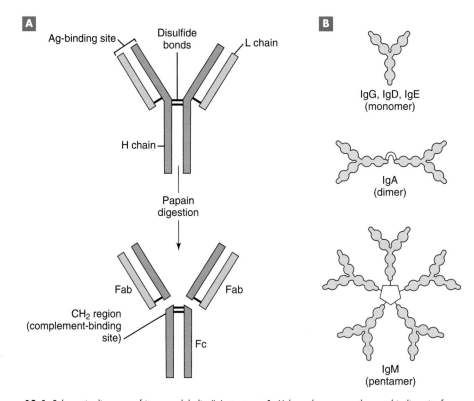

13-4: *Schematic diagrams of immunoglobulin (Ig) structure.* **A,** *Y-shaped monomers have a binding site for antigen (Ag) at the end of each arm. Papain digestion yields two Fab fragments, which bind antigen, and an Fc fragment, which binds to receptors on macrophages, mast cells, and basophils.* **B,** *Dimeric IgA and pentameric IgM have a higher antigen-binding valency than monomeric IgG, IgD, and IgE.*

(1) The variable regions are responsible for the antigen specificity of an antibody molecule.

(2) The total number of possible different antigen-binding specificities that can be produced in each person is estimated at 10^9 to 10^{11}.

c. Complement-binding sites are located on heavy chains in CH_2 domains just below the hinge region.

3. Immunoglobulin classes (Fig. 13-4B)
   - Sequence differences in the Fc region of the heavy chains define five immunoglobulin classes, or isotypes, which exhibit class-specific functional properties.

   a. Immunoglobulin (Ig) M: the predominant secreted antibody produced during a primary immune response
      - Exists as a pentamer that strongly activates the complement system

   b. IgG: the predominant secreted antibody produced during a secondary immune response
      - Promotes phagocytosis by macrophages
      - Crosses the placenta

   c. IgA: present in external secretions (e.g., tears, saliva, colostrum, mucous secretions of the gastrointestinal and respiratory tracts) as dimeric secretory IgA

   d. IgD: mostly membrane-bound antibody on unstimulated B cells
      - Functions primarily in B-cell activation

   e. IgE: the only Ig that triggers immediate (type I) hypersensitivity reactions (Fig. 13-5)

C. Monoclonal antibody is secreted by all the plasma cells derived from a single B cell (i.e., a clone of plasma cells).
   - Each molecule of a monoclonal antibody has the same antigen-binding specificity.

D. Humoral immunodeficiency diseases
   1. X-linked agammaglobulinemia: complete absence of mature B cells, plasma cells, and antibodies
      - Marked by recurrent pyogenic infections beginning after 6 months of age
   2. Selective IgA deficiency: normal levels of all isotypes except IgA
      - Marked by recurrent sinopulmonary infections and an increased incidence of allergy, gastrointestinal diseases (e.g., celiac disease), and certain autoimmune diseases

E. Multiple myeloma
   - This neoplastic disease results from bone marrow–based clonal proliferation of B cells that mature into abnormal but recognizable plasma cells.
   - Clinical manifestations include widespread osteolytic lesions, bone pain, pathologic fractures, hypercalcemia, and Bence Jones (light chain) proteinuria.

Immunoglobulin (Ig) isotypes:

- IgM: pentamer; complement activation; primary response
- IgG: most abundant antibody in the blood; promotes phagocytosis; secondary response
- IgA: dimer; in external secretions
- IgD: membrane form predominant
- IgE: type I hypersensitivity reactions (allergy and systemic anaphylaxis)

Immunoglobulin E-induced release of histamine, prostaglandins, and other mediators may cause localized allergic reactions (e.g., runny nose, itchy eyes, skin rash) or systemic anaphylaxis, a shocklike, potentially fatal state.

Selective immunoglobulin A deficiency is the most common immunodeficiency disorder.

Bence Jones protein is a monoclonal antibody light chain produced by multiple myeloma cells and excreted in urine.

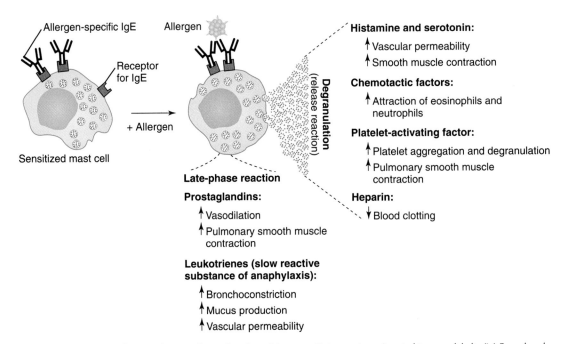

13-5: *Mechanism of immediate (type I) hypersensitivity reactions. Secreted immunoglobulin (Ig) E produced after the first exposure to an allergen binds to mast cells and basophils, which have receptors for the Fc portion of IgE antibodies. On subsequent exposure to the same allergen, cross-linking of receptor-bound IgE molecules by an allergen induces degranulation, releasing preformed mediators. These act to increase (↑) or decrease (↓) various parameters, leading to localized allergic symptoms (e.g., runny nose, itchy eyes, skin rash) or systemic anaphylaxis. After the release reaction, mast cells synthesize and release prostaglandins and leukotrienes, which mediate the late-phase reaction.*

IV. Lymphoid Tissues
   A. Diffuse lymphatic tissue comprises scattered clusters of plasma cells, macrophages, and lymphocytes in connective tissue (stromal) areas and other sites.
      1. Cutaneous-associated lymphoid tissue: found in the papillary layer of the dermis
      2. Lamina propria–associated lymphoid tissue
         a. Mucosal-associated lymphoid tissue
         b. Bronchial-associated lymphoid tissue
         c. Gut-associated lymphoid tissue
   B. Lymph follicles (nodules), which are not enclosed by a capsule, occur singly or in aggregates and are sites of B-cell localization and proliferation.
      1. Structure of follicles
         a. Primary follicles are round, tightly packed accumulations of virgin B cells and dendritic reticular cells that have not been exposed to an antigen.
         b. Secondary follicles arise from primary lymph follicles that have been exposed to a non–self-antigen.

Mucosal-associated lymphoid tissue, bronchial-associated lymphoid tissue, and gut-associated lymphoid tissue are diffuse types of lymphoid tissue associated with the lamina propria in the general mucosae, the bronchi, and the gut, respectively.

- Secondary follicles are not present before birth or after birth in individuals who are kept in a germ-free environment.
  (1) Corona: a dark peripheral region composed largely of densely packed B lymphocytes
  (2) Germinal center: a central, lighter-staining region composed largely of B lymphoblasts, memory B cells, plasma cells, and dendritic reticular cells, which trap antigen on their surface
  2. Aggregated lymph follicles are located beneath the epithelium but are in contact with the epithelium at several sites, including the following:
    a. The palatine, pharyngeal, and lingual tonsils
    b. Peyer's patches in the submucosa of the ileum (see Chapter 14)
      - These are the major sites of antibody production in children.
    c. The appendix

V. Lymphoid Organs
  - In primary lymphoid organs (thymus and bone marrow), lymphocyte precursors mature into immunocompetent cells, each programmed to recognize a specific antigen.
  - In secondary lymphoid organs (lymph nodes and spleen), trapped antigen stimulates clonal expansion of mature B and T cells (and memory cells).
  A. Bone marrow: maturation of B cells (see Chapter 12)
  B. Thymus: maturation of T cells (Fig. 13-6)
    - The connective tissue capsule of the thymus extends trabeculae into the parenchyma, dividing the organ into incomplete lobules, each composed of

Adenoids are formed by hypertrophy of the pharyngeal tonsils in the posterior wall of the nasopharynx.

The primary lymphoid organs are the thymus (T-cell maturation) and bone marrow (B-cell maturation).

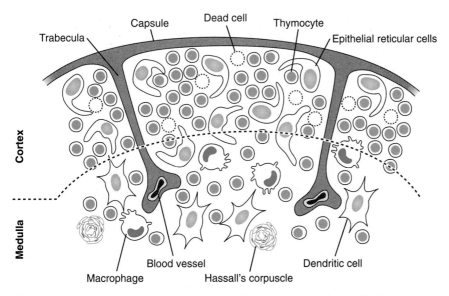

13-6: *Schematic cross-section of a portion of the thymus. The cortex is densely populated with immature T cells (thymocytes) and epithelial reticular cells. Some of these wrap around many thymocytes, forming large, multicellular complexes. As they mature, thymocytes move toward the medulla. Only approximately 5% of thymocyte progeny survive and reach the medulla.*

a distinguishable outer, darker region (cortex) and an inner, lighter region (medulla).

- Efferent lymphatic vessels but no afferent lymphatics serve the thymus; thus, lymph does not circulate through the organ.

1. Thymic cortex
   - Basic dyes, such as hematoxylin and eosin, densely stain the thymic cortex, which is filled with epithelial reticular cells and T cells in various stages of differentiation.
     a. Epithelial reticular cells secrete thymosin and other protein factors that promote maturation of T cells.
        - These cells, which are of endodermal origin (pharyngeal pouch), have long processes that surround the capillaries and form a meshwork in which T cells are closely packed.
     b. T-cell maturation occurs as lymphoblasts (thymocytes) in the outer cortex proliferate and become programmed to recognize a specific antigen as they migrate toward the inner cortex.
        - T cells that are programmed against self-antigens or are unable to recognize self-MHC molecules undergo programmed cell death, called *apoptosis* (>95% of thymocyte progeny do not survive).
        - Mature, immunocompetent T cells that remain recognize non–self-antigen in the context of MHC molecules.

2. Thymic medulla
   - The medulla is lighter staining than the cortex because the cells are relatively loosely packed.
     a. Mature T cells exit the medulla, via postcapillary venules and efferent lymphatic vessels, and circulate to secondary lymphoid organs.
     b. Hassall's corpuscles, found predominantly in the thymic medulla, are concentric arrays of squamous epithelial cells containing keratohyaline granules.
        - They are probably derived from nearby third branchial–pharyngeal cleft ectoderm during embryogenesis.

3. Blood–thymus barrier in the thymic cortex
   a. Function: prevents antigens in the bloodstream from reaching the developing T cells in the thymic cortex
      - The barrier is leaky during fetal life, allowing for the development of immunologic tolerance to self-antigen.
   b. Components: Endothelium → endothelial basal lamina (may house pericytes) → perivascular space → basal lamina of the reticular cell → reticular cell → thymic parenchymal cells

4. Thymic involution
   - The thymus reaches its maximal size during puberty and gradually atrophies by apoptosis thereafter.

5. DiGeorge syndrome
   - This disorder, marked by agenesis of the thymus and parathyroid glands, results from congenital failure of the third and fourth pharyngeal pouches to develop.

Maturing T cells are programmed to recognize specific antigens as they move from the outer thymic cortex to the deeper cortex. Cells that recognize self-antigens are destroyed, so that the individual exhibits tolerance to these antigens.

- Clinical manifestations include a severe reduction in the T-cell count, markedly depressed cell-mediated immunity, and hypocalcemia.

6. Histophysiology of the thymus gland
   - All cells of the body, including CD8 lymphocytes, have class I MHC surface molecules on them. CD4 lymphocytes bear class II MHC surface molecules, which are found on cells of the immune system, but not on general, or non–immune system, body cells.
   - As T lymphocytes differentiate in the inner cortex, they extensively rearrange the composition of their antigen receptors on the cell surface.

     The cell-to-cell variability in this receptor production process creates some sequences that "recognize" self–class I MHC molecules. Consequently, because these self–class I MHC molecules are found on all cells of the body, the newly differentiated T lymphocytes that can recognize self–class I MHC molecules would destroy those cells containing self–class I MHC molecules unless these types of T lymphocytes are somehow eliminated.

     These self-reactive T lymphocytes must be killed off or inactivated before they gain access to the circulation and lymphoid tissues body-wide, where they would attack a wide variety of self-antigens.

     In this way, a large amount of programmed cell death (apoptosis) or "negative immunologic selection" is occurring in the deeper regions of the cortex of the thymus. This process effectively removes all T lymphocytes that developed a means by which to recognize self–class I MHC molecules.
   - The "few" CD8 lymphocytes that survive the negative selection process complete their differentiation and gain access to the circulation. From there, they populate lymphoid tissues throughout the body by leaving the thymus and entering blood capillaries in the medullary region of the gland. Failure to remove all of the CD8 lymphocytes that react to self–class I MHC molecules is believed to be responsible for the lymphocytes involved in autoimmune diseases.

C. Lymph nodes (Fig. 13-7)
   - A connective tissue capsule surrounding the lymph nodes is pierced by many afferent lymphatic vessels and sends trabecular extensions inward.
   - Reticular fibers form a supporting meshwork in which lymphocytes, macrophages, and dendritic cells can be found.

   1. Outer cortex: rich in B cells that are organized into primary and secondary lymph follicles
   2. Paracortex: a high concentration of T cells, but no lymph follicles
      a. Postcapillary venules, which are lined by cuboidal to low columnar epithelium, are present in the paracortex.
      b. Circulating B and T cells in the blood can pass through these "high-endothelial" venules to enter the parenchyma of a node.
   3. Medulla: a central, lighter area containing some B and T cells and plasma cells
   4. Hilum: a region where arteries enter a node and veins and efferent lymphatic vessels exit from it

The secondary lymphoid organs are the lymph nodes and spleen. These are the sites of antigen-stimulated activation and clonal expansion of T and B cells.

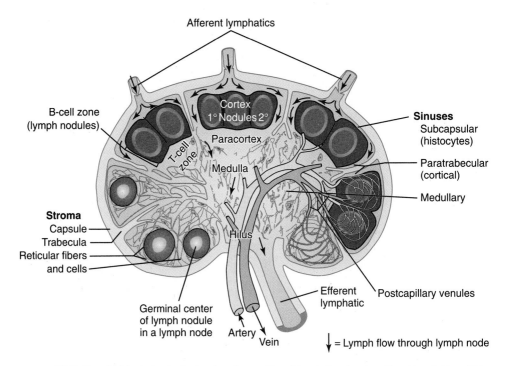

Afferent lymphatics

B-cell zone
(lymph nodules)

Cortex
1° Nodules 2°

Paracortex

Sinuses
Subcapsular
(histocytes)

T-cell zone

Medulla

Paratrabecular
(cortical)

Medullary

Stroma
Capsule
Trabecula
Reticular fibers
and cells

Hilus

Germinal center
of lymph nodule
in a lymph node

Artery
Vein

Efferent
lymphatic

Postcapillary venules

↓ = Lymph flow through lymph node

13-7: Histophysiologic sketch of a lymph node as a filter of lymph. Lymph enters afferent lymphatics, which pierce the capsule and drain into the subcapsular sinus → paratrabecular sinus → medullary sinus → efferent lymph vessels. Clonal expansion of B cells occurs in the outer cortex and of T cells in the paracortex.

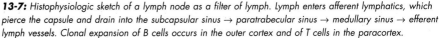

5. Sinuses: endothelium-lined spaces lying just below the capsule, along the trabeculae, and in the medulla
   • These spaces are bridged by reticular cells stretched out on reticular fibers (cobweb appearance); they also contain macrophages and lymphocytes.
6. Filtration of lymph as it passes through a node largely removes antigens and cellular debris carried in the lymph.
   • Malignant cells metastasizing to and through a node follow the same pathway as lymph (see Fig. 13-7).

D. Spleen
   • A mesothelium-lined connective tissue capsule contains some smooth muscle fibers and sends trabeculae into the splenic parenchyma.
   • During fetal life, the spleen functions as a hematopoietic organ.
1. The white pulp of the spleen is the site of clonal expansion of antigen-stimulated lymphocytes.
   a. The B-cell area contains secondary lymph follicles in which the central arteriole of the germinal centers is "off center."
   b. The T-cell area consists of numerous T lymphocytes located around the central arteries of the white pulp, forming the periarterial lymphatic sheath.

The splenic red pulp is involved in the filtration of blood. The splenic white pulp has both T-cell and B-cell areas, plus a marginal zone in which interaction between B and T cells occurs frequently.

2. The marginal zone of the spleen forms a sinusoidal interface between the red pulp and the white pulp.
   a. Antigen-presenting cells are abundant in the marginal zone.
   b. Lymphocytes first encounter antigen here, and activated T_H cells help in the activation of B cells.
3. The red pulp of the spleen, which constitutes 80% of the organ, functions to filter the blood.
   a. Cords of Billroth (Fig. 13-8)
      (1) These cords, forming the red pulp parenchyma, contain fixed and free macrophages, reticular cells and fibers, and various types of blood cells.
      (2) Terminal capillaries open into the substance of the cords, delivering blood directly to them (i.e., open circulation = not contained by endothelium).
      (3) Aged, defective RBCs are destroyed by macrophages in the cords of Billroth.

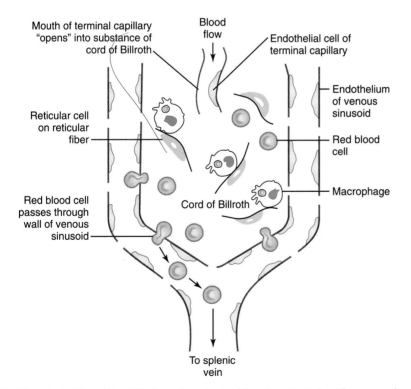

13-8: *Schematic depiction of blood filtration in the red pulp of the spleen. Terminal capillaries open directly into the red pulp parenchyma, which is divided into the cords of Billroth by venous sinusoids. As the blood and its formed elements pass through a cord, defective and aged red blood cells are phagocytosed and degraded by macrophages in the cord. Red blood cells and other elements in the "filtered" blood pass from a cord through the highly permeable endothelial wall of the venous sinusoids, thereby regaining access to the bloodstream.*

b. Venous sinusoids
   (1) Splenic sinusoids are lined by endothelial cells that are separated by paracellular gaps and have a discontinuous basement membrane (see Fig. 11-3).
   (2) Healthy RBCs pass from the cords of Billroth into the sinusoids, which serve as storage sites for RBCs.

E. Lymphomas: tumors of the lymphoid system, which all present with enlarged, painless, firm lymph nodes

1. Hodgkin's disease: a type of malignant lymphoma characterized by the presence of Reed-Sternberg cells, which are giant neoplastic cells that typically have two large, vacuolated nuclei, each with prominent nucleoli
   • Neoplastic lymph nodes develop in localized areas either above or below the diaphragm.
   • Other clinical manifestations include fever, night sweats, weight loss, leukocytosis, and pruritus.

2. Non-Hodgkin's disease: a large group of malignant lymphomas characterized by neoplastic transformation of B cells (most common), T cells, or histiocytes
   • Painless enlargement of one or more lymph nodes is the most common initial feature; generally, it is more disseminated than Hodgkin's disease.
   • The incidence increases with age.

Reed-Sternberg cells are large, generally binucleated neoplastic cells (owl's eye appearance) that are seen in Hodgkin's disease.

14

Digestive System

TARGET TOPICS

- The common histologic plan of the gastrointestinal tract and characteristic regional specializations
- Myenteric (Auerbach's) and submucosal (Meissner's) plexuses
- Gut-associated lymphoid tissue and secretory immunoglobulin A
- Secretions from the gastric and intestinal glands
- Hormones produced by the enteroendocrine cells and their

  functions in the gastrointestinal tract
- Histophysiologic organization and ultrastructure of the liver
- Pancreatic exocrine secretions
- Oral lesions, Plummer-Vinson syndrome, gastroesophageal reflux disease, peptic ulcer disease, Hirschsprung's disease, cirrhosis of the liver, gallstones, pancreatitis, gastrointestinal tract neoplasms

---

I. Introduction
- The digestive system consists of a continuous hollow tube extending from the lips to the anus, plus several extramural glands whose secretions are delivered to the lumen.
  A. Basic histologic plan of the alimentary canal (Fig. 14-1)
  - The wall of the alimentary canal (esophagus → anus) consists of four major layers throughout its length.
    1. Mucosa: three distinct sublayers
      a. The epithelium lining the lumen may have secretory, absorptive, and/or protective functions.
      b. The lamina propria of loose areolar connective tissue lies below the luminal epithelium.
        - Various glands and gut-associated lymphatic tissue are present in the lamina propria.
      c. The muscularis mucosa comprises one to three layers of smooth muscle.

General plan of the gut wall:
- Mucosa (epithelium, lamina propria, muscularis mucosa)
- Submucosa (connective tissue)
- Muscularis externa (two or three smooth muscle layers)
- Adventitia (retroperitoneal portions) or serosa (intraperitoneal portions)

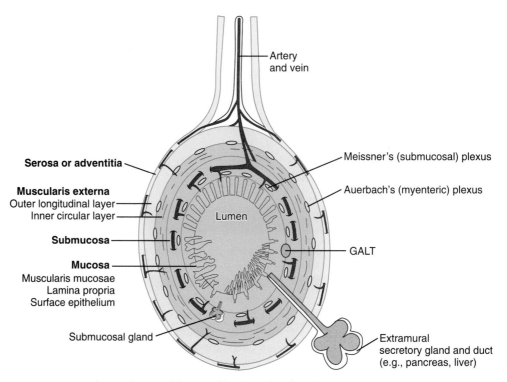

14-1: *Schematic diagram of the general histologic plan of the alimentary canal. The mucosa consists of the surface epithelium, the lamina propria, and usually a thin layer of smooth muscle (muscularis mucosa) adjacent to the submucosa, which is inside the muscularis externa. Serosa covers the intraperitoneal regions; adventitia covers the retroperitoneal regions. The extent of mucosal folding varies in different regions. It is relatively simple in the colon, as shown here, and more complex in the stomach and small intestine. GALT, gut-associated lymphatic tissue.*

Submucosal (Meissner's) autonomic plexuses control local secretion from the gut wall.

Myenteric (Auerbach's) autonomic plexuses control gut motility.

2. Submucosa: dense, irregular connective tissue
   • The submucosal autonomic plexuses or ganglia (Meissner's) are located here.
3. Muscularis externa: inner circular and outer longitudinal layer of smooth muscle
   • The myenteric autonomic plexuses or ganglia (Auerbach's) lie between the muscle layers.
4. Outermost layer: either a serosa or an adventitia (fibrosa)
   a. The serosa consists of a mesothelial lining and a layer of submesothelial connective tissue.
      • Forms the visceral peritoneum, which is a reflection of the serosal lining of the abdominal wall (parietal peritoneum)
      • Covers the intraperitoneal portions of the alimentary canal, the surface of the gallbladder exposed to the peritoneal cavity, and the surface of the colon facing the peritoneal cavity
   b. The adventitia (fibrosa) consists of dense, irregular connective tissue containing adipose tissue.
      • Blends with the connective tissue around adjacent organs

- Covers retroperitoneal portions of the alimentary canal, the surface of the gallbladder embedded in the liver, and the surface of the colon facing the posterior body wall

B. Turnover of luminal epithelium
  1. High rates of cell loss and cell birth characterize mucosa.
  2. Pap smear cytology can be performed on desquamated cells captured by swabs or lavages (e.g., gastric lavage).
  3. The gastrointestinal toxicity of radiation and chemotherapy agents results from the high rate of cell division.
     - Common clinical signs of toxicity are bloody diarrhea and ulcers in the oral cavity and esophagus. If these signs occur, therapy may be discontinued or lessened.

C. Innervation
  - Peristalsis depends on innervation to the smooth muscles of the digestive tract.
  1. Sympathetic postganglionic fibers from a sympathetic chain pass through the gut wall to the glands and smooth muscle.
  2. Parasympathetic preganglionic fibers arrive on the cell bodies of parasympathetic postganglionic neurons in ganglia in the gut wall; postganglionic fibers pass to glands and smooth muscle.
     a. Meissner's (submucosal) plexuses regulate local secretions, blood flow, and absorption.
     b. Auerbach's (myenteric) plexuses coordinate the muscular activity of the gut wall.

D. Gut-associated lymphoid tissue
  - The luminal surface of the lining epithelium is coated with secretory immunoglobulin A (IgA), forming a first line of defense against antigens in the gastrointestinal tract.
  1. Isolated lymph follicles (nodules)
     a. M cells, specialized squamous epithelial cells interspersed within the luminal epithelium, take up dietary antigens from the lumen and transport them to lymph follicles in the underlying lamina propria (Fig. 14-2).
     b. Antigen-stimulated B cells within follicles differentiate into IgA-secreting plasma cells, which move through the adjacent lamina propria.
  2. Diffuse lymphatic tissue of the lamina propria (lymphocytes, macrophages, and IgA-secreting plasma cells)
  3. Aggregated lymph follicles
     a. Waldeyer's ring of tonsils of the oropharynx
     b. Peyer's patches in the submucosa of the ileum

II. Oral Cavity
  - The histology of the oral cavity (lips → pharynx) is highly modified from the basic plan described earlier.
  A. Lips
     1. Core of skeletal muscle, the orbicularis oris

> Secretory immunoglobulin A, the intragut antibody, is produced by Peyer's patches and other gut-associated lymphoid tissue and then transported across the intestinal epithelium to protect against intraluminal antigens.

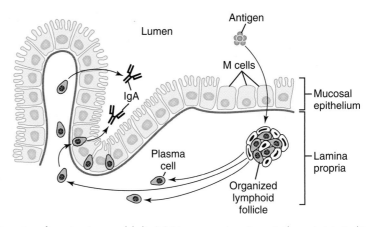

14-2: *Formation of secretory immunoglobulin (Ig) A in response to antigens in the gastrointestinal tract. M cells are specialized epithelial cells that transport antigens from the lumen to the underlying lamina propria. B lymphocytes, which are present within isolated or aggregated lymphoid follicles (e.g., Peyer's patches), interact with the antigen and differentiate into plasma cells that secrete IgA. As IgA is transported across the mucosa into the lumen, it acquires a protective secretory piece.*

  2. Anterior surface, covered by dermis and epidermis (e.g., hair follicles)

  3. Posterior surface, covered by a nonkeratinized stratified squamous epithelium, or oral epithelium, and a lamina propria (no muscularis mucosa)

 B. Teeth

  • From the inside to the outside, a tooth contains the following structural components:

  1. Pulp: connective tissue containing blood vessels and nerves located within the pulp cavity

   • Inflammation of the pulp produces the classic "toothache."

  2. Dentin: mineralized layer around the pulp cavity that forms the bulk of the tooth; harder than bone, but not as hard as enamel

  3. Enamel: relatively thin, mineralized layer that forms the external surface of the tooth crown; hardest substance in the body, containing 98% hydroxyapatite by weight

   • Acid injury from self-induced vomiting wears away the enamel layer.

  4. Cementum: mineralized layer that forms the external surface of the root of the tooth (the part within the bony socket) and is similar in composition to bone.

   • Like bone, the cementum layer extends the connective tissue fibers (Sharpey's fibers) into adjacent tissue.

 C. Tongue

  1. A skeletal muscle core, with fibers running in three different geometric planes, is characteristic of the tongue.

  2. The mucosa of the tongue lacks underlying submucosa on the dorsal surface and muscularis mucosa throughout.

   a. The ventral (inferior) surface is covered by oral epithelium (nonkeratinized stratified squamous epithelium).

    b. The dorsal (superior) surface is covered by stratified squamous epithelium that contains some keratin (parakeratinized).

   3. Lingual papillae are variously shaped structures with a connective tissue core that projects from the dorsal surface of the anterior two thirds of the tongue.

    a. Taste buds (see Chapter 19) are present in fungiform and circumvallate papillae but not in filiform papillae.

    b. The glands of von Ebner produce a serous secretion that continuously rinses out the trenches surrounding circumvallate papillae, so that any change in ingested food can be detected quickly by cleansed taste buds.

D. Hard palate

   • The mucosa of the hard palate is firmly attached to the palatine bone.

   1. The superior or nasal mucosa is lined by respiratory epithelium (pseudostratified ciliated columnar epithelium).

    • Contains considerable adipose tissue and seromucous glands

   2. The lingual mucosa is lined by parakeratinized stratified squamous epithelium.

    • Contains purely mucous glands

E. Soft palate

   1. Contraction of the skeletal muscle core raises the soft palate against the wall of the pharynx, closing the choanae (posterior nares) and thereby preventing food from entering the nasal cavity during swallowing.

   2. The mucosa is similar to that of the lingual mucosa of the hard palate.

   3. The uvula, the posterior tip of the soft palate, is covered with oral epithelium.

F. Pharynx

   • A common chamber for food and air, the pharynx is continuous with the nasal and oral cavities and with the lumen of the esophagus.

   1. Pharyngeal mucosa

    a. Respiratory epithelium where only air is present

    b. Oral epithelium where food may be present

   2. Pharyngeal constrictor muscles, which consist of skeletal muscle beneath mucosa

G. Disorders of the oral cavity

   1. Oral leukoplakia is marked by thickened, slightly raised white patches in the mucous membrane of the lips, tongue, and lining of the cheeks.

    • The use of smokeless tobacco and pipe smoking are risk factors.

    • Biopsy should be performed on patches to rule out squamous cell dysplasia or cancer.

   2. Oral cancer, most commonly squamous cell carcinoma, usually develops on the lips, tongue, and floor of the mouth and can spread to the lymph nodes.

   3. Herpetic stomatitis is characterized by fluid-filled, painful blisters (cold sores) on the lips or near the nostrils.

    • Outbreaks result from acute infection of the oral mucosa by herpes simplex virus type I (HSV1), which remains latent in the trigeminal ganglion.

Squamous cell carcinoma is the most common type of oral cancer. It is associated with smoking and excess alcohol intake.

Cold sores are fluid-filled blisters, usually on the lips or near the nostrils. They are caused by herpes simplex virus type I.

TABLE 14-1:
Selected Histologic Features of the Alimentary Canal

Region*	Surface Epithelial Cells	Glands	Regional Specialization
Esophagus	Stratified squamous nonkeratinized	Mucous glands in lamina propria and submucosa	Skeletal and smooth muscle in muscularis externa
Stomach	Mucous columnar	Gastric glands in lamina propria open into gastric pits	Rugae (mucosal folds) Three smooth muscle layers in muscularis externa
Small intestine	Enterocytes (columnar with microvilli) and goblet cells	Brunner's submucosal mucous glands (only in duodenum); crypts of Lieberkühn in mucosa; mucus-secreting goblet cells	Villi (mucosal folds) Plicae circulares (large folds of mucosa and submucosa) Peyer's patches in ileum
Large intestine Cecum Colon Rectum	From cecum to rectum, number of enterocytes decreases and number of goblet cells increases	Mucus-secreting goblet cells	*Taeniae coli* in muscularis externa of cecum and colon Crypts with few secretory Paneth cells
Anal canal	Proximal: similar to rectum; distal: stratified squamous nonkeratinized; at anus: stratified squamous keratinized (skin)	Sebaceous glands; mucus-producing circumanal glands	Anal columns of Morgagni (longitudinal mucosal folds) Anal valves (transverse mucosal folds) Anal sphincters

*All regions possess four basic tunics: mucosa, submucosa, muscularis externa, and serosa or adventitia.

Canker sores are whitish ulcers with a red border found in the mucosa of the lips, cheeks, and gums. They have a noninfectious etiology.

4. Aphthous stomatitis is characterized by small, whitish ulcers with a red border (canker sores) in the mucosa of the lips, cheeks, and gums.

III. Alimentary Canal

- The major regional specializations to the basic histologic plan of the alimentary canal are summarized in Table 14-1.

A. Esophagus

1. Mucosa
   - The surface is covered by oral epithelium (nonkeratinized stratified squamous epithelium), and it has a highly developed muscularis mucosa.
   - It exhibits mucosal folds when no food is passing through.

2. Muscularis externa
   a. Upper third of the esophagus: skeletal muscle only
   b. Middle third of the esophagus: a mixture of skeletal and smooth muscle
   c. Lower third of the esophagus: smooth muscle only

3. Mucous glands
   a. Esophageal glands in the submucosa
   b. Esophageal cardiac glands in the lamina propria
4. Esophageal disorders
   a. Plummer-Vinson syndrome is marked by a triad of cervical esophageal webs, iron deficiency anemia, and glossitis.
      (1) The growth of webs, which make swallowing solid foods difficult, is linked to a lack of iron. The webs disappear when iron deficiency is corrected.
      (2) Carcinoma of the oropharynx and upper esophagus are possible complications.
   b. Esophageal varices occur in patients with alcoholic cirrhosis, which compromises venous return from the liver to the hepatic vein.
      (1) Blood uses an alternate route, leading to distention of veins (varices) in the submucosa of the lower esophagus.
      (2) Vomiting may cause esophageal varices to rupture.
   c. Gastroesophageal reflux disease (GERD) results from an incompetent lower esophageal sphincter.
      (1) Heartburn is a common early symptom; difficulty swallowing and bleeding occur in more advanced cases.
      (2) In chronic cases, backflow of acidic stomach contents may lead to metaplasia of normal esophageal squamous epithelium to the gastric or intestinal type, producing Barrett's esophagus.
   d. Achalasia is the combined lack of peristalsis in the body of the esophagus and failure of the lower esophageal sphincter to relax.
      • This condition results from degeneration of the myenteric ganglion cells in the esophageal wall.
   e. Esophageal adenocarcinoma is the most common cancer of the esophagus. Barrett's esophagus is an important risk factor.
   f. Squamous cell carcinoma arises primarily in the lower two thirds of the organ and metastasizes to the regional lymph nodes.
      • Risk factors include cigarette smoking, heavy alcohol use, achalasia, and esophageal webs.

B. Stomach
   • A bolus of food from the esophagus is acidified and broken down in the stomach, forming chyme, a low pH viscous fluid that exits the pylorus into the duodenum.
1. The gastric mucosa is covered by simple epithelium composed of mucous columnar cells.
   a. Insoluble mucus secreted from the surface cells prevents damage to the lining from acidic luminal contents.
   b. The longitudinal mucosal folds (rugae) are most prominent in the empty stomach.
   c. Gastric pits are epithelial recesses into which gastric glands open.
2. The muscularis externa deviates from the basic histologic plan by the presence of three (not two) layers, with the addition of an inner oblique smooth muscle layer.

> Chronic gastroesophageal reflux disease may cause Barrett's esophagus, which predisposes to esophageal adenocarcinoma of the distal esophagus.

3. Gastric glands are simple branched tubular glands.
   - These glands consist of an isthmus, which opens into the bottom of a gastric pit; a neck; and a base (fundus), which traverses the lamina propria (Fig. 14-3).
   a. Mucous neck cells secrete soluble mucus.
   b. Stem cells (in the neck) proliferate and differentiate to replace all other cells of the gland, pit, and surface epithelium.
   c. Chief (zymogenic) cells (in the base) are typical protein-secreting cells with basal rough endoplasmic reticulum (RER) and apical secretory granules.
      - They secrete pepsinogen, which is converted into the proteolytic enzyme pepsin on exposure to the low pH of the stomach lumen.

Parietal cells produce intrinsic factor and HCl; chief cells produce pepsinogen.

   d. Parietal (oxyntic) cells (in the base) are large, triangular cells with eosinophilic cytoplasm, an extensive intracellular canalicular system, many microvilli at the apical surface, and many mitochondria.
      (1) They secrete intrinsic factor, which is necessary for absorption of vitamin B_{12} by the terminal ileum.
      (2) They manufacture HCl by transporting hydrogen and chloride ions across the canalicular membranes.

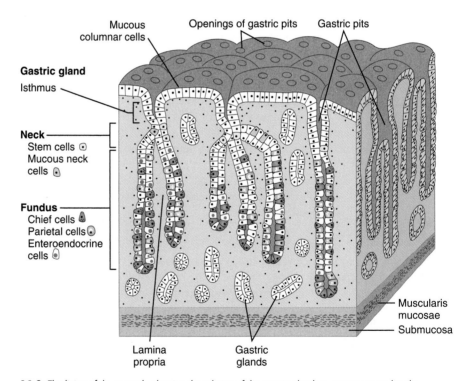

14-3: *The lining of the stomach, showing the relation of the gastric glands to gastric pits and to the underlying muscularis mucosae. The glands are most developed in the fundic region, where gastric pits form approximately one fifth of the mucosa and the glands themselves form approximately four fifths. Fundic glands, shown here, possess all of the different cell types found in the gastric glands, whereas cardiac and pyloric glands contain only mucus-producing cells and stem cells.*

(3) They are located primarily in the body and fundus of the stomach.
e. Enteroendocrine cells (in the base) belong to the population of diffuse neuroendocrine cells found throughout the body.
(1) They are also known as APUD (amine precursor uptake and decarboxylation) cells.
(2) They are oriented with the apex of the cell directed toward the basal lamina and the nucleus close to the free (luminal) surface.
(3) They secrete hormones toward capillaries in the lamina propria (Table 14-2)
C. Small intestine (Fig. 14-4)
1. Intestinal specializations that increase the surface area for absorption
a. Microvilli: projections from the apical surface of the columnar absorptive cells (enterocytes)
b. Villi: folds of the inner two mucosal layers (epithelium and lamina propria)
(1) Diffuse lymphatic tissue and lacteals (blind-ending lymphatic capillaries) are located within the lamina propria.
(2) Absence of villi, which greatly increase the absorption area of the small bowel, leads to malabsorption of nutrients.
c. Plicae circulares (Kerckring's valves): large permanent folds of mucosa and submucosa
• They begin in the lower duodenum, with most found in the jejunum; they decrease in size and amount in the ileum.
2. Glands whose secretions enter the intestinal lumen
a. Brunner's glands: submucosal glands that secrete alkaline mucus; present only in the duodenum
b. Unicellular mucous glands (goblet cells) within the luminal epithelium
c. Crypts of Lieberkühn: simple tubular glands within the intestinal mucosa that open between adjacent villi and extend to the muscularis mucosa (see Fig. 14-4)

TABLE 14-2: Some Hormones Secreted by Enteroendocrine Cells of the Gastrointestinal Tract

Hormone	Site of Secretion	Function*
Cholecystokinin	Small intestine	Stimulates secretion of pancreatic enzymes and gallbladder contraction; Inhibits gastric emptying
Gastrin	Stomach and duodenum	Stimulates secretion of hydrochloric acid and pepsinogen
Motilin	Small intestine	Increases gut motility
Secretin	Small intestine	Stimulates bicarbonate secretion by pancreas
Serotonin	Stomach through colon	Stimulates smooth muscle; Inhibits gastric secretion
Somatostatin	Stomach through colon	Inhibits nearby neuroendocrine cells
Vasoactive intestinal peptide	Stomach through colon	Increases gut motility and intestinal ion/water secretion

*Some of these substances have additional physiologic effects in other parts of the body.

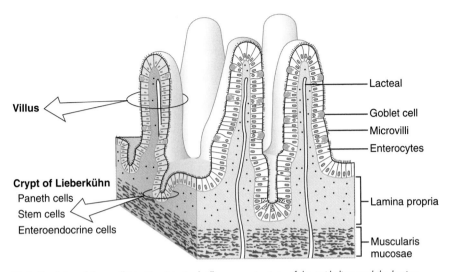

14-4: *The lining of the small intestine. Intestinal villi are evaginations of the epithelium and the lamina propria; each villus contains a single lacteal. The crypts of Lieberkühn are invaginations of the epithelium into the lamina propria.*

d. Extramural glands: pancreas, gallbladder, and liver
  • They empty their exocrine secretions into the duodenum.
3. Cells of the intestinal lining
  a. Enterocytes are tall, columnar, highly absorptive cells that constitute the primary cell type of the surface epithelium.
    (1) They are covered with closely packed microvilli on the apical surface facing the intestinal lumen, forming the brush border, which contains disaccharidases (see Fig. 4-4).
    (2) They possess junctional complexes that prevent paracellular movement of material across the intestinal epithelium.
  b. Goblet cells, which are interspersed among the enterocytes, increase in number from the duodenum to the rectum.
    • They are filled with mucigen granules in the apical portion of the cell.
  c. Enteroendocrine (APUD) cells are hormone-producing cells similar to those in the gastric lining (see Table 14-2).
  d. Paneth cells, at the base of the crypts of Lieberkühn, contain prominent eosinophilic granules.
    (1) They secrete digestive enzymes and lysozyme, an antibacterial enzyme.
    (2) They phagocytose some microorganisms and help regulate intestinal flora.
  e. Stem cells near the base of the crypts of Lieberkühn can replace all the other cells of the intestinal lining.
    • Daughter cells migrate upward to the tip of the villus and then desquamate by the trillions.

Enteroendocrine (APUD) cells located in the gastrointestinal tract produce serotonin, gastrin, motilin, cholecystokinin, secretin, and vasoactive intestinal peptide.

4. Absorption of monosaccharides and amino acids
    a. Transport proteins in the apical surface of the enterocytes mediate the uptake of monosaccharides and amino acids from the intestinal lumen.
    b. Absorbed materials are actively transported across the basal surface into the lamina propria, where they enter the circulation.
5. Absorption of lipids
    a. Bile salts help organize lipid digestion products into micelles, which are endocytosed at the apical surfaces of enterocytes.
    b. Within the smooth endoplasmic reticulum of the enterocytes, fatty acids and glycerol are resynthesized into triglycerides.
    c. Chylomicrons are formed in the Golgi and then released by exocytosis at the lateral cell membrane below the junctional complex (zonula occuldens, zonula adherens, and macula adherens).
        • They contain diet-derived triglycerides, cholesterol, protein, and fat-soluble vitamins.
        (1) Released chylomicrons pass between cells, cross the basal lamina, and enter the lacteals in the lamina propria (see Fig. 14-4).
        (2) The contents of the lymphatic vessels eventually reach the thoracic duct, which joins the blood circulation.
6. Peptic ulcers: inflammatory lesions in the mucosal lining of the stomach or duodenum that penetrate the muscularis mucosa
    a. *Helicobacter pylori,* the most common cause of peptic ulcers, produces urease.
    b. Ammonia, resulting from the action of urease on urea, damages the mucous barrier, leading to acid injury of the mucosa, submucosa, and underlying muscle layer.

> Gastric and duodenal ulcers are most commonly caused by *Helicobacter pylori.*

D. Large intestine
    • The primary functions are to absorb water and electrolytes and to lubricate feces with mucus.
    1. Surface features
        a. From the cecum to the anal canal, enterocytes decrease and goblet cells increase in number.
        b. Crypts are present (with few, if any, Paneth cells), but villi and plicae circulares are absent.
    2. Muscularis externa in the cecum and colon
        a. The outer longitudinal layer forms three strong, flat strips, the taeniae coli.
        b. Myenteric (Auerbach's) ganglia are located between the taeniae coli and the subjacent circular layer of smooth muscle.
    3. Hirschsprung's disease (congenital megacolon) is caused by congenital absence of autonomic ganglia (aganglionosis).
        • Paralysis in the aganglionic segment largely prevents passage of material through it, leading to distention of the bowel (megacolon) and possibly perforation if untreated.

> Congenital megacolon (Hirschsprung's disease) is due to the absence of autonomic ganglia; a proximal, distended section is innervated.

E. Anal canal
    1. The upper portion is continuous histologically and grossly with the rectum.
        a. Anal columns (of Morgagni): longitudinal folds of the anal mucosa

      b. Anal valves: small, transverse folds connecting the distal ends of the anal columns; the pectinate line of gross anatomy

      c. Anal sinuses: troughs between adjacent folds

  2. The lower portion (distal to the anal valves) is covered by nonkeratinized stratified squamous epithelium that is continuous with the skin of the anus.

  3. Anal sphincters

      a. Internal sphincter = circular smooth muscle of the muscularis externa

        • Is under involuntary feedback control

      b. External sphincter = skeletal muscle

        • Maintains continuous tonus, thus keeping the orifice closed, but the degree of tonus is under voluntary control

  4. Hemorrhoids: varicose veins either above or below the anorectal line

    • External hemorrhoids thrombose; internal hemorrhoids bleed.

F. Ulcerative colitis and Crohn's disease are chronic inflammatory diseases that exhibit a familial tendency and affect various portions of the gastrointestinal tract.

  • They are of unknown etiology, but may result from cytokines and inflammatory mediators released subsequent to inappropriate activation of the immune system.

IV. Extramural Glands of the Digestive System

  • Exocrine secretions critical to the digestive process enter the oral cavity from the salivary glands and enter the small intestine from the liver, gallbladder, and pancreas.

A. Major salivary glands

  1. Components of saliva

      a. Water and glycoproteins clean and lubricate the oral cavity.

      b. IgA, lysozyme, and lactoferrin provide defense against pathogens.

      c. Salivary amylase begins the digestion of carbohydrates.

  2. Neoplasms of the salivary glands

      a. Pleomorphic (mixed) adenoma (benign): the most common salivary gland tumor, occurring much more frequently in women than in men

        • Presents as a smooth, painless, hard, slow-growing mass, most often in the parotid gland

      b. Mucoepidermoid carcinoma: the most common malignant tumor of the salivary glands; may be indolent or aggressive

B. Liver

  1. Hepatic functions

      a. Synthesis and release of bile into the canaliculi between the individual hepatocytes (exocrine function)

      b. Synthesis and release directly into the blood of several plasma proteins (e.g., albumin, prothrombin, fibrinogen, lipoproteins) and glucose (gluconeogenesis)

      c. Storage of metabolites, particularly glycogen (stored carbohydrate) and triglycerides (stored lipid)

Salivary gland acini:
- Parotid glands: mostly serous
- Sublingual glands: mostly mucous
- Submandibular glands: both (mixed)

d. Biochemical degradation of toxic substances (e.g., alcohol) and certain endogenous metabolites (e.g., estrogen)

e. Metabolic activation of certain substances that are inactive in the body until chemically transformed by liver enzymes

- Examples include cyclophosphamide, a chemotherapeutic drug, and indirect-acting carcinogens (e.g., vinyl chloride, aflatoxin B_1, and benzpyrene).

2. Histophysiologic organization of the liver (Fig. 14-5)

- The basic structural-functional unit of the liver parenchyma has been described in three ways.

a. The classic hepatic lobule emphasizes the release of plasma proteins and glucose into the blood.

(1) Shape: hexagon

(2) At the center: a single central vein

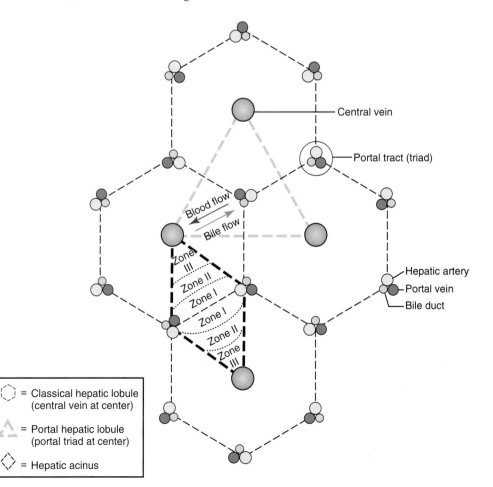

14-5: *Schematic representation of the classic lobule, portal lobule, and acinus of the liver. Each portal tract, or triad, contains branches of the hepatic artery, portal vein, and bile duct. Note that blood flows from the triads toward the central veins, whereas bile drains in the opposite direction toward the triads.*

(3) At the periphery: six portal tracts (triads or canals), each containing branches of the hepatic artery, portal vein, and bile duct

b. The portal lobule emphasizes the release of bile.
   (1) Shape: triangle
   (2) At the center: a portal tract
   (3) At the periphery: three "surrounding" central veins at points of the triangle

c. The acinus emphasizes the gradient of metabolic activity within the liver.
   (1) Shape: diamond
   (2) At the center: a vascular backbone with contributions from vessels in each of the two portal tracts
   (3) At the periphery: two central veins at the ends of a long axis and two portal tracts at the ends of a short axis

3. Blood flow to and from the liver
   a. The portal vein from the small intestine, spleen, and pancreas brings nutrient-rich blood to the liver.
   b. The common hepatic artery brings oxygen-rich blood to the liver.
   c. Arterial and venous blood mix in the hepatic sinusoids.
   d. The hepatic vein, formed by coalescence of the central veins, carries blood from the liver to the inferior vena cava to the right side of the heart.

4. Bile flow
   a. The direction of bile flow is toward the periphery of the classic hepatic lobule, opposite the direction of blood flow (see Fig. 14-5).
   b. Bile flows through the canaliculi between the adjacent hepatocytes → ductules (canals of Hering) in portal canals → larger bile ducts

5. Metabolic zones of the hepatic acini
   • Oxygen is lost from blood as it flows from branches of the hepatic artery through the acinar sinusoids toward the two central veins associated with an acinus.
   • The resulting oxygen gradient divides each half of an acinus into three functional zones (see Fig. 14-5).
   a. Zone 1 (closest to the arterial center): highest oxygen saturation, nutrient levels, and metabolic activity
      • This zone is most resistant to injury, and hepatocytes here are the first to begin the regenerative process after a partial hepatectomy.
   b. Zone 2: anatomically and physiologically intermediate between zones 1 and 3
   c. Zone 3 (closest to the central vein): lowest oxygen saturation, nutrient levels, and metabolic activity

6. Hepatic ultrastructure (Fig. 14-6)
   a. Hepatic sinusoids arise near the periphery of the classic lobule and course between the cords of hepatocytes, draining toward the central vein.
      • Lined by sinusoidal endothelial cells and phagocytic Kupffer cells

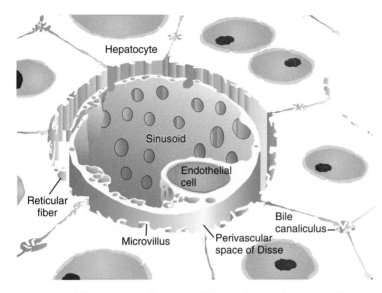

14-6: *Three-dimensional depiction of the ultrastructure of the liver showing the relation of hepatocytes to a blood sinusoid. Materials readily move from the sinusoidal lumen into the space of Disse because the endothelium contains paracellular gaps and is underlain by a discontinuous basement membrane (see Fig. 11-3). Hepatocytes secrete bile into the canaliculi, which drain toward triads at the periphery of a classic lobule.*

    b. The space of Disse is a perivascular space between the sinusoid endothelium and the adjacent hepatocytes.
- Contains the reticular fibers, lipocytes (Ito cells) that store vitamin A, and blood plasma minus formed elements

    c. Hepatocytes, the liver's parenchymal cells, freely exchange material with the contents of the space of Disse.
       (1) Microvilli are present on those surfaces facing the space of Disse.
       (2) Bile canaliculi are delineated as tiny grooves between the abutting surfaces of adjacent hepatocytes and are sealed laterally by zonulae occludens.
       (3) Basophilic cytoplasmic regions contain RER and free polysomes.
       (4) Acidophilic cytoplasmic regions contain mitochondria and peroxisomes, which break down hydrogen peroxide produced by normal metabolic activity.
       (5) Unstained cytoplasmic regions contain multiple Golgi bodies, glycogen inclusions (periodic acid-Schiff–positive), and lipid droplets.

  7. Cirrhosis of the liver: chronic disease marked by death of hepatocytes and their replacement by fibroblasts and collagen fibers, producing cirrhotic scarring and regenerative nodules, consisting of hepatocytes entrapped by the fibrous tissues
    a. Cardiac cirrhosis: cirrhotic changes initially confined to zone 3 of the acini (i.e., around the central veins)

- Caused by sluggish blood flow in the hepatic vein, central veins, and sinusoids resulting from right-sided heart failure
    b. Biliary cirrhosis: cirrhotic changes initially confined to zone 1 of the acini (i.e., in the portal tract regions).
    - Caused by autoimmune destruction of the bile ducts in the triads
8. Viral hepatitis: inflammation of the liver caused by several different viruses that are distinguished by immunologic tests
9. Liver cancers
    a. Metastatic cancer: the most common type of cancer to involve the liver
    b. Hepatocellular carcinoma: malignancy of the hepatocyte; the most common primary liver cancer
        (1) Clinical features include jaundice, abdominal distention, ascites, and increased α-fetoprotein level.
        (2) Predisposing factors are cirrhosis associated with chronic hepatitis B and C infection, hemochromatosis, and cirrhosis associated with alcoholism.
C. Gallbladder
    1. Functions of the gallbladder
        a. Storage and concentration of bile
        b. Release of bile in response to the presence of fat in the duodenum
            - Cholecystokinin secreted by enteroendocrine cells in the duodenum stimulates contraction of the gallbladder and release of its contents.
    2. Tunics of the gallbladder
        - The muscularis mucosa and submucosa are absent.
        a. Mucosa
            (1) Simple columnar epithelium with microvilli and junctional complexes
            (2) Richly vascularized lamina propria
        b. Muscularis externa: thin, with three indistinct layers
        c. Serosa on the external surface facing the peritoneal cavity; fibrosa or adventitia on the external surface facing the liver
    3. Gallstones (cholelithiasis): concretions, usually of cholesterol, that form in the gallbladder or bile duct
        a. Primary causes are too much cholesterol in the bile and too little bile salt.
        b. A common disorder, seen especially in women over age 40 years, gallstones generally are asymptomatic.
D. Exocrine pancreas
    - The endocrine secretions of the pancreas, which have no role in digestion, are discussed in Chapter 18.
    1. Pancreatic acinar cells
        - These pyramidal serous cells contain basally located nuclei and RER, a prominent Golgi complex, and apical secretory granules.
    2. Duct system of the pancreas
        a. Centroacinar cells located within the acini form the beginning of the duct system.

b. The main pancreatic duct converges with the common bile duct just before emptying into the duodenum.

3. Pancreatic secretions
   a. Digestive enzymes are synthesized and stored in the acinar cells. Their release is stimulated by cholecystokinin.
   b. Bicarbonate-rich alkaline fluid is released by the ductal epithelial cells in response to secretin.
      • This fluid raises the pH of chyme to an optimal level for pancreatic enzyme function.

4. Acute pancreatitis: inflammation of the pancreas, most often occurring in middle-aged or older patients who abuse alcohol and have biliary tract obstruction (e.g., gallstones)
   a. Clinical features include midepigastric pain radiating to the back and elevated serum lipase and amylase levels.
   b. Histologic features include pancreatic edema and white areas containing saponified fatty acids released by the action of excess lipase on adjacent adipose tissue (enzymatic fat necrosis).

Secretin stimulates the release of sodium bicarbonate from the pancreatic ductal epithelium, whereas cholecystokinin causes the release of enzymes from the serous acini.

Pancreatic enzymes delivered to the duodenum include lipase, amylase, trypsinogen, pepsinogen, DNAase, and RNAase.

Urinary System

I. Introduction
- The urinary system comprises the paired kidneys and ureters and the unpaired bladder and urethra.
  - A. Functions of the kidneys
    1. Production of urine
    2. Synthesis of endocrine hormones
       - a. Renin, which participates in the regulation of blood pressure
       - b. Erythropoietin, which promotes erythrocyte production
       - c. Vitamin D, which is involved in the mineralization of bone
         - Conversion of inactive 25-(OH) provitamin D to active 1,25-(OH)$_2$ vitamin D (calcitriol) in the kidneys is stimulated by parathyroid hormone, which promotes the synthesis of 1α-hydroxylase in the proximal tubules.
    3. Removal of metabolic waste products (e.g., urea, NH$_3$, and creatinine)
    4. Maintenance of the volume and composition (e.g., pH, electrolytes) of blood and tissue fluid
  - B. Uriniferous tubule: a continuous tubular structure that has regional specializations and constitutes the functional unit of the kidney
    - Each uriniferous tubule consists of a nephron and the collecting tubules into which it drains.

Uriniferous tubule (functional unit of the kidney) = nephron + collecting tubules.

Nephron components: renal (malpighian) corpuscle → proximal convoluted tubule → loop of Henle → distal convoluted tubule

1. The nephron includes the renal corpuscle, proximal convoluted tubule (PCT), loop of Henle, and distal convoluted tubule (DCT).
2. The collecting tubules extend from the arched collecting tubules to the papillary duct.

II. Gross Anatomy of the Kidney (Fig. 15-1)
   - The kidney is a bean-shaped organ that contains mostly parenchyma (little stroma) and is covered by a fibrous capsule.
   A. Renal hilum: an indentation on the medial border of the kidney where the capsule is discontinuous
      - The site where blood vessels, nerves, and the ureter enter and leave
      - Expands interiorly to form the renal sinus
   B. Renal pelvis: the expanded upper end of the ureter located within the renal sinus
      1. Major calyces: intercommunicating branches of the renal pelvis
      2. Minor calyces: subdivisions of the major calyces
   C. Renal cortex: the dark, highly vascular surface layer that contains the renal corpuscles and has a granular appearance
   D. Renal medulla: the lighter interior layer that contains mostly tubules, giving it a striate appearance
      1. Renal (medullary) pyramid: a pyramidal-shaped division of the medulla bordered by the renal columns of Bertin, which are extensions of cortical tissue into the medulla

Renal corpuscles are located in the cortex. The tubules are located primarily in the medulla, which receives only 10% of the blood delivered to the kidneys.

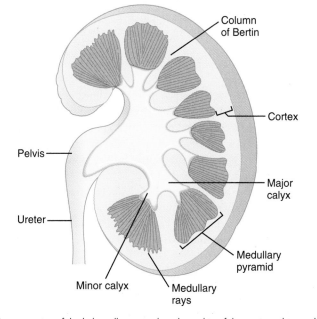

15-1: *General organization of the kidney illustrating the relationship of the ureter, pelvis, and calyces. Renal corpuscles, where filtrate is produced, are located in the outer cortical layer. Tubules in the medullary rays carry the filtrate from the cortex into the medullary pyramids, which exit into the minor calyces.*

- Each kidney has 10 to 18 renal pyramids.
- The tips of two or three pyramids extend into a minor calyx as a renal papilla.

2. Medullary rays: radial extensions of medullary tissue into the cortex

E. Renal lobe: a renal pyramid and its overlying cortex

F. Renal lobule: a central medullary ray and the surrounding nephrons that drain into it
- The boundaries of the lobules are imaginary lines located midway between adjacent medullary rays. Interlobular arteries and veins aid in defining the boundaries of the renal lobules.

III. Uriniferous Tubules and Urine Production
- The general structure of the uriniferous tubule and the characteristics of the simple epithelium lining the wall are illustrated in Figure 15-2.

A. Renal (malpighian) corpuscle
- Filtration of blood occurs in the renal corpuscle, which consists of a tuft of capillaries, the glomerulus, surrounded by Bowman's capsule (Fig. 15-3A).
- Nephrons are classified into two types, depending on the location of the renal corpuscle: cortical nephrons (≈85% of the total) and juxtamedullary nephrons (≈15% of the total).

> Juxtamedullary nephrons have a long loop of Henle. Their corpuscles are located near the medulla–cortex boundary. They play a major role in establishing the interstitial osmotic gradient.

1. Glomerulus
   a. The endothelial cells of the glomerular capillaries have large fenestrae but lack the thin diaphragms that typically span the openings in fenestrated capillaries.
   b. Blood flows from the afferent arteriole through the glomerular capillary network to the efferent arteriole.
   c. Mesangial cells, similar to pericytes, are located around the glomerular capillaries.
      - These cells are phagocytic and help support capillary loops.

2. Bowman's capsule
   a. A visceral layer is formed of highly modified epithelial cells, called podocytes, which are primarily responsible for synthesis of the glomerular basement membrane (Fig. 15-3B).
      (1) Pedicels: secondary (foot) processes extending from the podocyte primary processes; they surround the glomerular capillaries and interdigitate with each other
      (2) Filtration slits: elongated spaces between adjacent pedicels; covered by a diaphragm (slit membrane)
      (3) Fused basal lamina of the glomerular endothelium and podocytes: the only continuous structure separating the podocytes and endothelial cells
   b. Bowman's (urinary) space is the narrow cavity between the visceral and parietal layers into which the glomerular filtrate drains.
      - This space is continuous with the proximal convoluted tubule at the urinary pole.
   c. A parietal layer composed of simple squamous epithelium forms the outer wall of Bowman's capsule.

> Cortical nephrons have relatively short loops of Henle. Their renal corpuscles are located in the outer cortex. These account for 85% of the total nephrons.

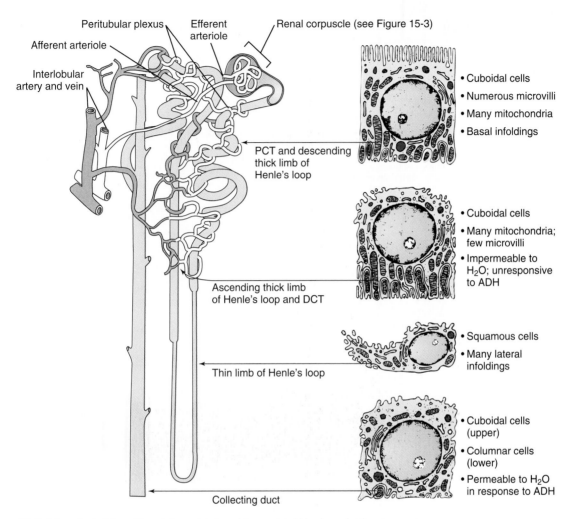

15-2: *Schematic depiction of the uriniferous tubule and its associated blood vessels. The microscopic appearance of the epithelial cells at various points shows their characteristic ultrastructure. The long, thin limb of Henle's loop in the juxtamedullary nephrons is surrounded by small vessels (vasa recta), which are not shown. ADH, antidiuretic hormone; DCT, distal convoluted tubule; PCT, proximal convoluted tubule.*

The labels in the figure are:

Peritubular plexus

Efferent arteriole

Renal corpuscle (see Figure 15-3)

Afferent arteriole

Interlobular artery and vein

PCT and descending thick limb of Henle's loop
- Cuboidal cells
- Numerous microvilli
- Many mitochondria
- Basal infoldings

Ascending thick limb of Henle's loop and DCT
- Cuboidal cells
- Many mitochondria; few microvilli
- Impermeable to H_2O; unresponsive to ADH

Thin limb of Henle's loop
- Squamous cells
- Many lateral infoldings

Collecting duct
- Cuboidal cells (upper)
- Columnar cells (lower)
- Permeable to H_2O in response to ADH

3. Formation of the glomerular filtrate
   - Selective movement of substances from the glomerular capillaries into Bowman's space forms the glomerular filtrate.
   a. Components of the renal filtration barrier (urinary membrane)
      (1) Fenestrated endothelium
      (2) Fused basal laminae of the endothelial cells and podocytes
      (3) Slit membrane
   b. Selectivity of the renal filtration barrier
      (1) Water, ions, and most molecules with a molecular weight <60 to 70 kDa pass into Bowman's space.

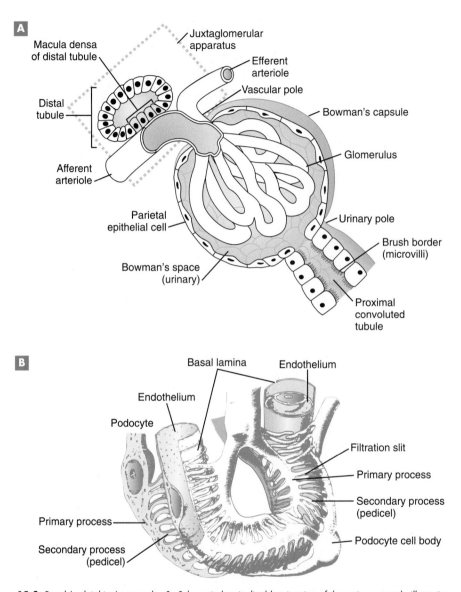

15-3: *Renal (malpighian) corpuscle.* **A,** *Schematic longitudinal hemisection of the entire corpuscle illustrating its main structural features. Near the vascular pole, the distal convoluted tubule abuts the afferent arteriole in the juxtaglomerular apparatus.* **B,** *Three-dimensional reconstruction of the interface between the glomerular endothelium and the podocytes in the visceral layer of Bowman's capsule. This interface constitutes the urinary membrane (renal filtration barrier).*

(2) Molecules with a molecular weight >60 to 70 kDa (e.g., albumin) are excluded and remain in the capillaries.

(3) Molecules carrying a large negative charge (e.g., albumin) also are excluded by negatively charged heparan sulfate in the fused basal lamina.

    c. Factors promoting the movement of fluid from the glomerular capillaries into Bowman's space
       (1) The total cross-sectional area of the efferent arteriole is less than that of the afferent arteriole, leading to increased hydrostatic pressure in the glomerulus.
       (2) The total hydrostatic pressure in the capillary network is higher than that in Bowman's space.
  4. Rate of filtrate and urine production per day
    a. Approximately 1700 liters of whole blood pass through the kidneys per day.
    b. Approximately 170 liters of glomerular filtrate are formed daily.
    c. Approximately 1.5 liters of urine are produced daily from the filtrate as it moves from Bowman's space through the remainder of the uriniferous tubules.
      • During the production of urine, water and solutes move in and out of the tubules by diffusion or active transport.
      (1) Reabsorption: material in the tubules (tubular fluid) → tissue fluid (interstitium) → blood in the surrounding capillaries
      (2) Secretion: material in the blood in the capillaries → tissue fluid → lumen of the tubules

B. Proximal convoluted tubule (PCT): ≈14 mm long
  • The distal portion, which is straight, also is called the thick descending limb of Henle's loop.
  1. The wall is composed of large, cuboidal epithelial cells marked by the following structures (see Fig. 15-2):
    a. Abundant microvilli (brush border), which contain carbonic anhydrase, on the apical surface facing the lumen
    b. Apical tubular invaginations (canaculi), vesicles, and granules, which function in transport of macromolecules into the cytoplasm
    c. Extensive infoldings of the basal plasmalemma, which increase its surface area
    d. Numerous mitochondria, which are compartmentalized in the basal portion of cells by basal infoldings and provide energy for the active transport of Na^+ ions and other solutes
  2. The filtrate remains isotonic as it passes through the PCT and the thick descending limb of Henle's loop, but it is reduced to approximately one fourth of its initial volume.
    a. Approximately two thirds of the water, Na^+, and Cl^- in the glomerular filtrate is reabsorbed in the PCT (Fig. 15-4).
    b. All of the glucose and amino acids in the filtrate normally are reabsorbed with the aid of carrier proteins in the plasma membrane of the tubular cells.
    c. Larger metabolites (e.g., proteins, polysaccharides) in the filtrate are endocytosed at the apical surface of the tubular cells and released into the interstitium by exocytosis at the basal surface.

> Filtrate remains isotonic in the proximal convoluted tubule, where much of the H_2O, Na^+, K^+, and Cl^-, and all of the glucose and amino acids are reabsorbed.

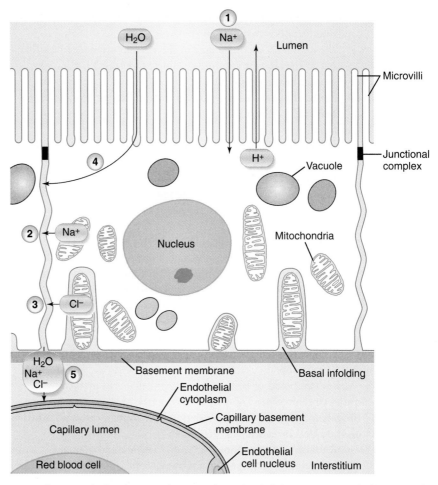

15-4: *Reabsorption of salt and water in the proximal convoluted tubule. 1, Na⁺ ions in the filtrate cross the apical surface of the tubular cells in exchange for H⁺ ions. 2, Na⁺/K⁺ pumps in the lateral membrane actively transport intracellular Na⁺ ions into the spaces between adjacent tubule cells basal to junctional complexes; Cl⁻ ions passively follow (3). Water reabsorption (4) is a consequence of the osmotic draw caused by the active transport of Na⁺ into the pericellular spaces. 5, Water, salt, and other solutes that pass into the interstitium readily enter the capillaries of the peritubular plexus, thus returning reabsorbed materials to the blood.*

    C. Thin segment of Henle's loop: ≈2 to 10 mm in length
- Long, thin segments in the juxtamedullary nephrons descend deeply into the medulla and are critical in establishing a gradient of increasing tonicity from the outer to the inner medulla.
    1. The wall is composed of squamous epithelial cells (see Fig. 15-2).
      a. Many lateral interdigitations between adjacent cells provide slits for the passage of small molecules (especially H₂O) by diffusion.
      b. The apical surface possesses sparse microvilli.

2. The filtrate becomes hypertonic as it passes through the thin descending limb of Henle's loop due to passive movement of H_2O into the interstitium.

D. Thick ascending segment of Henle's loop: ≈ 9 mm in length

    1. The wall is composed of cuboidal epithelial cells similar to those of the proximal convoluted tubule but with few microvilli (see Fig. 15-2).

    2. The filtrate becomes hypotonic as it passes through the thick segment of Henle's loop.

        a. Cl- is actively transported from the lumen to the interstitium, and Na^+ and K^+ follow passively.

        b. Because the thick segment is impermeable to H_2O, reabsorption of Na^+, K^+, and Cl- decreases the tonicity of the filtrate and increases the tonicity of the interstitium.

        c. Increased interstitial tonicity drives the diffusion of H_2O out of the thin segment of Henle's loop.

E. Distal convoluted tubule (DCT): ≈ 5 mm in length

    1. The wall (simple cuboidal epithelium) is histologically similar to that of the thick ascending segment of Henle's loop and also is impermeable to H_2O.

    2. The filtrate becomes increasingly hypotonic as it passes through the DCT.

        a. Na^+, Cl^-, Ca^{2+}, and PO_4^{3-} are reabsorbed from the DCT lumen.

        b. K^+, H^+, and NH_3 are secreted into the DCT lumen.

F. Collecting tubules and ducts

    1. Arched collecting tubule: a short segment, lined by simple cuboidal epithelium, connecting the distal convoluted tubule of a nephron and the collecting tubule into which it drains

    2. Collecting duct: a straight tubule formed by the convergence of the arched tubules from multiple nephrons

        a. The upper (cortical) portion has cuboidal epithelium and lies within a medullary ray.

        b. The lower (medullary) portion has columnar epithelium and lies within a medullary pyramid.

    3. Papillary ducts of Bellini: large collecting tubules, with simple columnar epithelium, formed by the convergence of smaller tubules within a pyramid.

      • They perforate the surface of the renal papilla at the area cribrosa, emptying urine into a minor calyx.

G. Regulation of urine concentration in response to blood osmolarity (Fig. 15-5)

    • Antidiuretic hormone (ADH), released from the posterior pituitary gland, increases the H_2O permeability of the collecting tubules.

    • Because capillary networks surrounding the tubules are freely permeable to H_2O and ions, changes in the tonicity of tubular fluid leads to corresponding changes in blood tonicity.

    1. Increased tonicity of the blood (hypertonic) → increased ADH release → increased H_2O reabsorption from the kidney tubules

---

Filtrate becomes hypertonic in the thin descending limb of Henle's loop.

Antidiuretic hormone controls the H_2O permeability of the collecting tubules: ↑ blood tonicity causes ↑ ADH secretion, which leads to ↑ H_2O reabsorption, resulting in ↓ blood tonicity.

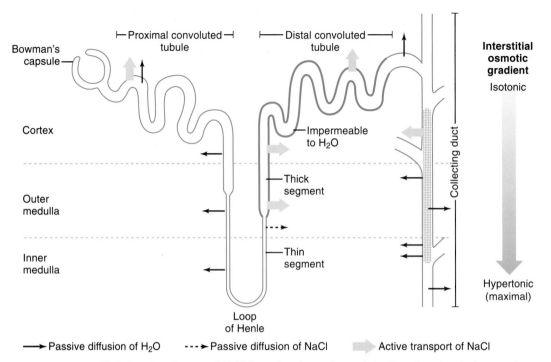

15-5: *Overview of water and NaCl fluxes along the uriniferous tubules. These fluxes largely determine the urine concentration. The interstitial osmotic gradient is established by differential permeability to H_2O and NaCl in the thin segment of Henle's loop and high permeability to urea in the distal portion of the collecting duct. The filtrate becomes hypotonic in the distal convoluted tubule due to active transport of NaCl out of the lumen and its impermeability to water. Antidiuretic hormone (ADH) controls the permeability of the collecting tubules for H_2O (shaded area). In the presence of ADH, H_2O is drawn osmotically from fluid in the collecting tubules as it passes through the increasingly hypertonic medullary interstitium, thereby concentrating the urine.*

- Result: more concentrated (hypertonic) urine and a decrease in the tonicity of the blood
2. Decreased tonicity of the blood (hypotonic) → decreased ADH release → decreased H_2O reabsorption from the kidney tubules
- Result: less concentrated (hypotonic) urine and an increase in the tonicity of the blood
H. Diseases affecting kidney function
1. Diabetes insipidus (DI): polyuria leading to dehydration and polydipsia
- Decreased release of ADH (central DI) or decreased responsiveness of the renal tubules to ADH (nephrogenic DI) reduces water reabsorption by the collecting tubules, resulting in a large volume of dilute (low-tonicity) urine.
2. Glomerulonephritis: inflammation of the glomeruli, impairing their ability to filter plasma
- Symptoms include proteinuria, hematuria, decreased urine production (oliguria), and periorbital edema.
- The acute form may occur secondary to group A streptococcal infection (e.g., tonsillitis).

Diabetes insipidus is caused by decreased release of antidiuretic hormone or decreased responsiveness of the tubules to antidiuretic hormone. Symptoms include polyuria, dehydration, and polydipsia.

3. Polycystic kidney disease: an inherited disorder in which cystic dilation of the tubules develops throughout both kidneys
   - Clinical manifestations include hematuria, hypertension, bilaterally enlarged kidneys, and pain in the lower back over the kidney area.
4. Nephrotic syndrome: any condition marked by massive proteinuria (>3.5 g in 24 hours), hypoalbuminemia, pitting edema, and hyperlipidemia resulting from damage to the glomeruli
   - This condition occurs in several diseases, including minimal change disease (lipoid nephrosis), a common childhood disorder in which the negative charge on the urinary membrane is lost.
5. Alport's syndrome: see Chapter 5, section V

IV. Juxtaglomerular Apparatus (see Fig. 15-3A)
   - This structure, located near the vascular pole of the renal corpuscle, functions in the regulation of blood pressure.
   A. Components of the juxtaglomerular apparatus
      1. Macula densa: specialized epithelial cells of the distal convoluted tubule where it contacts the afferent arteriole
      2. Juxtaglomerular cells: myoepithelial cells derived from smooth muscle in the tunica media of the afferent arteriole
   B. Renin-angiotensin-aldosterone system (Fig. 15-6)
      1. Renin, an enzyme secreted by the juxtaglomerular cells in response to a decrease in blood pressure, converts angiotensinogen to angiotensin I in the circulation.
      2. Angiotensin-converting enzyme, located in the endothelial cells of the pulmonary capillaries, hydrolyzes angiotensin I to angiotensin II.
      3. Angiotensin II increases blood pressure directly by stimulating vasoconstriction and indirectly by stimulating aldosterone secretion.
         - In the kidneys, aldosterone promotes Na^+ reabsorption, increasing blood tonicity.

Angiotensin-converting enzyme inhibitors, which prevent the formation of angiotensin II, reduce vasoconstriction and aldosterone secretion, thereby lowering blood pressure.

V. Blood Supply of the Kidney
   A. Arterial division
      - Renal artery → interlobar arteries (between the pyramids) → arcuate arteries (between the cortex and medulla) → interlobular arteries (between two medullary rays) → afferent arterioles → glomerular capillaries → efferent arterioles (see Fig. 15-2)
   B. Secondary capillary networks
      1. The peritubular plexuses, which arise from the efferent arterioles of the cortical nephrons, supply the cortical parenchyma and then drain into the interlobular veins.
      2. The vasa recta, which arise from the efferent arterioles of the juxtamedullary nephrons, are important in reabsorption.
         - Arteriolae rectae (descend into the medulla) → capillary network surrounding Henle's loop → venulae rectae (ascend toward the arcuate veins at the corticomedullary boundary)

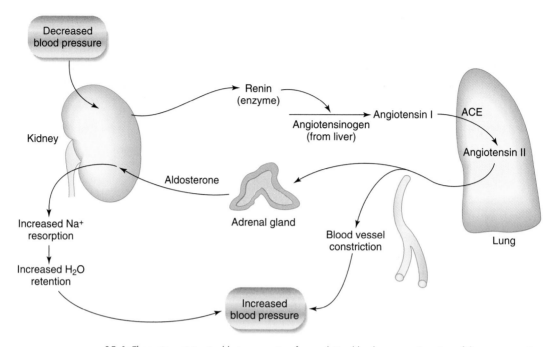

15-6: *The renin-angiotensin-aldosterone system for regulating blood pressure. Secretion of the enzyme renin from the juxtaglomerular apparatus in response to a drop in renal blood flow leads to formation of angiotensin II in the lung. Angiotensin II is a vasoconstrictor and also promotes the synthesis and release of aldosterone, which increases Na+ and H_2O reabsorption in the kidney. Angiotensin-converting enzyme (ACE), which cleaves angiotensin I to angiotensin II, is found primarily in the lungs.*

    C. Venous division
- Stellate veins (in the outer cortex) → interlobular veins (midway between two medullary rays) → arcuate veins (between the cortex and medulla) → interlobar veins (between the pyramids) → renal vein

  VI. Excretory Passages
- Distal to the renal papilla, a closed system of spaces and ducts collects, stores, and conveys urine to the body surface.

    A. Components
      1. Inside the kidneys: Minor calyx → major calyx → renal pelvis
      2. Outside the kidneys: Ureter → bladder → urethra

    B. Histology of the urine-conducting system
- With a few exceptions, the wall of the excretory passages is composed of the following layers:

      1. Transitional epithelium underlain by a lamina propria
- From the upper to the lower portions of the urethra, the epithelium changes from transitional to stratified squamous.

      2. Tunica muscularis, containing two or three smooth muscle layers
- The external sphincter of the urethra is composed of striated muscle.

3. Tunica adventitia of fibroelastic tissue
   - This layer is absent in the renal calyces and the pelvis.
C. Bladder cancer
   - The most common cancer of the urinary tract, bladder cancer is a transitional cell carcinoma marked by hematuria and multiple, recurring tumors.
   - Risk factors include cigarette smoking, aniline dyes, cyclophosphamide, and infection with *Schistosoma haematobium,* which causes squamous cell carcinoma.

Bladder cancer is a transitional cell carcinoma (the most common urinary tract cancer). It causes hematuria and multiple tumors that tend to recur.

Male Reproductive System

I. Introduction
   A. Testes (paired gonads) produce male gametes (spermatozoa).
      1. Tunica albuginea: connective tissue capsule surrounding each testis
         - The mediastinum testis (thickened posterior region of the capsule) extends incomplete connective tissue septa that divide the testis into numerous lobules, each containing two to four seminiferous tubules.
      2. Seminiferous (germinal) tubules: highly convoluted tubules (30 to 70 cm long)
         - The seminiferous epithelium lining the tubules is a specialized glandlike epithelium where spermatogenesis (formation of spermatozoa from spermatogonia) occurs.
      3. Intratesticular ducts that convey spermatozoa to the surface of the testis
         a. Tubuli recti: straight terminal portions of the seminiferous tubules lined by simple columnar epithelium
         b. Rete testis: an anastomosing network of channels lined by simple cuboidal epithelium and located at the mediastinum
            - The tubuli recti drain into the rete testis.
   B. Extratesticular ducts conduct spermatozoa outside the body.
   C. Specialized glands release secretions that provide nutritive and lubricative elements to semen.
      1. Seminal vesicles
      2. Prostate gland
      3. Bulbourethral (Cowper's) glands

D. Glandular functions of the testes

1. Exocrine function: Production of a holocrine cytogenic secretion containing spermatozoa occurs within the seminiferous epithelium.
2. Endocrine function: Synthesis and secretion of hormones is carried out by Leydig cells within the interstitium and by Sertoli cells within the seminiferous epithelium.

II. Spermatogenesis

A. Composition of the seminiferous epithelium (Fig. 16-1)

1. Spermatogenic cells

a. Before puberty, the only spermatogenic cells present are undifferentiated, basally located spermatogonia that are mitotically inactive.

b. After puberty, when spermatogenesis begins, spermatogenic cells are present in a gradient from basal undifferentiated cells to differentiated spermatids ready for release as mature spermatozoa into the lumen.

> Spermatogenesis = spermatocytogenesis + meiosis + spermiogenesis.

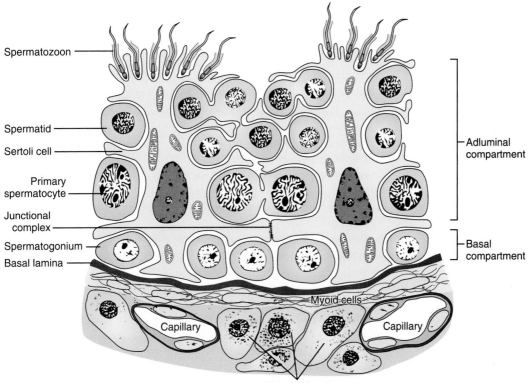

16-1: *The seminiferous epithelium and surrounding interstitial tissue. The spermatogenic cells are arranged in a basal → lumen gradient from the least differentiated (spermatogonia) to the most differentiated (spermatids). The epithelium is divided into two compartments by tight junctions between adjacent Sertoli cells, forming the blood–testis barrier. The basal compartment is occupied by spermatogonia and the adluminal compartment by developing spermatocytes, which are enveloped by Sertoli cells.*

2. Sertoli cells are tall, columnar cells that extend from the basement membrane to the lumen.
   - These cells support, protect, and nurture the germ cells within the seminiferous epithelium; they also secrete inhibin and androgen-binding protein.
   - They are nondividing cells that remain after degeneration of the germ cells in the senescent gonad.
   a. Tight junctions (zonulae occludens) between adjacent Sertoli cells divide the epithelium into a basal compartment containing spermatogonia and an adluminal compartment containing cells in the later stages of spermatogenesis.
   b. The blood–testis barrier results from the tight junctions between Sertoli cells.
      (1) Tissue fluid must pass through the Sertoli cells to reach the developing sperm in the adluminal compartment.
      (2) Proteins from the developing sperm in the adluminal compartment cannot reach the bloodstream, thereby preventing a possible immune response.

B. Stages in spermatogenesis (Fig. 16-2)
   - Formation of spermatozoa does not occur in synchrony in all tubules, but rather in wavelike cycles of the seminiferous epithelium involving the following stages:
   1. Spermatocytogenesis: Spermatogonia → primary spermatocytes (mitotic divisions)
   2. Meiosis: Primary spermatocytes → spermatids (meiotic divisions)
   3. Spermiogenesis: Spermatids → mature spermatozoa (series of morphologic and physiologic changes)

C. Mitotic division of spermatogonia
   1. Division of type A spermatogonia (stem cells) occurs in two forms.
      a. Dark (Ad) cells divide to replenish themselves or differentiate to form pale cells.
      b. Pale (Ap) cells undergo multiple mitotic divisions with incomplete cytokinesis and mature into type B spermatogonia (see Fig. 16-2, top).
   2. Type B spermatogonia undergo further mitotic divisions, and then a cluster of linked cells, having replicated their deoxyribonucleic acid (DNA) in the S phase, enter meiosis as primary spermatocytes.

D. Meiotic division of spermatocytes (see Fig. 3-6B)
   - Each primary spermatocyte gives rise to four spermatids. A group of primary spermatocytes derived from a single type A spermatogonium and linked by intercellular bridges undergoes meiosis in synchrony (see Fig. 16-2, middle).
   1. Primary spermatocytes are diploid cells with 4C DNA content that undergo reductional division to form secondary spermatocytes.
      - Crossing over and recombination of maternal and paternal chromatids can occur, producing new genetic combinations.

Before entering into cell division (mitosis or meiosis), spermatogonia or primary spermatocytes must replicate their deoxyribonucleic acid (S phase).

B spermatogonia → spermatozoa takes about 64 days. Of the total duration, approximately one fourth of the time (16 days) is spent in spermiogenesis.

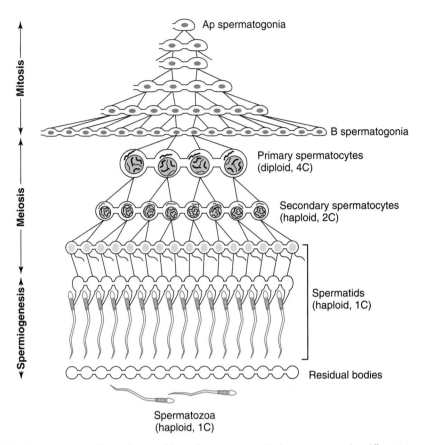

Ap spermatogonia

B spermatogonia

Primary spermatocytes
(diploid, 4C)

Secondary spermatocytes
(haploid, 2C)

Spermatids
(haploid, 1C)

Residual bodies

Spermatozoa
(haploid, 1C)

Mitosis

Meiosis

Spermiogenesis

16-2: *Spermatogenesis. Mitotic division of the earliest spermatogonia that are committed to differentiation (Ap cells) yields daughter cells that are connected by intercellular bridges. These bridges, which persist through subsequent mitotic and meiotic divisions, are shed as part of residual bodies during the final phase of spermatid maturation to yield separate spermatozoa. Meiotic division of each primary spermatocyte, a diploid cell with 4C DNA, produces four haploid spermatids, each with 1C DNA.*

    2. Secondary spermatocytes are haploid cells with 2C DNA that rapidly undergo equational division (without any intervening DNA synthesis) to form haploid spermatids with 1C DNA.
- Fusion of sperm and egg during fertilization restores the diploid chromosome number and 2C DNA in the zygote.
- Each spermatid (and subsequent gamete) contains either an X or a Y chromosome; thus, the male gamete determines the sex of the zygote (see Fig. 3-7).

E. Transformation of spermatids into mature spermatozoa
- A group of spermatids linked by intercellular bridges and nestled within the apical cytoplasm of the Sertoli cells undergo spermiogenesis in synchrony as shown in Figure 16-3.

F. Characteristics of spermatozoa (Fig. 16-4)
    1. Morphologically mature spermatozoa released into the tubular lumen at the end of spermiogenesis are immotile and incapable of fertilization.

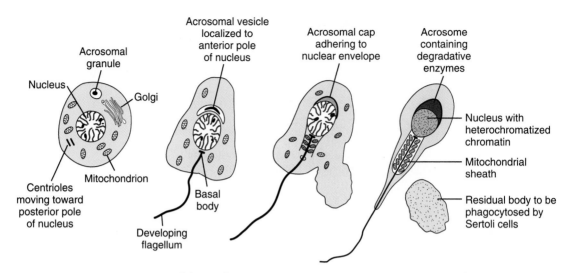

16-3: *Principal changes that occur in a spermatid during spermiogenesis. Elements of the Golgi complex are incorporated into the acrosomal granule, and the Golgi complex disappears. The centrioles initiate the formation of the basal body and flagellum. The mitochondria gather as a sheath around the upper portion of the flagellum. In the final stage, excess cytoplasm and intercellular bridges connecting spermatids are discarded, forming residual bodies that are phagocytosed. Finally, the morphologically mature but nonmotile spermatozoa are released, tail first, into the lumen of the seminiferous tubule.*

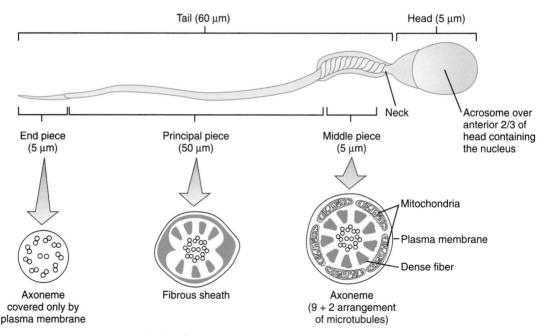

16-4: *Morphology of a mammalian spermatozoon showing features that are visible by light microscopy (top) and the ultrastructure of the tail regions (bottom). Note that the various regions are not to scale; the principal piece is much longer than the other regions.*

2. Sperm motility is activated in the epididymis.
   • Males with immotile cilia syndrome or Kartagener's syndrome are infertile because their sperm are incapable of motility.
3. Fertilization capability is acquired during capacitation of sperm within the uterine tube of the female.
4. Enzymes within the acrosome that are released during fertilization facilitate entry of the sperm nucleus into the oocyte.

G. Temperature requirement for sperm production
   1. A temperature of 35°C, slightly below the core body temperature, is necessary for spermatogenesis to occur. This temperature is achieved because the testes are housed within the scrotal chamber.
   2. Cryptorchidism, failure of one or both the testes to descend, results in impaired spermatogenesis if the testis is not surgically moved into the scrotal sac before 2 years of age.

Before it is capable of fertilization, a spermatozoon must undergo capacitation and the acrosome reaction, which releases enzymes that assist entry into the oocyte.

III. Transport of Spermatozoa and Production of Semen
   A. Ducts through which sperm move from the rete testis
      • Ductuli efferentes → duct of epididymis → ductus (vas) deferens → ampulla of the ductus deferens → ejaculatory duct → urethra
   B. Mechanism of sperm movement
      1. The secretion of fluid by the Sertoli cells into the lumen of the seminiferous tubule and its reabsorption in the ductuli efferentes create a current that moves sperm from the rete testis to the ductus epididymis.
      2. The ductus epididymis and ductus deferens are storage regions. Weak peristaltic movements in these ducts move spermatozoa distally.
      3. Muscular contractions of the ductus epididymis, ductus deferens, and urethra force the release of spermatozoa during ejaculation.
   C. Composition of semen
      • Semen = sperm + secretions from the testis, ductal system, and accessory glands.
      • Erotic stimulation promotes the release of secretions from the accessory glands.
      1. The seminal vesicles secrete a viscous fluid that is rich in fructose, which provides energy for movement of the sperm flagella.
         • Seminal fluid also contains factors that promote the coagulation of semen and prevent agglutination of spermatozoa.
      2. The prostate gland secretes a thin fluid that is rich in acid phosphatase and contains prostaglandins.
      3. The bulbourethral (Cowper's) glands secrete a mucuslike material that lubricates the urethra, augmenting the mucous secretions of the glands of Littre within the penis.
   D. Penis
      • The male copulatory organ contains three masses of erectile tissue surrounded by tunica albuginea, a thick connective tissue sheath containing collagen and elastic fibers.
      1. Corpora cavernosae: paired dorsal bodies containing irregular vascular spaces

- Cavernous spaces are lined by continuous endothelium and separated by strands of smooth muscle.
- Engorgement of these spaces with blood during erection is under parasympathetic control.

2. Corpus cavernosum urethrae (corpus spongiosum): a single ventral body surrounding the urethra and containing regular vascular spaces
  - Vascular spaces are lined by continuous endothelium and separated by septa that contain more elastic fibers and less smooth muscle than the corpora cavernosae

3. Glans penis: the dilated distal end of the corpus spongiosum that is lined by stratified squamous epithelium
  - It contains smooth muscle, sebaceous glands, and numerous sensory receptors.

E. Sequence of events at ejaculation
  - Secretion from Cowper's and Littre's glands → prostate secretion → release of spermatozoa from the epididymis and vas deferens → seminal vesicle secretions → release of semen.

IV. Hormonal Control of the Male Reproductive System (Fig. 16-5)
  A. Pituitary hormones that promote testicular hormone production
    - Release of these hormones is stimulated by gonadotropin-releasing hormone (GnRH) from the hypothalamus.
    1. Luteinizing hormone (LH) stimulates Leydig cells to secrete testosterone.
      - LH is also known as interstitial cell–stimulating hormone (ICSH) in males.
    2. Follicle-stimulating hormone (FSH) stimulates the Sertoli cells to secrete inhibin and produce androgen-binding protein.
  B. Effects of testicular hormones
    1. Testosterone
      a. Promotes the development of secondary sex characteristics
      b. Stimulates spermatogenesis
      c. Maintains the function of the ducts and accessory glands
      d. Acts on the hypothalamus to reduce the release of GnRH, thereby exerting negative feedback on LH and FSH secretion.
    2. Androgen-binding protein
      a. Binds testosterone and helps transport it across the seminiferous epithelium to the tubular lumen
      b. Helps maintain a high local concentration of testosterone, which promotes spermatogenesis
    3. Inhibin
      - Acts on the anterior pituitary to decrease FSH secretion

V. Disorders of the Male Reproductive System
  A. Testicular cancers
    1. Seminoma is one of several germ cell neoplasms, all of which are malignant.

Leydig cells in the testicular interstitium secrete testosterone in response to stimulation by luteinizing hormone from the pituitary gland.

Sertoli cells produce androgen-binding protein and inhibin in response to follicle-stimulating hormone from the pituitary gland.

Most testicular cancers are malignant and derived from germ cells. These include seminoma, embryonal carcinoma, choriocarcinoma, yolk sac carcinoma, and teratoma.

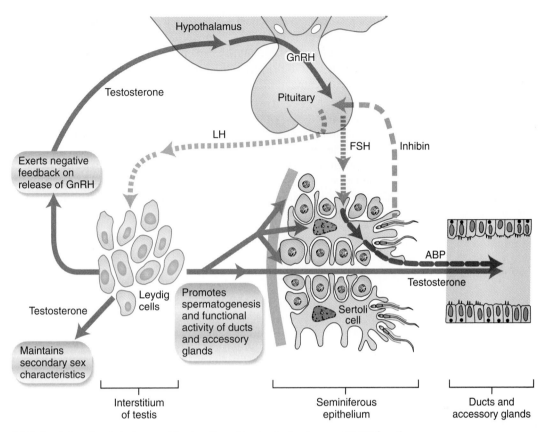

16-5: *Regulation of testicular hormonal function. Gonadotropin-releasing hormone (GnRH) from the hypothalamus stimulates the secretion of follicle-stimulating hormone (FSH) and luteinizing hormone (LH) from the anterior pituitary. FSH promotes the production of androgen-binding protein (ABP) and inhibin by Sertoli cells. LH stimulates Leydig cells to secrete testosterone, which has several effects that are critical to male reproductive function. Testosterone also acts on the hypothalamus to inhibit GnRH secretion.*

    a. This neoplasm usually presents as painless testicular enlargement; it may metastasize before the original tumor can be felt.

    b. The highest incidence is in men between 35 and 40 years of age and those with undescended (cryptorchid) testes.

    c. Seminomas are less aggressive and more sensitive to radiation than other types of germ cell neoplasms.

  2. Leydig cell and Sertoli cell tumors generally are benign but may cause endocrine abnormalities (e.g., gynecomastia, precocious puberty).

B. Varicocele: varicosity of the venous plexus of the spermatic cord (more common in the left cord than in the right cord)

  • Marked by soft, elastic, often painful swelling in the scrotum

  • Associated with reduced spermatogenesis due to increased temperature

C. Hydrocele: accumulation of fluid in the scrotum or along the spermatic cord

  • May be caused by swelling of the testis or obstruction in the cord

> The most common risk factor for seminoma of the testis is an undescended testis (cryptorchidism).

Benign prostatic hyperplasia is the most common cause of urinary tract obstruction in males.

Prostatic adenocarcinoma is the most common malignancy of men, with onset beginning after 50 years of age and the peak incidence occurring at approximately 75 years of age. Prostate-specific antigen is a tumor marker.

- Congenital form due to failure of the canal between the trunk cavity and the scrotum to close completely before birth
D. Benign prostatic hyperplasia: usually hyperplasia of the glandular cells or smooth muscle cells in the periurethral zone of the prostate gland
  - Marked by nocturia, difficulty initiating a urine stream, and urinary frequency
  - Not a precancerous disorder
E. Prostatic adenocarcinoma: origin usually in the peripheral zone of the prostrate; metastasis to bone common
  - Marked clinically by an enlarged, firm, nodular prostate on digital rectal examination
  - Often associated with elevated serum levels of acid phosphatase and prostate-specific antigen (PSA)

Female Reproductive System

I. Introduction
  A. Organs of the female reproductive system
    1. Ovaries
       a. Exocrine function: maturation and release of the developing ova
       b. Endocrine function: synthesis and secretion of several hormones (e.g., estrogen, progesterone)
    2. Oviducts
    3. Uterus
    4. Vagina and external genitalia
    5. Breasts
  B. Menstrual cycle: hormone-induced histophysiologic changes in the ovaries and uterus that accompany oocyte maturation
    1. Menarche: occurrence of the first menses
    2. Menopause: the period during which cyclical changes become intermittent and eventually cease
       • During the postmenopausal period, there is a slow, progressive involution of the female reproductive system.
  C. Pregnancy-induced changes
    1. Cessation of the menstrual cycle

2. Formation of the placenta, a temporary structure that secretes the hormones needed to maintain pregnancy and permits the exchange of materials between the maternal and the fetal blood supply
3. Development of secretory cells in the breasts in preparation for postnatal lactation

II. Ovaries
   A. General histologic features of the ovary
      1. Simple squamous to cuboidal epithelium (a continuation of the peritoneum) covers the external surface.
         a. This epithelium is sometimes incorrectly referred to as *germinal epithelium.*
         b. Surface-derived tumors of the ovary come from this epithelium.
      2. The tunica albuginea of fibrous connective tissue lies under the surface epithelium.
      3. The cortex contains ovarian follicles in various stages of maturation.
      4. The medulla, a vascular, highly cellular connective tissue, is not well defined.
   B. Embryonic formation of the primordial follicles
      1. Primordial germ cells (oogonia) migrate from the yolk sac endoderm into the ovaries early in the embryonic period.
      2. The oogonia proliferate by mitosis until 20 to 28 weeks' gestation, resulting in 3 million oogonia per ovary.
         a. After ceasing mitosis, the oogonia enter and become arrested in prophase I of meiosis; these arrested cells, called *primary oocytes,* are diploid ($2n$) and have 4C deoxyribonucleic acid (DNA) [46 chromosomes, 92 chromatids].
         b. No additional primary oocytes are formed later in life.
      3. Primordial follicles consist of one primary oocyte surrounded by a single layer of squamous epithelial (follicular) cells and a basal lamina.
         • Apoptosis (programmed cell death) of the primordial follicles reduces their number to ≈200,000 per ovary at menarche.
   C. Maturation of the ovarian follicles (Fig. 17-1)
      • At menarche, groups of 10 to 15 primordial follicles begin to grow at the start of each menstrual cycle, although only one of each cohort develops into a mature (graafian) follicle and ovulates.
      • Follicle maturation is marked by progressive morphologic changes in the oocyte, the surrounding follicular cells, and the adjacent stroma.
      1. Unilaminar primary follicle
         a. Simple squamous epithelium of primordial follicle changes to a single layer of cuboidal follicular cells.
         b. Differentiation of the primary oocyte begins, marked by increases in the size and number of mitochondria, Golgi, rough endoplasmic reticulum (RER), and polysomes, which augment the synthetic capacity of the oocyte.
         c. The zona pellucida, synthesized by both the oocyte and the follicular cells, begins to form around the oocyte.

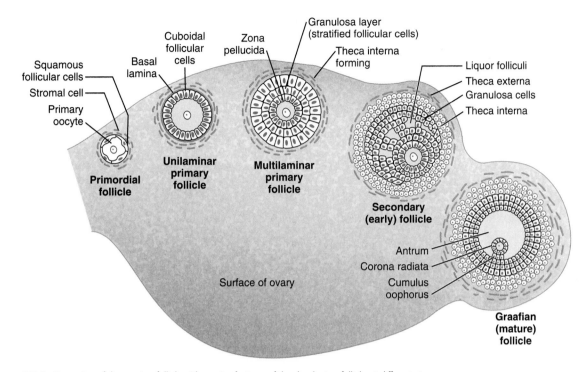

17-1: *Maturation of the ovarian follicles. The major features of the developing follicle at different stages are depicted diagrammatically. The primary oocyte within a maturing follicle completes meiosis I and is arrested at metaphase II (haploid secondary oocyte) within a graafian follicle shortly before ovulation. Completion of the second meiotic division occurs during fertilization. (Adapted from Bergman RA, Afifi AK, Heidger PM Jr: Saunders Text and Review Series: Histology. Philadelphia: WB Saunders, 1996, p 284.)*

- During fertilization, sperm bind to the zona pellucida.
2. Multilaminar primary follicle
   a. Stratification of cuboidal follicular cells occurs, forming the granulosa layer.
   b. Stromal cells begin to form the thecal layer around the follicle.
3. Secondary (antral) follicle
   a. Spaces filled with fluid (liquor folliculi) appear between granulosa cells and eventually coalesce into a single large space, the antrum.
   b. The cumulus oophorus, a mound of granulosa cells extending into the antrum, attaches the oocyte to the follicular wall.
      - Granulosa cells adjacent to the zona pellucida constitute the corona radiata, which accompanies the oocyte during ovulation.
   c. The theca interna, a secretory stromal layer adjacent to the granulosa cells, secretes 17-ketosteroids (e.g., androstenedione).
      (1) Androstenedione is enzymatically converted to testosterone.
      (2) Follicle-stimulating hormone (FSH) stimulates enzymatic conversion of these androgens to estrogen in the granulosa cells.

(3) The subsequent increase in the estrogen level induces the expression of receptors for luteinizing hormone (LH) by the granulosa cells.

   d. The theca externa, a fibrous, vascular stromal layer peripheral to the theca interna, has no endocrine function.

4. Graafian follicle

- A mature ovarian follicle, which visibly bulges on the ovarian surface, exists for 1 to 2 days before ovulation.

   a. The primary oocyte completes the first meiotic division within the mature follicle shortly before ovulation, forming a large secondary oocyte and a small polar body.

   b. The secondary oocyte, a haploid cell ($1n$) with 2C DNA (23 chromosomes, 46 chromatids), enters the second meiotic division but is arrested in metaphase II at the time of ovulation.

5. Atretic follicles

- Follicles in all stages are continually undergoing atresia.
- No scar is evident when the atretic process is complete.

D. Ovulation and fate of the secondary oocyte

- A surge of LH, induced by an increasing level of estrogen acting on the hypothalamo-hypophyseal system, triggers the release of the secondary oocyte surrounded by its corona radiata from the graafian follicle (Fig. 17-2).

1. The ovulated secondary oocyte is briefly contained in the peritoneal cavity and normally is caught by the fimbria of the oviduct.

2. In the absence of fertilization, the ovulated oocyte dies in approximately 24 hours.

3. During fertilization, the oocyte completes meiosis II.

E. Corpus luteum

- The collapsed remains of the ovulated graafian follicle (corpus hemorrhagicum) are transformed into the corpus luteum, a temporary endocrine gland whose cells become luteinized by exposure to LH.

1. Luteal cells

- Have abundant smooth endoplasmic reticulum and other cytoplasmic structures associated with steroid secretion

   a. Granulosa lutein cells (derived from the granulosa cells) produce most of the body's progesterone.

   b. Theca lutein cells (derived from the theca interna cells) produce estrogen and some progesterone.

2. Fate of the corpus luteum in the absence of fertilization

   a. An increasing progesterone level progressively inhibits LH production.

   b. A subsequent decrease in LH leads to atrophy of the corpus luteum.

   c. The resulting decrease in progesterone and estrogen sets the stage for menstruation and the onset of another menstrual cycle.

3. Fate of the corpus luteum in pregnancy

   a. Human chorionic gonadotropin (hCG), produced by syncytiotrophoblast cells of the implanting embryo, maintains the corpus luteum and its hormonal synthesis early in pregnancy.

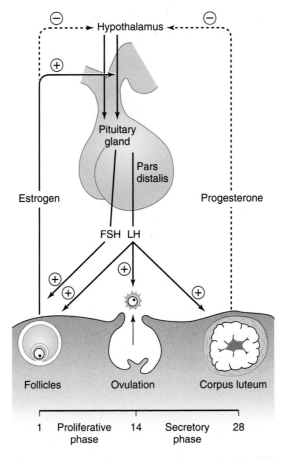

17-2: *Hormonal control of ovarian function. Estrogen produced by the developing follicle acts to inhibit follicle-stimulating hormone (FSH) and stimulate luteinizing hormone (LH) release, leading to a surge of LH and a proper FSH/LH ratio at midcycle that triggers ovulation. Progesterone produced by the corpus luteum acts on the hypothalamus to decrease LH release. The scale at the bottom refers to the days in the menstrual cycle.*

- Detection of hCG is the basis of some pregnancy tests.
  b. Luteal-derived progesterone and estrogen sustain pregnancy for 2 to 3 months, after which the placenta becomes the main source of these hormones.
    - Bilateral oophorectomy (ovariectomy) at this stage will not terminate a pregnancy.
  c. Relaxin, produced by the corpus luteum, relaxes the uterine smooth muscle during pregnancy and facilitates parturition.
4. Corpus albicans: scarred remains of the corpus luteum after it degenerates following menstruation or pregnancy

III. Oviduct (Fallopian Tube)
  A. Regions of the oviduct
    1. Infundibulum: the funnel-shaped free end with fingerlike projections (fimbria) that "sweep" the ovarian surface at the time of ovulation
    2. Ampulla: the dilated region proximal to the infundibulum where fertilization usually occurs
    3. Isthmus: the nondilated region proximal to the ampulla
    4. Pars intramuralis: the part coursing through the uterine wall
  B. Oviduct wall
    1. Mucosa
      a. Simple columnar epithelium (tallest during the proliferative phase of the menstrual cycle)
        (1) Ciliated cells beat their cilia toward the uterus, assisting in transport of the zygote.
        (2) Secretory cells produce viscous liquid film that supplies nourishment for the ovum, zygote, and early embryo.
      b. Lamina propria: edematous during the premenstrual phase
    2. Muscularis (two smooth muscle layers)
      a. Contractions facilitate contact between male and female gametes and movement of the zygote to the uterus.
      b. Estrogen stimulates contraction; progesterone inhibits contraction.
    3. Serosa
  C. Ectopic pregnancy
    • Implantation of the early embryo in the wall of the oviduct or another extrauterine site (e.g., intestinal surface) that cannot support fetal development
    • Clinically marked by amenorrhea, pelvic pain and tenderness, tissue mass (usually in the fallopian tube), an elevated hCG level, and hemorrhage into the peritoneal cavity, if not surgically treated

IV. Uterus
  A. Uterine wall
    1. Perimetrium: external uterine covering that is serosa or adventitia, depending on the peritoneal reflections
    2. Myometrium: vascularized smooth muscle tunic of the uterus
      a. The thickness increases during pregnancy due to estrogen-stimulated hypertrophy and hyperplasia of the smooth muscle cells.
      b. Progesterone and relaxin depress uterine contractions.
      c. Oxytocin and prostaglandin ($PGF_{2\alpha}$) stimulate contractions, especially during parturition.
    3. Endometrium: the mucosal lining of the uterus, composed of a simple columnar epithelium, a highly vascular lamina propria, and endometrial glands
      a. The functional layer (superficial 80%) undergoes hormone-induced changes during the menstrual cycle and is sloughed during menses.
        • Coiled (spiral) arteries extend into this layer.
      b. The basal layer (deep 20%) is never sloughed.

Layers of the uterine wall:

• Perimetrium: the external layer
• Myometrium: the smooth muscle layer that thickens during pregnancy
• Endometrium: the inner mucosal lining

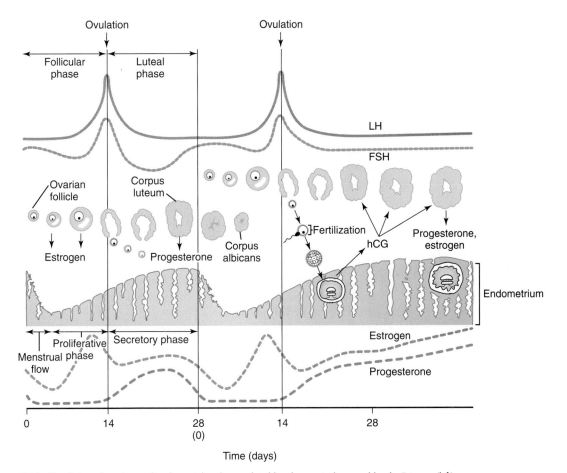

17-3: Correlation of ovarian and endometrial cycles regulated by changes in hormonal levels. Estrogen (left) secreted from the developing ovarian follicles promotes rebuilding of the functional layer of the endometrium (proliferative phase), which is sloughed during menstrual flow. High estrogen levels cause a surge of luteinizing hormone (LH), triggering ovulation from one follicle. Rising levels of progesterone secreted from the corpus luteum mediate further changes in the endometrium (secretory phase). In the absence of fertilization and implantation (left), the corpus luteum atrophies due to negative feedback by progesterone on LH release, causing a drop in the amount of progesterone and estrogen available to the endometrium. Degeneration of the functional layer occurs rapidly (ischemic phase), followed by menstruation. As progesterone and estrogen levels fall, pituitary secretion of follicle-stimulating hormone (FSH) and LH increases and the cycle begins again. If fertilization and implantation occur (right), human chorionic gonadotropin (hCG) secreted by the implanted embryo "rescues" the corpus luteum. Continued secretion of progesterone and estrogen by the corpus luteum under stimulation of hCG maintains pregnancy for 2 to 3 months; placental estrogen and progesterone then take over. (Adapted from Randall D, Burggren W, French K: Eckert Animal Physiology: Mechanisms and Adaptations, 4th ed. New York: WH Freeman, p 341.)

- Regeneration of the functional layer occurs from the intact bases of the endometrial glands in the basal layer.
B. Changes in the endometrium during the menstrual cycle (Fig. 17-3, left)
    1. Menses: days 1 to 4
        - The functional layer sloughs, generating the flow of menstrual blood, which does not clot due to the fibrinolytic activity of plasmin.

2. Proliferative phase: days 5 to 14
   - This is the most variable phase of the cycle.
   a. Estrogen secreted from the developing ovarian follicles stimulates rebuilding of the functional layer.
   b. Ovulation, which signals the end of this phase, is marked by an increase in body temperature (progesterone effect) and the presence of subnuclear vacuoles in the glandular cells.

3. Secretory phase: days 15 to 26
   - Progesterone secreted from the corpus luteum prepares the estrogen-primed endometrium for implantation.
   a. Endometrial glands become coiled, secrete glycoprotein material into the lumen, and accumulate glycogen within their cells.
      - As the secretory phase progresses, glycogen moves from the base to the apex of the endometrial gland cells.
   b. The spiral arteries become more highly coiled and elongate to almost reach the endometrial surface.
   c. The endometrial stroma becomes highly edematous in the late secretory phase in the absence of fertilization and implantation.

4. Ischemic (premenstrual) phase: days 27 to 28
   - An abrupt drop in estrogen and progesterone after atrophy of the corpus luteum leads to progressive degeneration.
   a. The coiled arteries spasmodically contract.
   b. Ischemia is followed by necrosis of the tissue distal to the contracted segment.
   c. Hemorrhage of the endometrial arteries marks the beginning of menses.

C. Cessation of the menstrual cycle during pregnancy (Fig. 17-3, right)
   1. After fertilization and implantation of the embryo (usually on day 21), hCG from the embryonic trophoblast maintains the corpus luteum.
      - Continued progesterone and estrogen secretion from the corpus luteum maintains the endometrium, which participates in the formation of the placenta.
   2. Feedback inhibition of FSH and LH release from the pituitary by progesterone and estrogen prevents the development of ovarian follicles and ovulation during pregnancy.

D. Uterine disorders
   1. Endometriosis: ectopic presence of non-neoplastic endometrial tissue in extrauterine sites (commonly the ovaries or oviducts)
      a. Ectopic tissue undergoes hormone-induced changes during the menstrual cycle.
      b. Dysmenorrhea (pain and excessive bleeding) occurs; infertility may result.
   2. Uterine fibroid (leiomyoma): a benign tumor of smooth muscle cells in the uterine wall
      a. This is the most common tumor in women, with a peak incidence at 35 to 45 years of age.

Endometrial phases are menses (days 1 to 4); the proliferative phase (days 5 to 14), ending with ovulation; the secretory phase (days 15 to 26); and the premenstrual phase (days 27 to 28).

Uterine leiomyoma (fibroid) is the most common benign tumor in women.

   b. Clinical features, which are dependent on tumor size, location, and number (multiple lesions are common), include abnormal uterine bleeding, pelvic discomfort, and infertility.

  3. Endometrial carcinoma: the most common malignancy of the female genital tract, with a peak incidence in postmenopausal women (55 to 65 years of age)

   a. Usually causes irregular vaginal bleeding

   b. Associated with hyperestrogenism (nulliparity, early menarche), obesity, hypertension, and diabetes mellitus

V. Uterine Cervix

 • The lower cylindrical part of the uterus does not undergo the extreme cyclical changes that are characteristic of the endometrium.

 A. Endocervix (proximal end)

  1. Simple, mucus-secreting columnar epithelium containing branched cervical (mucous) glands

  2. Variations in the cervical mucus

   a. At midcycle, the mucus is watery and copious, facilitating the movement of sperm through the cervical os.

   b. Postovulation and during pregnancy, the mucus is viscous and less copious, inhibiting the entrance of sperm and microorganisms.

 B. Portio vaginalis (distal end protruding into the vagina)

  1. The stratified squamous parakeratinized epithelium contains five histologically distinct cell types.

   • Estrogen stimulates cytodifferentiation: Basal cells → parabasal cells → intermediate cells → precornified cells → cornified cells (surface)

  2. The features of the exfoliated cells on Pap smear reflect the stage of the menstrual cycle.

   a. During the proliferative phase, more mature cells (precornified and cornified) predominate (estrogen effect).

   b. During the secretory phase, intermediate cells predominate (progesterone effect).

 C. Cervical cancer: invasive squamous cell carcinoma that evolves from the progression of cervical intraepithelial neoplasia (CIN)

  • Preinvasive CIN changes can be detected on Pap smear.

  • Risk factors include infection with human papilloma virus (HPV16, HPV18), early age at first coitus, multiple high-risk sex partners, use of birth control pills, and cigarette smoking.

VI. Vagina

 A. Vaginal wall

  1. Mucosa

   a. Stratified squamous parakeratinized epithelium

    (1) Glycogen accumulated by the superficial cells is deposited in the vaginal lumen as cells desquamate.

    (2) The epithelium is thickest during the proliferative phase.

Pap smear of exfoliated cervical cells, which reflect the stage of the menstrual cycle, is useful in detecting cervical cancer but not very effective in detecting endometrial carcinoma.

Invasive cervical carcinoma is preceded by neoplastic changes (cervical intraepithelial neoplasia) that can be detected on Pap smear. Infection with human papilloma virus (HPV16, HPV18) is associated with cervical intraepithelial neoplasia and invasive carcinoma in most cases.

b. Lamina propria: rich in elastic fibers; no glands; highly vascularized

2. Muscularis: mostly longitudinal smooth muscle, with some circular smooth muscle closest to the lamina propria

3. Adventitia: rich in elastic fibers

B. Vaginal lumen

1. Lactobacilli in the normal bacterial flora metabolize glycogen from desquamated cells, releasing lactic acid.
   - The resulting low pH of the vaginal lumen inhibits the growth of pathogenic bacteria.

2. Variations in glycogen content during the menstrual cycle cause changes in the luminal pH.

   a. The highest glycogen level occurs at midcycle (lowest luminal pH; least susceptible to infection)

   b. The lowest glycogen level occurs during the late secretory phase (highest luminal pH; most susceptible to infection)

VII. External Genitalia

Clitoromegaly is a sign of excess androgens in a woman.

A. Clitoris: two bodies of erectile tissue, containing many sensory nerve endings and blood vessels that terminate in the rudimentary glans clitoris
   - Developmentally and structurally homologous to the penis

B. Labia minora: folds of skin with a core of dense, irregular connective tissue

C. Labia majora: longitudinal folds of skin containing considerable adipose tissue and a thin layer of smooth muscle
   - Developmentally homologous to the scrotum

D. Vulvovaginal (Bartholin's) glands: mucus-secreting glands that empty into each side of the vaginal vestibule
   - Homologous to the bulbourethral (Cowper's) glands in the male

VIII. Fertilization

A. Fusion of the sperm and oocyte cytoplasm

1. Sperm penetrates the corona radiata and binds to the zona pellucida.

2. The sperm plasma membrane fuses with the acrosome membrane, forming channels through which acrosomal enzymes are released (acrosomal reaction).

3. Released enzymes degrade the acrosome, permitting the acrosomal process, an extension of the sperm head, to penetrate the zona pellucida.

4. Plasma membranes of the oocyte and the sperm head fuse, and the sperm nucleus enters the oocyte cytoplasm.

5. The oocyte exocytoses enzymes that reduce its sperm-binding capacity (cortical reaction), helping to prevent the entry of multiple sperm.

B. Formation of the zygote and initial cleavage

1. After fertilization, the secondary oocyte completes meiosis II, forming a second polar body and a large mature gamete, the ovum, containing female and male pronuclei.

   a. Female pronucleus: 1C DNA, haploid ($1n$), one sex chromosome (X)

   b. Male pronucleus: 1C DNA, haploid ($1n$), one sex chromosome (X or Y)

2. DNA replication occurs in each pronucleus, yielding a diploid zygote (2*n*, 4C DNA) with 46 chromosomes (92 chromatids) housed in the two pronuclei.
3. The membranes of the pronuclei break down, and all the duplicated chromosomes align at the metaphase plate of the first cleavage division.
4. Completion of mitosis produces a two-cell embryo with 46 chromosomes in each cell (2*n*, 2C DNA).
   a. 22 autosomes from the maternal parent
   b. 22 autosomes from the paternal parent
   c. 1 sex chromosome from the maternal parent (X)
   d. 1 sex chromosome from the paternal parent (X or Y)
C. Errors of fertilization
   1. Polyspermy results from the entry of two sperm into the oocyte.
      a. The zygote has two male and one female pronuclei.
      b. The resulting triploid embryo is nonviable, and spontaneous abortion ensues.
   2. Polygyny results when a second polar body fails to form during meiotic division of the secondary oocyte.
      a. The zygote has two female and one male pronuclei.
      b. The resulting triploid embryo is nonviable, and spontaneous abortion ensues.

Two major errors of fertilization yield a nonviable, triploid embryo:

- Polyspermy occurs when two sperm fertilize the egg (responsible for a partial mole).
- Polygyny occurs when a secondary oocyte fails to emit a second polar body after fertilization.

IX. Placenta
   • A temporary organ consisting of maternal and fetal components, the placenta forms after successful implantation of the embryo into the uterine wall.
   • The maternal portion synthesizes and secretes estrogen and progesterone.
   • The fetal portion synthesizes and secretes hCG and human placental lactogen (hPL).
   A. Implantation
      1. The embryo travels through the oviduct and reaches the uterus in approximately 3 days, when it is at the morula stage.
      2. Shedding of the zona pellucida at the blastocyst stage exposes trophoblast cells, which mediate penetration of the endometrium, usually at 7 days' postovulation (day 21 of the menstrual cycle).
      3. The trophoblast differentiates into two layers.
         a. Cytotrophoblast: the inner stem cell layer
         b. Syncytiotrophoblast: the outer layer, arising from the cytotrophoblast; a true syncytium containing cell organelles for hormone synthesis (hCG and hPL)
      4. By day 11 postovulation, the blastocyst is deeply embedded within the endometrium and the syncytiotrophoblast faces spaces (lacunae) filled with maternal blood.
   B. The endometrium during pregnancy (Fig. 17-4)
      • In response to implantation, the endometrial stromal cells enlarge and become filled with glycogen and lipid, forming decidual cells.

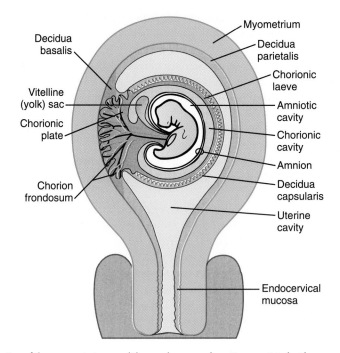

17-4: *Overview of the pregnant uterus and the membranes and cavities associated with pregnancy. The portion of the chorion containing villi (chorion frondosum) and the decidua basalis of the endometrium form the placenta.*

1. The decidua basalis, which faces the invading trophoblast in the region of vascular apposition (chorion frondosum), constitutes the maternal portion of the placenta.
   - During the fourth and fifth months, septa from the decidua basalis grow into the chorion frondosum, dividing the placenta into 10 to 35 chambers (cotyledons).
2. The decidua capsularis overlies the embryo within the uterine cavity.
3. The decidua parietalis constitutes the remainder of the decidualized endometrium.
   - Fusion of the decidua capsularis and the decidua parietalis at midpregnancy obliterates the uterine cavity.
C. The fetal portion of the placenta (chorion frondosum)
   - Villi, which develop as extensions from the chorionic plate, extend into the intervillous space (old lacunar spaces formed by the syncytiotrophoblast at implantation).
1. Structure of mature (tertiary) villi
   a. The outer syncytiotrophoblast layer has both absorptive and secretory functions.
      (1) The absorptive function is indicated by the numerous pinocytic vessels and microvilli on the surface bathed in maternal blood.

The syncytiotrophoblast, the outer layer of the fetal portion of the placenta (chorion frondosum), produces human chorionic gonadotropin and human placental lactogen.

(2) The secretory function is indicated by the well-developed endoplasmic reticulum and Golgi complex and the abundant mitochondria.

  b. The inner cytotrophoblastic layer functions primarily to supply cells to the syncytiotrophoblast.
- This layer becomes discontinuous as pregnancy proceeds, allowing the syncytiotrophoblast to sit on the basement membrane.

  c. The mesodermal connective tissue core contains fetal blood vessels and macrophages (Hofbauer cells).

2. Types and distribution of mature villi (Fig. 17-5)

  a. Anchoring (stem) villi are large villi attached to the decidua basalis.
- Cytotrophoblastic cells of the anchoring villi form an outer cytotrophoblastic shell, which is separated from maternal cells by a fibrinoid deposit.

  b. Floating (free) villi branch from the anchoring villi and float in the intervillous space, which is filled with maternal blood.

3. Placental membrane

  a. Function: a sievelike barrier through which substances can move between maternal blood in the intervillous space and fetal blood within the capillaries of the villi

  b. Components in the maternal to fetal direction:
- Syncytiotrophoblast → cytotrophoblast → basement membrane of the trophoblast epithelium → basement membrane of the fetal capillary → fetal capillary endothelium

D. Metabolic exchange across the placental membrane

1. Blood flow and gas exchange (see Fig. 17-5)

  a. Maternal arteries and veins open into the intervillous space within each cotyledon.

  b. Highly oxygenated maternal arterial blood under high hydrostatic pressure spurts toward the chorionic plate and falls over the villi.

  c. Fetal red blood cells in the capillaries of the villi take up oxygen from the maternal blood and release carbon dioxide.
- The high oxygen affinity of fetal hemoglobin facilitates gas exchange.

  d. Deoxygenated maternal blood enters the veins and is returned to the maternal lungs.

2. Other substances transported

  a. Nutrients, electrolytes, and hormones

  b. Metabolic waste products from the fetus

  c. Immunoglobulin G maternal antibodies (passive immunization of the fetus)

  d. Drugs (e.g., alcohol producing fetal alcohol syndrome) and infectious agents

  e. A small amount of blood cells
- Fetal blood cells can be separated from the maternal blood and grown in vitro for fetal karyotyping as an alternative to amniocentesis or placental biopsy.

> Fetal hemoglobin has a higher affinity for oxygen than adult hemoglobin, facilitating the transfer of oxygen from maternal red blood cells to fetal red blood cells.

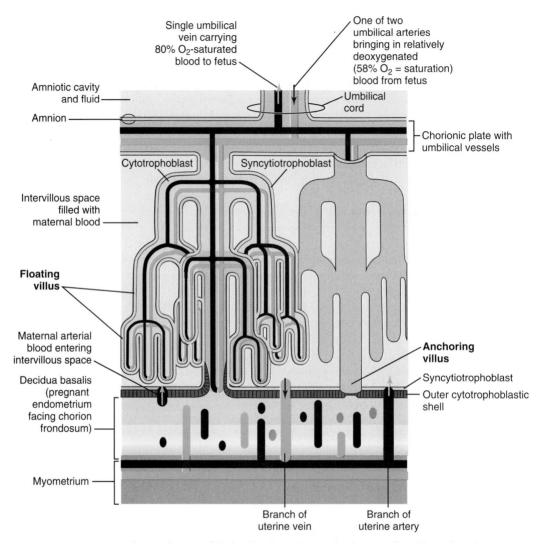

Single umbilical vein carrying 80% O$_2$-saturated blood to fetus

One of two umbilical arteries bringing in relatively deoxygenated (58% O$_2$ = saturation) blood from fetus

Amniotic cavity and fluid

Amnion

Umbilical cord

Chorionic plate with umbilical vessels

Cytotrophoblast

Syncytiotrophoblast

Intervillous space filled with maternal blood

Floating villus

Maternal arterial blood entering intervillous space

Decidua basalis (pregnant endometrium facing chorion frondosum)

Anchoring villus

Syncytiotrophoblast

Outer cytotrophoblastic shell

Myometrium

Branch of uterine vein

Branch of uterine artery

17-5: *Schematic depiction of the fetal blood vessels within the chorionic villi and their relationships to maternal blood in the intervillous space and the decidua basalis of the endometrium. When an anchoring villus contacts the decidua basalis, the cytotrophoblast "breaks through" the syncytiotrophoblast to form the outer cytotrophoblastic shell. Note that branches of the two umbilical arteries carry deoxygenated blood into the villi, whereas branches of the single umbilical vein carry oxygenated blood out of the villi.*

    3. Mechanisms of transport across the placental membrane
      a. Simple and facilitated diffusion
      b. Active transport
      c. Pinocytosis
  E. Placenta and fetal membranes in twins
    1. Fraternal (dizygotic) twins
      • Two amnions, two chorions, two placentas (may be fused)

2. Identical (monozygotic) twins
   a. Division of the embryonic disk or inner cell mass (96% of cases)
      - One or two amnions, one chorion, one placenta
   b. Earlier division of the embryo at the two-cell stage to the morula (4% of cases)
      - Two amnions, two chorions, two placentas (same as for fraternal twins)
   c. Late but incomplete division of the embryo (<0.2% of cases)
      - One amnion, one chorion, one placenta (conjoined twins)
F. Placental abnormalities
   1. Placenta accreta: trophoblastic invasion into the uterine wall due to the absence of a decidual layer
      - Results in massive hemorrhage at parturition as a result of improper separation
   2. Placenta previa: implantation in the lower segment of the uterus, overlying the cervical os
      - Associated with painless bleeding during the last trimester
   3. Abruptio placentae: premature detachment of the placenta, with a retroplacental clot
      - Often causes shock, oliguria, and disseminated intravascular coagulation in the mother and may lead to fetal death
   4. Hydatidiform mole: an abnormal enlargement of the chorionic villi early in pregnancy, resulting in a mass of cysts resembling a cluster of grapes
      - Clinically manifests as a marked increase in hCG, vaginal bleeding, an enlarged uterus, extreme nausea, and edema during the first trimester.
      - No embryo is present in complete mole (46,XX, with both X chromosomes of paternal origin).
      - A triploid embryo is present in partial mole (69,XXY).
   5. Choriocarcinoma: malignancy arising from the trophoblastic cells of fetal membranes
      - May develop from complete hydatidiform mole or after a normal pregnancy or abortion

X. Mammary Glands
   A. Anatomy of the mammary gland (Fig. 17-6)
      1. Lobes
         a. Each gland consists of 15 to 25 lobes, separated by dense connective tissue septa.
         b. Each lobe houses compound tubuloalveolar glands draining into the intralobular ducts → interlobular ducts → lactiferous sinus → lactiferous duct → nipple.
      2. Lactiferous sinuses and ducts
         a. Stratified cuboidal or columnar epithelium lines are the largest; simple cuboidal lines are the smallest.
         b. Epithelium is surrounded by loose, areolar connective tissue outside of which is dense, irregular connective tissue with adipose cells.

Placenta accreta is a connection between the fetal placenta and the uterine wall with partial or complete absence of the decidua basalis. Hemorrhage occurs on separation.

Placenta previa is attachment of the placenta to the lower uterus so it covers the os. Painless bleeding occurs.

Abruptio placentae is separation of the placenta from the uterine wall with a retroplacental clot.

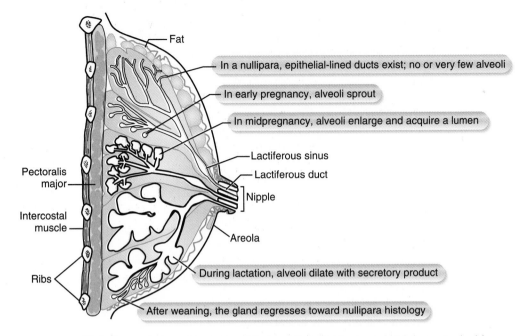

17-6: *Gross and microscopic anatomy of the breast illustrating hormone-induced changes in glandular morphology at different stages of pregnancy. Some sprouting of alveoli occurs during the secretory phase of the menstrual cycle.*

3. Alveoli
   - The dilated ends of the intralobular ducts are lined by simple cuboidal epithelium and surrounded by a discontinuous layer of stellate myoepithelial cells.
   a. In the nulliparous female
      - Few, if any, alveoli are present; some may develop and the breast may enlarge during the secretory phase of the menstrual cycle.
   b. During pregnancy
      - The alveoli undergo intense growth and development stimulated by hormones (estrogen, progesterone, and placental lactogen).
   c. During lactation
      - Alveolar epithelial cells contain cytoplasmic fat droplets and secretory granules filled with milk proteins. The lumens of the alveoli are distended with secretion.
   d. During weaning
      - The alveoli revert to the nulliparous state.
B. Production and secretion of milk
   1. Prolactin, secreted from the anterior pituitary, stimulates milk production.
      - Breastfeeding keeps prolactin levels high, thereby prolonging milk production in the postpartum period.
   2. Oxytocin stimulates contraction of the stellate myoepithelial cells, causing release of the secretion into the ducts.

- Release of oxytocin from the posterior pituitary is stimulated by suckling.
3. Colostrum, the first secretion from the breast in the postpartum period, contains less fat and more protein (e.g., antibodies) than later milk.
4. Milk secretion occurs by two mechanisms.
   a. Apocrine secretion: lipid droplets
   b. Merocrine secretion (exocytosis): milk proteins, lactose, and antibodies
C. Breast cancer
   - Ninety percent of cases arise in the ductal, not the glandular, epithelium.
   - The upper, outer quadrant is the most common location, because most breast tissue is located in that quadrant.
1. Noninfiltrating intraductal carcinoma is confined within the basement membrane (carcinoma in situ).
2. Infiltrating ductal carcinoma involves penetration of the basement membrane by malignant ductal epithelial cells.
   - It is usually accompanied by reactive fibrosis (scirrhous carcinoma) and even some calcification, giving the mass a stony, hard consistency.

Most breast cancers arise from ductal epithelium and are located in upper, outer quadrant.

Endocrine System

TARGET TOPICS

- Histology of the major endocrine organs
- Mechanisms for regulating hormone secretion
- Secretory cells of the pituitary gland
- Synthesis, storage, and release of thyroid hormones
- Regional secretory activity of the adrenal gland
- Secretory cells of the islets of Langerhans
- Primary effects of the major hormones

I. Introduction
- Endocrine signaling molecules (hormones) travel in the bloodstream (the functional "duct") from their site of secretion to target cells.
- Binding of hormone molecules to specific receptors expressed by target cells elicits specific responses within those cells.
  - A. Components of the endocrine system
    1. Several ductless glands (e.g., thyroid, adrenal, pituitary)
    2. Clusters of cells within certain organs (e.g., pancreas, ovary, testis)
    3. Scattered endocrine cells within the digestive and respiratory systems (see Table 14-2)
  - B. Major cytologic specializations of endocrine cells
    1. Polarity
       - The apex of the cell is oriented toward the blood vessel.
    2. Organelles
       a. Steroid hormone–producing cells: prominence of the smooth endoplasmic reticulum (SER)
       b. Protein or polypeptide-producing cells: prominence of the rough endoplasmic reticulum (RER)
       c. Glycoprotein-producing cells: well-developed SER and RER
  - C. Hormone storage by endocrine cells
    1. Little or no storage (released immediately after synthesis): steroid sex hormones (e.g., estrogen, testosterone)

2. Intracellular storage (cytoplasmic granules): protein and peptide hormones (e.g., insulin, oxytocin, prolactin)
3. Extracellular storage (follicles): thyroid hormones

D. Regulation of endocrine hormone secretion
1. Neural control
- Sensory input to the brain triggers nerve impulse to endocrine cells and stimulates secretion.
  a. Infant suckling at the nipple → oxytocin release
  b. Intense emotions (anger, fear) → catecholamine release
2. Direct feedback control (non-neural)
- Effect of hormone action regulates secretion by endocrine cells. Examples include:
  a. Increase in blood glucose → insulin secretion increases → blood sugar falls → insulin secretion decreases
  b. Decline in blood glucose → glucagon secretion increases → blood sugar increases → glucagon secretion decreases
  c. Decline in blood Ca^{2+} → parathyroid hormone secretion increases → blood Ca^{2+} increases → parathyroid hormone secretion decreases
3. Indirect feedback control (non-neural)
  a. The effect of hormone action or hormone level controls the release of hypothalamic hormones, which in turn regulate secretion by endocrine cells.
  b. The hypothalamo-hypophyseal-ovary axis is one example:
   - The estrogen level in the blood falls → gonadotropin-releasing hormone secretion from the hypothalamus increases → luteinizing hormone secretion increases → estrogen secretion from the ovaries increases → the estrogen level in the blood rises → gonadotropin-releasing hormone secretion decreases (Box 18-1)

II. Pituitary Gland (Hypophysis)
A. Structural and functional divisions of the hypophysis (Fig. 18-1)
1. The adenohypophysis (anterior pituitary) arises from the oral ectoderm (Rathke's pouch) and is divided into three parts:
  a. The pars distalis contains several types of endocrine cells.
  b. The pars tuberalis surrounds the infundibulum and carries portal veins of the hypophyseal portal system.
  c. The pars intermedia is rudimentary in humans.
2. The neurohypophysis (posterior pituitary) arises from the neural ectoderm and is divided into two parts:
  a. The pars nervosa contains the axon terminals of neurosecretory cells whose cell bodies lie in the hypothalamus.
  b. The infundibulum connects the pars nervosa to the hypothalamus and carries the axons of the hypothalamic neurosecretory cells.
B. Hypophyseal portal system
1. Components (see Fig. 18-1)
  a. The primary capillary plexus in the median eminence arises from the superior hypophyseal arteries.

Mechanisms for controlling hormone secretion:
- Neural impulses to the secreting cells (e.g., oxytocin, catecholamines)
- Direct feedback control on the secreting cells (e.g., insulin, glucagon)
- Indirect feedback control via the hypothalamus on the secreting cells (e.g., estrogen, thyroid hormones)

BOX 18-1

HORMONE ABBREVIATIONS

Hypothalamic Regulatory Hormones

CRH = corticotropin-releasing hormone
GnRH = gonadotropin-releasing hormone
PIF = prolactin-inhibiting factor (dopamine)
PSF = prolactin-stimulating factor
SRH = somatotropin-releasing hormone
TRH = thyrotropin-releasing hormone

Other Hormones

ACTH = adrenocorticotropic hormone
ADH = antidiuretic hormone (vasopressin)
FSH = follicle-stimulating hormone
GH = growth hormone
LH = luteinizing hormone
PTH = parathyroid hormone
T_3 = triiodothyronine
T_4 = thyroxine
TSH = thyroid-stimulating hormone

  b. The secondary capillary plexus surrounds the endocrine cells of the pars distalis.
  c. Portal veins (one to three) in the pars tuberalis carry blood from the primary to the secondary plexus.
 2. Hypothalamic regulation of the anterior pituitary
  • Finely tuned feedback regulatory systems, involving the hypophyseal portal system, control hormone secretion from the adenohypophysis.
  • The hypothalamo-hypophyseal-thyroid axis illustrated in Figure 18-2 is one example. The hypothalamo-hypophyseal-ovary axis is another example (see Fig. 17-2).
  a. Releasing hormones (see Box 18-1), which are produced in the cell bodies of hypothalamic neurosecretory cells, are released from axon terminals in the median eminence and enter the primary capillary plexus.
  b. After transport by portal veins to the secondary capillary plexus, the hormones enter tissue fluid and act on specific endocrine cells in the anterior pituitary to control their secretion.
  c. Blood levels of hormones (or other physiologic factors) in turn control the secretory activity of hypothalamic cells.
 C. Secretory activity of the adenohypophysis
  • In humans, the pars distalis is the primary source of anterior pituitary hormones, although the pars tuberalis contains some endocrine cells.

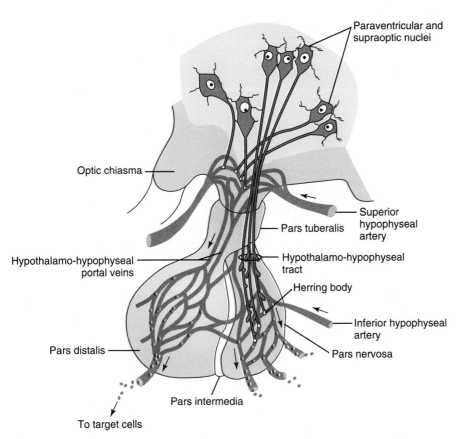

Optic chiasma

Hypothalamo-hypophyseal portal veins

Pars distalis

Pars intermedia

To target cells

Paraventricular and supraoptic nuclei

Superior hypophyseal artery

Pars tuberalis

Hypothalamo-hypophyseal tract

Herring body

Inferior hypophyseal artery

Pars nervosa

18-1: *Drawing of the hypophysis showing its relationship to the hypothalamus and to vascularization.*

- Secretory cells, classified as acidophils or basophils, are filled with hormone-containing secretory granules of varying size, abundance, and staining properties.
1. Acidophil secretions
   a. Mammotrophs → prolactin
   b. Somatotrophs → growth hormone (somatotropin)
2. Basophil secretions
   a. Corticotrophs → adrenocorticotropic hormone
   b. Gonadotrophs → follicle-stimulating hormone and luteinizing hormone
   c. Thyrotrophs → thyroid-stimulating hormone
3. Exocytosis of the secretory granules is stimulated or inhibited by hypothalamic hormones delivered by the hypophyseal portal system (see Box 18-1).
4. Actions of the anterior pituitary hormones (Table 18-1)
   - With the exception of prolactin and growth hormone, the anterior pituitary hormones directly or indirectly promote the production of other hormones.

The anterior pituitary hormones and their target organs are as follows: adrenocorticotropic hormone, adrenal cortex; thyroid-stimulating hormone, thyroid gland; follicle-stimulating hormone, ovary and testis; luteinizing hormone, ovary and testis; growth hormone, all tissues; prolactin, breast.

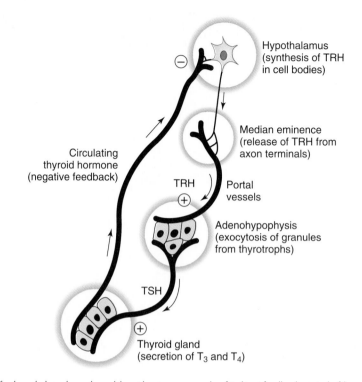

18-2: *The hypothalamo-hypophyseal-thyroid axis, an example of indirect feedback control of hormone secretion from the adenohypophysis. Synthesis and secretion of thyrotropin-releasing hormone (TRH) is stimulated by low blood levels of thyroid hormones (T_3 and T_4). TRH promotes the secretion (+) of thyroid-stimulating hormone (TSH) from endocrine cells in the adenohypophysis. TSH acts on the thyroid gland to stimulate the secretion of T_3 and T_4, leading to a rise in the blood level of these hormones, which inhibits (–) TRH-producing hypothalamic cells.*

D. Secretory activity of the pars nervosa (see Table 18-1)
   1. Pituicytes are stromal cells analogous to the glial cells of the central nervous system.
   2. The distal ends of the hypothalamic neurosecretory cells constitute the parenchyma of the pars distalis (see Fig. 18-1).

The posterior pituitary hormones and their target organs are as follows: antidiuretic hormone (vasopressin), kidney and smooth muscle; oxytocin, breast and uterus.

      a. Cell bodies, located in the paraventricular and supraoptic nuclei of the hypothalamus, synthesize either oxytocin or antidiuretic hormone (vasopressin).
      b. Hormones are transported down the long axons of these neurons, the hypothalamo-hypophyseal tract, to axon terminals where secretory granules accumulate, forming Herring bodies.
   3. Hormone release is under neural control.

III. Thyroid Gland
   A. Thyroid follicles are spherical structures lined by follicular epithelial cells and filled with colloid, a viscous gel composed primarily of iodinated thyroglobulin.

TABLE 18-1:
**Major
Hypophyseal
Hormones in
Humans**

Hormone	Regulated by*	Target Organ/Tissue: Major Effects†
Anterior Pituitary (Pars Distalis)		
ACTH	↑ CRH ↓ Somatostatin	Adrenal cortex: synthesis/secretion of glucocorticoids, androgens, estrogens
FSH	↑ GnRH ↓ Testosterone, estrogen, inhibin	Ovary: maturation of follicle; synthesis of estrogen Testis: secretion of androgen-binding protein and inhibin by Sertoli cells
LH	↑ LH, high estrogen ↓ Progesterone, testosterone	Ovary: final maturation of follicles; ovulation; formation of corpus luteum Testis: synthesis/secretion of testosterone by Leydig cells
TSH	↑ TRH ↓ Somatostatin	Thyroid gland: synthesis/secretion of thyroid hormone (T_3, T_4)
GH (somatotropin)	↑ SRH, hypoglycemia, stress, exercise ↓ Somatostatin, hyperglycemia	Liver: secretion of IGF-1, which stimulates growth (epiphyseal plates and soft tissue) All tissues: RNA and protein synthesis, tissue growth, transport of glucose and amino acids into cells
Prolactin	↑ PSF ↓ PIF (dopamine)	Mammary gland: production/ secretion of milk; breast development
Posterior Pituitary (Pars Nervosa)		
ADH (vasopressin)	↑ High blood osmolarity ↓ Low blood osmolarity	Kidney collecting ducts: water resorption Vascular smooth muscle: contraction
Oxytocin	↑ Suckling, cervical dilation ↓ Progesterone, alcohol	Mammary glands: milk ejection (milk letdown) Uterine smooth muscle: contraction

*↑, stimulation of secretion; ↓, inhibition of secretion.
†In all cases, the indicated effect is stimulated by the corresponding hormone.
ACTH, adrenocorticotropic hormone; ADH, antidiuretic hormone's CRH, corticotropin-releasing hormone; FSH, follicle-stimulating hormone; GH, growth hormone; GnRH, IGF = 1, LH, luteinizing hormone; PIF, prolactin-inhibiting factor (dopamine); PSF, prolactin-stimulating factor; RNA, ribonucleic acid; SRH, somatotropin-releasing hormone; T_3, triiodithyronine; T_4, thyroxine; TSH, thyroid-stimulating hormone.

- Colloid functions as an extracellular storage site for thyroid hormones.
B. Follicular cells are derived from the endoderm of the thyroglossal duct.
  1. They have low cuboidal to squamous morphology when synthesizing and releasing thyroglobulin into the colloid (Fig. 18-3A).
     a. Iodide from the blood is imported and transported to the follicular lumen.
     b. Thyroid peroxidase in the apical membrane iodinates the tyrosine residues of thyroglobulin extracellularly.
  2. They have tall columnar morphology when liberating thyroid hormones from thyroglobulin (Fig. 18-3B).

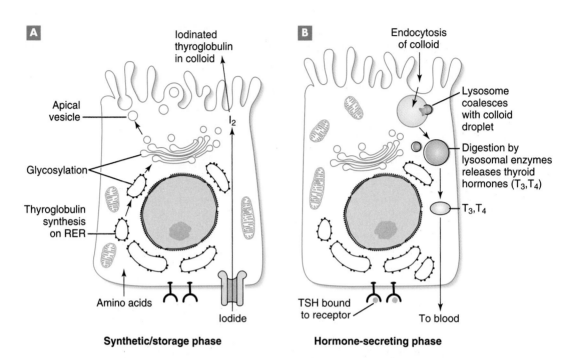

18-3: *Synthesis, storage, and secretion of thyroid hormone by follicular cells. **A,** Follicular cells produce iodinated thyroglobulin, the major component of the viscous colloid that fills the lumen of thyroid follicles. Oxidation of iodide to iodine (I_2) and iodination of thyroglobulin are catalyzed by an enzyme localized near the apical membrane. **B,** In the presence of thyroid-stimulating hormone (TSH), follicular cells release thyroid hormones from thyroglobulin and secrete T_3 and T_4 (major fraction) from the basal surface into the blood. RER, rough endoplasmic reticulum.*

a. Under stimulation by thyroid-stimulating hormone, colloid is endocytosed.
b. Lysosomal enzymes degrade iodinated thyroglobulin, releasing primarily T_4, the prohormone form of the more biologically active T_3.
c. T_3 and T_4 (major fraction) are released from the basal surface and enter the capillaries.
   • T_4 is deiodinated in the peripheral tissues (e.g., liver, kidney, heart) to T_3.
   • The major effect of the thyroid hormones is to accelerate the basal metabolic rate, which leads to an increase in heat production.

Thyroid-stimulating hormone promotes the production of thyroglobulin and the release of T_3 and T_4.

C. Parafollicular cells, also known as clear (C) cells, are derived from the endoderm of the ultimobranchial body, a diverticulum of the fifth pharyngeal pouch.
   1. Location: C cells are interspersed between the follicular cells and the basal lamina at the periphery of the follicles, with their apex oriented away from the follicular lumen; they never reach the lumen.
   2. Secretion: In response to an increase in the blood Ca^{2+} level, C cells secrete calcitonin, which suppresses bone reabsorption, leading to a decrease in blood Ca^{2+}.

IV. Parathyroid Glands
- The parenchyma of the inferior and superior parathyroid glands is derived from the endoderm of the third and fourth pharyngeal pouches, respectively.

Parathyroid hormone excess → hypercalcemia and hypophosphatemia

  A. The chief (principal) cells secrete parathyroid hormone.
    1. Active cells have dark cytoplasm with numerous granules and well-developed Golgi and RER.
    2. Inactive cells have light cytoplasm with few granules and less prominent Golgi and RER.
      - The normal ratio of inactive to active cells is 3:1.
  B. Parathyroid hormone secretion is stimulated by a decline in the blood Ca^{2+} level.
    - Parathyroid hormone raises the blood Ca^{2+} level by promoting the release of osteoclast-activating factor from the osteoblasts, decreasing Ca^{2+} excretion by the kidneys, and, with vitamin D, promoting the intestinal absorption of Ca^{2+}.

Parathyroid hormone deficiency → hypocalcemia and hyperphosphatemia

V. Adrenal Glands
  A. Structural and functional divisions of the adrenal glands
    1. The cortex is derived from the mesodermal root of the dorsal mesentery.
      - The parenchyma is divided into three regions that synthesize and secrete different steroid hormones.
    2. The medulla is derived from the neural crest cells.
      - Parenchymal cells secrete catecholamines (epinephrine and norepinephrine).
  B. Secretory activity of the adrenal cortex (Fig. 18-4)
    1. Zona glomerulosa: a superficial region constituting approximately 15% of the cortical volume
      a. Parenchymal cells are arranged in clumps or glomerular masses.
      b. Mineralocorticoids secreted by these cells (e.g., aldosterone) regulate the balance of electrolytes and water via their action on the renal tubules (see Fig. 15-6).
        - Atrial natriuretic peptide increases the secretion of water and sodium in the kidneys, antagonistic to the effect of aldosterone.

Regions of the adrenal cortex from outside to inside:

- Zona glomerulosa → aldosterone (mineralocorticoids)
- Zona fasciculata → cortisol (glucocorticoids)
- Zona reticularis → androgens and estrogens

    2. Zona fasciculata: the middle region, constituting approximately 78% of the cortical volume
      a. Parenchymal cells are arranged in cords that project radially inward from the zona glomerulosa.
      b. Glucocorticoids secreted by these cells (e.g., cortisol) primarily regulate carbohydrate metabolism but have numerous other effects.
    3. Zona reticularis: the deepest region, constituting approximately 7% of the cortical volume
      a. Parenchymal cells are arranged in anastomosing cords between the zona fasciculata and the medulla.
      b. Androgens and estrogens are produced in this zone in both sexes, supplementing those produced in the gonads.

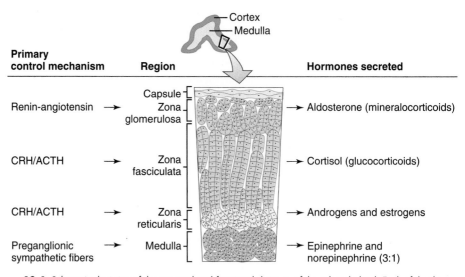

Primary control mechanism	Region	Hormones secreted
Cortex		
Medulla		
Renin-angiotensin →	Capsule, Zona glomerulosa	→ Aldosterone (mineralocorticoids)
CRH/ACTH →	Zona fasciculata	→ Cortisol (glucocorticoids)
CRH/ACTH →	Zona reticularis	→ Androgens and estrogens
Preganglionic sympathetic fibers →	Medulla	→ Epinephrine and norepinephrine (3:1)

18-4: *Schematic depiction of the structural and functional divisions of the adrenal gland. Each of the three zones of the cortex secretes characteristic hormones, as does the medulla. CRH/ACTH refers to the hypothalamo-hypophyseal-adrenal axis involving corticotropin-releasing hormone (CRH) and adrenocorticotropic hormone (ACTH). See Figure 15-6 for renin-angiotensin control of aldosterone secretion.*

The adrenal medulla, derived from the neural crest cells, produces epinephrine and norepinephrine in a 3:1 ratio.

C. Secretory activity of the adrenal medulla
  1. Chromaffin cells are modified postganglionic sympathetic neurons that synthesize, store, and secrete catecholamines.
    a. Norepinephrine-producing cells (25% of the total) contain heterogeneous granules, with a very electron-dense core surrounded by a pale halo.
    b. Epinephrine-producing cells (75% of the total) contain small, homogeneous, electron-dense granules.
  2. Catecholamine release is triggered by stimulation from preganglionic sympathetic axons that synapse on chromaffin cells.
    a. Neural stimulation, and hence secretion, increases in situations of fear, anger, and stress.
    b. A subsequent fight-or-flight response, mediated by epinephrine and norepinephrine, is marked by increased heart rate, blood pressure, and glycogenolysis.

The fight-or-flight response is mediated by epinephrine and norepinephrine: ↑ heart rate, ↑ blood pressure, ↑ glycogenolysis.

VI. Pancreatic Islets of Langerhans
  • The pancreas contains clusters, or islets, of endodermal-derived endocrine cells scattered among its exocrine secretory acini (see Chapter 14).
  • The islets are most numerous in the tail of the pancreas.
  A. Alpha (A, α) cells secrete glucagon, which promotes the breakdown of glycogen to glucose in the liver.
    • Glucagon has a hyperglycemic effect that is antagonistic to insulin.
  B. Beta (B, β) cells secrete insulin, which acts on the plasma membrane of most cells to increase the transport of glucose from the blood into the cells.
    • Insulin has a hypoglycemic effect that is antagonistic to glucagon.

C. Delta (D, δ) cells secrete somatostatin, which acts in two ways.
1. Paracrine effect: inhibition of glucagon and insulin release from the A and B cells of the pancreas
2. Endocrine effect: inhibition of growth hormone release from the pars distalis

VII. Pineal Gland (Epiphysis Cerebri)
A. Pinealocytes (parenchymal cells) are derived from the neural ectoderm.
- Produce melatonin from serotonin
- Possess long cellular processes that terminate in bulbous expansions near capillaries
B. Melatonin secretion is stimulated by neural impulses originating in areas of the central nervous system and reaching the pineal gland via postganglionic sympathetic fibers.
C. Circadian fluctuation in melatonin levels
- Under normal light–dark conditions, the blood melatonin level is threefold higher during the night than during the day.
D. Antigonadotropic effect of melatonin
1. Destruction of the pineal gland during childhood causes precocious sexual development.
2. Administration of melatonin to a child delays the onset of puberty.

VIII. Summary of Major Nonpituitary Hormones (Table 18-2)

Secretions of the pancreatic islet cells:
- α cells → glucagon
- β cells → insulin
- δ cells → somatostatin

The hypoglycemic effect of insulin is antagonistic to the hyperglycemic effect of glucagon.

The melatonin level is highest during the nocturnal phase; it is lowest during the diurnal phase.

TABLE 18-2:
Major Nonpituitary Hormones

Target Organ/Tissue: Origin/Hormone	Regulated by*	Major Effects†
Thyroid Gland		
T_3, T_4	↑ TSH ↓ Somatostatin, high thyroid hormones (T_3, T_4)	Most cells: ↑ basal metabolic rate, cardiac output, and nutrient utilization
Calcitonin	↑ High blood Ca^{2+} ↓ Low blood Ca^{2+}	Bones: ↓ resorption
Parathyroid Glands		
PTH	↑ Low blood Ca^{2+} ↓ High blood Ca^{2+}, very low blood Mg^{2+}	Bones: ↑ resorption Kidneys: ↓ Ca^{2+} excretion Intestine: ↑ Ca^{2+} absorption (with vitamin D)
Adrenal Glands		
Aldosterone (mineralocorticoids)	↑ Angiotensin II, low blood volume ↓ Fluid overload	Distal kidney tubules: ↑ reabsorption of Na^+ (and thus of H_2O) and K^+ secretion

continued

TABLE 18-2:
Major Nonpituitary Hormones—cont'd

Target Organ/Tissue: Origin/Hormone	Regulated by*	Major Effects†
Adrenal Glands—cont'd		
Cortisol (glucocorticoids)	↑ ACTH, stress ↓ High cortisol	Liver: ↑ gluconeogenesis to raise blood sugar Adipose tissue: ↑ breakdown of triglycerides Various tissues: anti-inflammatory effects
Epinephrine and norepinephrine	↑ Sympathetic stimulation in response to fear, anger, stress	Most tissues: ↑ cardiac output, vasoconstriction, glycogenolysis (hyperglycemic effect), and lipolysis
Pancreatic Islets		
Glucagon (α cells)	↑ Low blood glucose ↓ High blood glucose, somatostatin	Liver: ↑ glycogenolysis (hyperglycemic effect) and gluconeogenesis Adipose tissue: ↑ lipolysis
Insulin (β cells)	↑ High blood glucose and amino acids ↓ Low blood glucose, somatostatin	Muscle and adipose tissue: ↑ uptake of blood glucose (hypoglycemic effect) and amino acids into cells; ↑ protein synthesis Adipose tissue: ↓ lipolysis; ↑ fat deposition
Somatostatin (δ cells)‡	↑ High hormone levels	Pancreatic α and β cells: ↓ secretion of glucagon and insulin Pars distalis: ↓ secretion of GH, TSH, and ACTH Gastrointestinal tract: ↓ secretion of gastrin and secretin
Pineal Gland		
Melatonin	↑ Light exposure	Gonads: ↓ development
Testis		
Testosterone (Leydig cells)	↑ LH ↓ High testosterone	Seminiferous tubules: ↑ spermatogenesis Other tissues: ↑ development and maintenance of male sex characteristics
Ovary		
Estrogen (follicles and corpus luteum)	↑ FSH ↓ High estrogen	Uterus: ↑ rebuilding of endometrium after menses Other tissues: ↑ development and maintenance of female sex characteristics

TABLE 18-2:
Major Nonpituitary Hormones—cont'd

Target Organ/Tissue: Origin/Hormone	Regulated by*	Major Effects†
Ovary—cont'd		
Progesterone (corpus luteum)	↑ LH ↓ High progesterone	Uterus: ↑ secretory phase of menstrual cycle; ↓ uterine contractions Breast: ↑ development of alveoli during pregnancy
Gastrointestinal Tract		
See Table 14-2		

*↑, Stimulation of hormone secretion; ↓, inhibition of secretion.
†↑, Stimulation of indicated effect; ↓, inhibition of indicated effect.
‡Also secreted by the hypothalamus.
ACTH, adrenocorticotropic hormone; FSH, follicle-stimulating hormone; GH, growth hormone; LH, luteinizing hormone; PTH, parathyroid hormone; T_3, triiodithyronine; T_4, thyroxine; TSH, thyroid-stimulating hormone.

Sense Organs

TARGET TOPICS

- Chambers and tunics of the eye
- Layers of the retina and their functions
- Accommodation for near and distant vision
- Structure and histophysiology of the vestibular organ
- Structure and histophysiology of the auditory organ
- Wilson's disease, glaucoma, lens defects, retinal disorders, Horner's syndrome, conjunctivitis, otitis media, hearing loss, Ménière's disease

I. Eye
  A. Tunics of the eye (Fig. 19-1)
    1. Retina (innermost tunic)
      a. Photosensitive region: posterior to the ora serrata
        (1) Optic disc: the region on the posterior aspect of the eye where the optic nerve exits
          • Possesses no photosensitive retina and constitutes the blind spot
        (2) Fovea centralis: located approximately 2.5 mm lateral to the optic disc in the area of the retina containing yellow pigment (macula lutea)
          • Contains only cones and exhibits the most acute vision
      b. Nonphotosensitive region: anterior to the ora serrata
        • Consists of two cell layers covering the iris, ciliary body, and ciliary processes
    2. Uvea (middle layer)
      a. Choroid: highly vascular connective tissue layer containing the melanocytes
        (1) The choriocapillaris, the inner choroid zone, contains small blood vessels that supply the cells of the retina.
        (2) Bruch's membrane, composed of the fused basal laminae of the choriocapillaris and the pigmented epithelium of the retina, constitutes the choroid's inner aspect.
      b. Ciliary body: a wedge-shaped expansion of the choroid peripheral to the lens

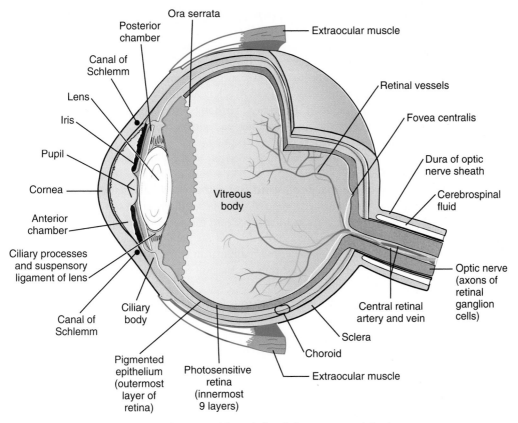

Posterior chamber
Ora serrata
Extraocular muscle
Canal of Schlemm
Lens
Iris
Pupil
Cornea
Anterior chamber
Ciliary processes and suspensory ligament of lens
Canal of Schlemm
Ciliary body
Pigmented epithelium (outermost layer of retina)
Photosensitive retina (innermost 9 layers)
Vitreous body
Extraocular muscle
Choroid
Sclera
Central retinal artery and vein
Optic nerve (axons of retinal ganglion cells)
Cerebrospinal fluid
Dura of optic nerve sheath
Fovea centralis
Retinal vessels

19-1: *General anatomy of the eyeball, including its tunics and chambers.*

(1) The ciliary processes project toward the lens.
(2) The suspensory ligaments of Zinn (zonula ciliaris) extend from the ciliary processes to just behind the equator of the lens, anchoring the lens in place.
(3) The ciliary muscle, a circular mass of smooth muscle innervated by parasympathetic neurons, changes the shape of the lens by relaxing and contracting.

c. Iris: the portion of the uvea anterior to the lens that separates the anterior and posterior chambers and contains a central aperture, the pupil
(1) Contraction of the dilator pupillae muscle (sympathetic stimulation) dilates the pupil.
(2) Contraction of the sphincter pupillae muscle (parasympathetic stimulation) constricts the pupil.

3. Fibrous tunic (outer layer)
a. Sclera: a dense, collagenous connective tissue that forms the external layer of the posterior five sixths of the eyeball and receives the insertions of the extraocular muscles

Sympathetic impulses → dilation of pupil. Parasympathetic impulses → constriction of pupil.

Congenital absence of the iris (aniridia) is commonly associated with Wilms' tumor, a rapidly developing carcinoma of the kidneys.

b. Cornea: the transparent, avascular anterior portion of the fibrous tunic, composed of the corneal epithelium, Bowman's (basement) membrane, the substantia propria (fibroblasts and collagen fibers), Descemet's (basement) membrane, and the corneal endothelium

c. Wilson's disease (hepatolenticular degeneration): abnormality of copper processing that can lead to a Kayser-Fleischer ring (brown or green coloration of the cornea), cirrhosis of the liver, and degeneration of neurons in the central nervous system

B. Chambers of the eye
1. Anterior chamber: located posterior to the cornea and anterior to the iris
2. Posterior chamber: located posterior to the iris and anterior to the lens
   a. Unpigmented epithelial cells of the ciliary retina secrete aqueous humor, a plasma-like fluid, into the posterior chamber.
   b. Aqueous humor flows through the pupil to the anterior chamber and then drains through a trabecular meshwork at the corneoscleral junction (limbus) into the canal of Schlemm and eventually into the episcleral veins.
3. Vitreal cavity: located posterior to the lens and bordered by the retina
   • Contains the vitreous body, a structureless gelatinous mass that is 99% water
4. Glaucoma: any condition characterized by increased intraocular pressure
   • Compromised drainage of aqueous humor from the anterior chamber is associated with most types of glaucoma.

C. Lens of the eye
   • The lens, a biconvex avascular structure located behind the iris, receives nourishment from the aqueous humor and vitreous body.
1. Structural components
   a. The capsule, the carbohydrate-rich external layer of the lens, contains type IV collagen and glycoproteins. It is underlain anteriorly by a simple cuboidal epithelium.
   b. Lens fibers—elongated, anucleated, six-sided cells (prisms)—fill the core of the lens.
   c. A cataract, an opacity of the lens or lens capsule that obstructs the passage of light, results in impaired vision or blindness.
2. Accommodation of the lens
   • Because of the natural elasticity of the lens, its shape can change to adjust to viewing objects at different distances.
   a. Distant vision
      (1) A thin, stretched lens can focus light rays from distant objects but not near objects.
      (2) When the ciliary muscle is relaxed, tension is placed on the suspensory ligament, causing the lens to flatten = accommodation for distant vision.
   b. Near vision
      (1) A thick, unstretched lens can refract (bend) light rays enough to focus on near objects.

Kayser-Fleischer ring is a golden brown or green discoloration at the outer margin of the cornea that is seen in Wilson's disease.

Glaucoma is marked by increased intraocular pressure caused by excess aqueous humor.

A cataract is an alteration in the lens core or capsule that interferes with light transmission. The most common type is associated with aging.

For near accommodation, the ciliary and sphincter muscles contract, the pupil becomes smaller, and the lens becomes thicker. For far accommodation, the ciliary and sphincter muscles relax, the pupil becomes larger, and the lens becomes thinner.

(2) When the ciliary muscle is contracted, tension on the suspensory ligament is released and the lens becomes more spherical = accommodation for near vision.

(3) Reading for long periods requires constant contraction of the ciliary muscle = tired eyes.

3. Lens defects affecting focusing of light
   a. Myopia (nearsightedness): inability to focus on distant objects
      • Entering light rays are brought into focus in front of the retina. It is corrected by a concave lens.
   b. Hyperopia (farsightedness): inability to focus on near objects
      • Entering light rays are brought into focus behind the retina. It is corrected by a convex lens.
   c. Presbyopia: inability to focus on near objects (hyperopia) due to decreased elasticity of the lens, which commonly occurs with aging. It is corrected by a convex lens.

D. Histology of the retina
   1. Retinal layers
      • The 10 named layers of the retina are shown in Figure 19-2.
      • The outer pigmented layer, adjacent to the choroid, is derived from the outer layer of the optic cup; all the other layers are derived from the inner layer of the optic cup.
   2. Photosensitive cells (first-order neurons)
      • Cell bodies of the rods and cones are located in the outer nuclear layer.
      • Except in the region of the fovea centralis, rods are much more numerous than cones.
      a. Rods are sensitive to low-intensity light and are responsible for black-and-white vision.

> The rods are used for low-light, black-and-white vision; the cones are used for high-light, acute vision and color perception.

         (1) The outer segment is filled with membranous lamellae that are not continuous with the covering plasmalemma. The lamellae contain photosensitive rhodopsin (visual purple).
         (2) The inner segment possesses numerous mitochondria as well as glycogen, rough endoplasmic reticulum, and Golgi complexes. It exhibits metabolic activity and protein synthesis.
         (3) Axons from as many as 100 rods synapse with a single bipolar cell in the outer plexiform layer.
         (4) *Dark adaptation* refers to the increase in the photosensitivity of rhodopsin that occurs when an individual moves from bright light to dim light; this process takes some time.
      b. Cones are sensitive to high-intensity light and produce greater visual acuity than rods; they are responsible for color vision.
         (1) The outer segment is filled with membranous lamellae that are continuous with the covering plasmalemma. The lamellae contain one of three different iodopsins, which differ in their sensitivity to red, blue, and green light.
         (2) The inner segment is a synthetic region with many mitochondria and protein-synthesizing organelles.

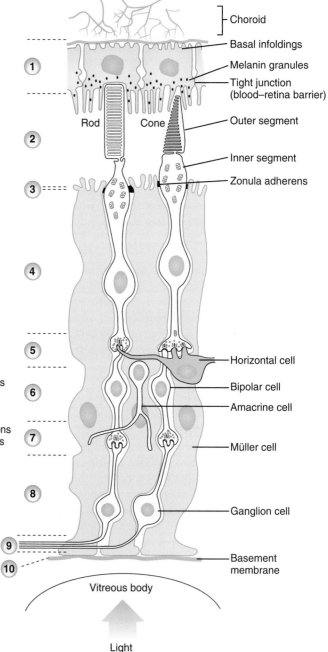

Pigmented epithelium: epithelial cells and Bruch's membrane (basement membrane)

Photoreceptor layer: inner and outer segments of rods and cones

External limiting membrane: adherens junctions between rods and cones and Müller cells

Outer nuclear layer: cell bodies of rods and cones (first-order neurons)

Outer plexiform layer: synapses between axons of rods and cones and dendrites of bipolar neurons and horizontal cells

Inner nuclear layer: cell bodies of bipolar cells (second-order neurons) and of horizontal, amacrine, and Müller cells

Inner plexiform layer: synapses between axons of bipolar cells and dendrites of ganglion cells

Ganglion cell layer: cell bodies of ganglion cells (third-order neurons)

Optic nerve layer: axons of ganglion cells

Internal limiting membrane: terminations of Müller cell processes and their basement membrane

19-2: Diagram of the 10 layers of the retina. Light enters through the internal limiting membrane, adjacent to the vitreous body, and passes through all of the intervening layers to the outer segments of rods and cones, which contain light-absorbing pigments. Absorption of light generates nerve impulses that are transmitted back through the layers via bipolar and ganglion cells, exiting the retina in the axons of ganglion cells (layer 9).

         (3) Each cone synapses with a single bipolar cell (in contrast, each rod may synapse with several bipolar neurons).

  3. Other retinal cells (see Fig. 19-2)

    a. Pigmented epithelial cells: the outer layer adjacent to the choroid

       (1) Synthesize melanin, which prevents reflection from the uvea and sclera

       (2) Have apical processes that surround and protect the photosensitive outer segments of the rods and cones

       (3) Phagocytose lamellae shed from the rods and cones and degrade them in the lysosomes

       (4) Are connected by tight junctions, forming the blood–retina barrier, which prevents blood from the choroid from reaching the retina

       (5) Esterify vitamin A, which is transported to the rods and cones and is used in the formation of photosensitive pigments

    b. Bipolar cells: second-order neurons with which rods and cones synapse

    c. Ganglion cells: multipolar third-order neurons whose long axons eventually are collected as the fibers of the optic nerve

    d. Horizontal cells: interneurons that connect the rods and cones with each other and with the bipolar neurons

    e. Amacrine cells: interneurons that connect the ganglion cells and bipolar neurons

    f. Müller cells: irregularly branched, neuroglial cells that extend to most layers of the retina

       (1) The zonulae adherens between the Müller cells and the rods and cones form the external limiting membrane.

       (2) The innermost terminations of the Müller cell processes and their basement membrane form the internal limiting membrane.

  4. Disorders of the retina

    a. Retinal detachment can result from seepage of vitreous fluid or blood through the retina, leading to separation of the pigmented epithelial layer from all the sensory layers.

      • Develops slowly, generally after age 40 years

      • Often initially marked by the appearance of numerous floating spots in front of the affected eye, later progressing to a shadow that gradually comes over the eye

    b. Macular degeneration entails a progressive breakdown of the macula lutea, leading to gradual loss of central vision (fine detail), usually with preservation of peripheral vision.

      • Initial symptoms include blurred vision, distortion of vertical straight lines, and worsening color vision.

    c. Retinoblastoma results from loss of function of the *RB* gene, a tumor-suppressor gene.

      • Most cases occur in young children; initial symptoms include a red, painful eye; leukokoria (cat's eye reflex); and squinting.

E. Accessory structures of the eye

  1. Eyelid

    a. The anterior surface is covered with skin.

> Retinal detachment is separation of the pigmented epithelium from the remaining retinal layers. The patient senses floating spots and then gradually an enlarging shadow over the eye.

(1) The glands of Zeiss are sebaceous glands associated with the eyelashes.

(2) The glands of Moll are sweat glands whose ducts open into the eyelash follicles.

b. The palpebral fascia (tarsal plate) constitutes the fibrous core of the eyelids.

(1) Sympathetic stimulation causes chronic contraction of the superior tarsal muscle attached to the fascia of the upper lid, causing elevation of the upper eyelid.

(2) Meibomian glands are sebaceous glands, not associated with hair follicles, that open in front of the free edge of the lid. Their secretion keeps a normal tear film in the eye.

c. The palpebral conjunctiva, a stratified columnar or squamous epithelium containing many goblet cells, lines the inner surface of the eyelids.

(1) The bulbar conjunctiva, covering the eyeball, is similar to and continuous with the palpebral conjunctiva.

(2) "Lost" contact lenses become lodged at junctions between two conjunctivae, the superior and inferior fornices.

d. Horner's ptosis (drooping of the upper lid) results from loss of sympathetic innervation to the superior tarsal muscle.

e. Horner's syndrome includes ptosis, miosis (small pupil), and anhydrosis (loss of sweating) on the affected side of the face.

- Both Horner's ptosis and Horner's syndrome may indicate invasion of lung carcinoma and destruction of the cervical sympathetic chain on the ipsilateral side.

f. A stye (hordeolum) is a localized inflammatory infection of one or more sebaceous glands (meibomian or zeisian) in the eyelid, commonly caused by staphylococci.

g. Conjunctivitis, inflammation of the palpebral or bulbar conjunctivae, is caused by infection or allergy.

- Common symptoms are thick discharge, sticky eyelids, and red eyes.

2. Lacrimal apparatus

a. The lacrimal gland is a tubuloalveolar exocrine gland.

- Serous acini produce tears, which contain lysozyme (a bactericidal substance).

b. Ducts drain into the fornices of the superior conjunctival sac, so that tears wash the anterior surface of the eye, keeping the cornea and conjunctiva moist.

c. Tears collected in the lacrimal ducts → sac → nasolacrimal duct.

II. Ear

A. Outer ear

1. Auricle

- A core of elastic cartilage is covered by thin skin (keratinized stratified squamous epithelium).

Horner's syndrome = ptosis (droopy upper eyelid) + miosis (contracted pupil) + anhydrosis (lack of sweating). It may be a sign of metastatic lung carcinoma.

2. External auditory meatus and canal
   a. The wall is composed of elastic cartilage in its outer third and bone in its inner two thirds.
   b. Stratified squamous epithelium lining the canal contains sebaceous glands and modified sweat glands (ceruminous glands).
      • Combined secretions form earwax.
3. Tympanic membrane (eardrum)
   • The eardrum delimits the external auditory canal medially and separates it from the middle ear.
   a. The core is formed of connective tissue (from the mesoderm) that is vascularized and innervated.
   b. The external surface is covered by thin skin derived from the ectoderm of the first branchial groove.
   c. The inner surface is covered by simple cuboidal epithelium derived from the first pharyngeal pouch.

B. Middle ear (tympanic cavity)
   1. The auditory (eustachian) tube, derived from the first pharyngeal pouch, connects the middle ear with the nasopharynx.
   2. The oval and round windows are membrane-covered regions in the bony surface of the middle ear, separating it from the inner ear.
   3. The auditory ossicles traverse the tympanic cavity and transmit movements of the tympanic membrane to the oval window. From lateral to medial:
      a. Malleus (attached to the tympanic membrane)
      b. Incus
      c. Stapes (the medial end inserted into the oval window)
   4. The tensor tympani and stapedius muscles insert into the malleus and stapes, respectively.
      • Reflex contraction of these muscles in response to loud sounds dampens vibrations of the auditory ossicles.

C. Inner ear
   1. Bony labyrinth: a complicated system of canals and chambers in the bone, including the semicircular canals, cochlea, scala vestibuli, and scala tympani
      • Filled with perilymph, which is high in sodium
   2. Membranous labyrinth: various membranous structures, suspended inside the bony labyrinth, that function as auditory or vestibular organs
      • Filled with endolymph, which is high in potassium
   3. Vestibular organ: patches of special sensory epithelium that responds to changes in position (Fig. 19-3)
      a. Maculae of the saccule and utricle
         (1) The epithelium contains columnar supporting cells and vestibular hair cells with numerous stereocilia and a single kinocilium on their apical surface.
         (2) Afferent nerve endings contact the hair cells.
         (3) The otolithic membrane, a gelatinous mass containing calcium carbonate crystals (otoliths), overlies the epithelium.

Surface layers of the eardrum: External = thin skin derived from the first branchial groove; internal = simple cuboidal epithelium derived from the first pharyngeal pouch.

Ossicles from the eardrum to the oval window: Malleus → incus → stapes. Fusion of the ossicles (otosclerosis) is one cause of conductive hearing loss.

The vestibular organ detects changes in position; it comprises the ampullae of the semicircular canals and the maculae of the saccule and utricle.

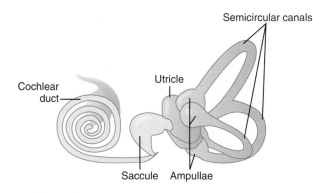

19-3: *Components of the membranous labyrinth. Sensory receptors in the saccule, utricle, and cristae ampullae of the semicircular ducts form the vestibular organ. The organ of Corti within the cochlear duct is the auditory organ.*

Linear acceleration of the head causes movement of the otolithic membrane in the saccule and utricle → stimulation of sensory hair cells.

Rotation of the head causes movement of the cupula in the semicircular ducts → stimulation of sensory hair cells.

       (4) Linear acceleration of the head displaces the otolithic membrane, causing bending of the stereocilia, which triggers a sensory impulse.

    b. Cristae ampullae of the semicircular ducts

       (1) The epithelium contains supporting cells, hair cells, and efferent nerve endings similar to those in the maculae.

       (2) The cupula, a gelatinous layer lacking otoliths, overlies the epithelium.

       (3) Rotation of the head displaces the cupula, causing bending of the stereocilia, which triggers a sensory impulse.

4. Auditory organ

    a. The cochlear duct (scala media) is an endolymph-filled, triangular structure that divides the bony cochlea into two perilymph-filled spaces: the scala vestibuli and the scala tympani (Fig. 19-4A).

       (1) The vestibular membrane forms the roof of the duct.

       (2) The basilar membrane forms the floor of the duct.

       (3) The stria vascularis forms the lateral aspect and participates in the formation of endolymph.

    b. The organ of Corti lies on the basilar membrane of the cochlear duct (Fig. 19-4B).

       (1) The inner and outer hair cells, the auditory receptor cells, have stereocilia (but no kinocilium) on their apical border.

       (2) Supporting cells of several types are associated with hair cells.

       (3) The tectorial membrane, a gelatinous mass, contacts the stereocilia of the hair cells.

D. Histophysiology of hearing

    1. Sound transmission from the environment to the organ of Corti occurs via the following pathway:

       • Air vibrations → external auditory canal → tympanic membrane → auditory ossicles → footplate of the stapes in the oval window → perilymph of the scala vestibuli → vestibular membrane → endolymph of the cochlear duct → basilar membrane and organ of Corti → perilymph of the scala tympani → round window

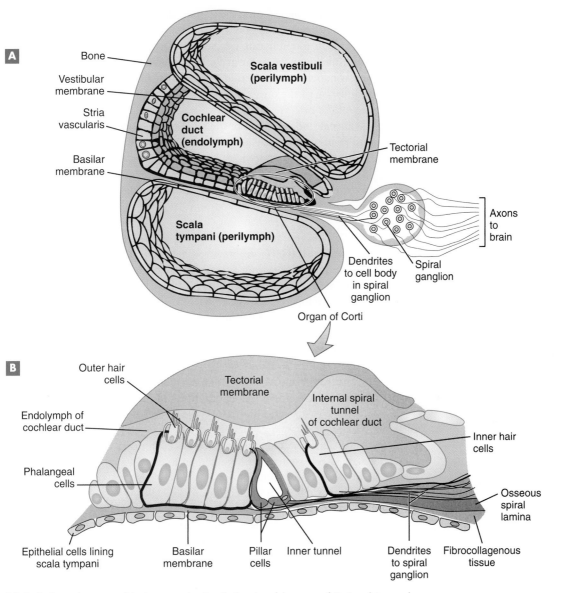

A Bone

Vestibular membrane

Stria vascularis

Basilar membrane

Scala vestibuli (perilymph)

Cochlear duct (endolymph)

Tectorial membrane

Scala tympani (perilymph)

Axons to brain

Dendrites to cell body in spiral ganglion

Spiral ganglion

Organ of Corti

B Outer hair cells

Endolymph of cochlear duct

Phalangeal cells

Epithelial cells lining scala tympani

Tectorial membrane

Internal spiral tunnel of cochlear duct

Inner hair cells

Osseous spiral lamina

Basilar membrane

Pillar cells

Inner tunnel

Dendrites to spiral ganglion

Fibrocollagenous tissue

*19-4: **A,** General structure of the inner ear showing the location of the organ of Corti and its neural projection to the spiral ganglion and beyond. **B,** Detailed structure of the organ of Corti.*

2. Displacement of the stereocilia on the hair cells of the organ of Corti, caused by deflection of the basilar membrane, is converted into an electric impulse (depolarization wave) that is conducted to the cell bodies of neurons in the spiral ganglion.

3. High-frequency sounds cause the greatest deflection of the basilar membrane toward the base of the cochlea, closer to the oval window.

4. Low-frequency sounds cause the greatest deflection of the basilar membrane toward the apex of the cochlea, where the scala vestibuli and scala tympani communicate via the helicotrema.
   - Thus, the lower the frequency of sound vibrations, the farther from the oval window is the deflection of the basilar membrane and the stimulation of the organ of Corti.

E. Disorders of the ear
   1. Otitis media (inflammation of the middle ear) commonly is caused by the spread of bacterial pathogens (most commonly *Streptococcus pneumoniae*) from the upper respiratory tract to the middle ear via the eustachian tube.
      - If the eustachian tube becomes blocked, outward bulging or perforation of the eardrum may occur due to pressure buildup.
   2. Conductive hearing loss is caused by a defect of the sound-conducting apparatus in the external auditory canal or middle ear.
      - Otitis media and otosclerosis (fusion of the ossicles) of the middle ear may cause this type of deafness.
   3. Neural deafness results from a lesion in any of the neuronal segments carrying impulses from the organ of Corti to the brain.
      - Disease, prolonged exposure to loud noises, and exposure to certain drugs may cause nerve deafness.
   4. Ménière's disease, a chronic disease of the inner ear, is caused by overproduction or decreased absorption of endolymph, leading to distention of the membranous labyrinth.
      - Hallmark symptoms are tinnitus, recurrent vertigo, progressive hearing loss, and a feeling of fullness in the ear.

Ménière's disease includes symptoms of tinnitus, recurrent vertigo, and progressive hearing loss due to excessive amounts of endolymph in the membranous labyrinth.

III. Olfactory Mucosa
   - The mucous membrane lining the roof of the nasal cavity consists of a pseudostratified columnar epithelium and an underlying lamina propria of loose, areolar connective tissue.

A. Cells composing the olfactory epithelium (Fig. 19-5A)
   1. Olfactory receptor cells are bipolar neurons.
      a. A single apical dendrite forms the expanded knoblike olfactory vesicle.
      b. Several modified cilia (olfactory hairs) project from the vesicle into the layer of fluid covering the epithelium.
      c. An unmyelinated axon emerges from the basal portion and enters the lamina propria. Bundles of axons join to form the olfactory nerve (cranial nerve [CN] I).
   2. Supporting (sustentacular) cells have many apical microvilli.
   3. Basal cells are mitotically active, replacing themselves and other cells of the epithelium.

B. Bowman's glands
   - These branched tubuloalveolar glands release a serous secretion via narrow ducts to the surface.
   - Odoriferous substances dissolved in these secretions interact with receptors on the olfactory hairs, generating an electric impulse.

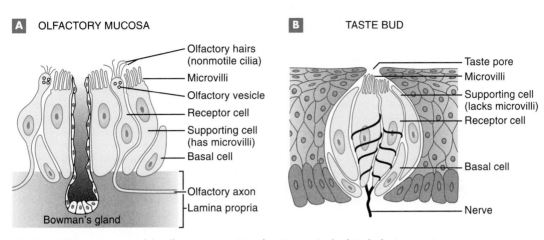

A OLFACTORY MUCOSA

Olfactory hairs (nonmotile cilia)
Microvilli
Olfactory vesicle
Receptor cell
Supporting cell (has microvilli)
Basal cell
Olfactory axon
Lamina propria
Bowman's gland

B TASTE BUD

Taste pore
Microvilli
Supporting cell (lacks microvilli)
Receptor cell
Basal cell
Nerve

19-5: A, *Cellular components of the olfactory mucosa. Ducts from Bowman's glands in the lamina propria project between the epithelial cells, delivering serous secretions to the surface. Olfactory hairs detect odoriferous substances dissolved in these secretions.* **B,** *Cellular components of the taste buds. Microvilli on the neuroepithelial receptor cells extend into the taste pore, which opens to the surface.*

IV. Taste Buds
- Taste buds are oval structures that extend across the epithelium of the lingual papillae; they are most numerous in fungiform and circumvallate papillae.
  A. Cells composing taste buds (Fig. 19-5B)
    1. Neuroepithelial (receptor) cells are elongated cells possessing numerous microvilli that extend into the taste pore, a small opening to the surface.
       a. Detect bitter, acid, sweet, or salt sensations by direct contact of the microvilli with dissolved substances
       b. Have synaptic vesicles near the sites of apposition with nerve terminals
    2. Supporting (sustentacular) cells lack microvilli.
    3. Basal cells are mitotically active and replace all supporting and receptor cells, which are continually lost.
  B. Nerve fibers
    - Sensory nerve endings of the facial (CN VII), glossopharyngeal (CN IX), and vagus (CN X) nerves enter the base of taste buds and wind around receptor cells.
    - Impulses from stimulated receptor cells are transmitted to nerve terminals across chemical synapses.

Common Laboratory Values

Test	Conventional Units	SI Units
Blood, Plasma, Serum		
Alanine aminotransferase (ALT, GPT at 30°C)	8–20 U/L	8–20 U/L
Amylase, serum	25–125 U/L	25–125 U/L
Aspartate aminotransferase (AST, GOT at 30°C)	8–20 U/L	8–20 U/L
Bilirubin, serum (adult): total; direct	0.1–1.0 mg/dL; 0.0–0.3 mg/dL	2–17 μmol/L; 0–5 μmol/L
Calcium, serum (Ca^{2+})	8.4–10.2 mg/dL	2.1–2.8 mmol/L
Cholesterol, serum	Rec: <200 mg/dL	<5.2 mmol/L
Cortisol, serum	8:00 AM: 6–23 μg/dL; 4:00 PM: 3–15 μg/dL 8:00 PM: ≤50% of 8:00 AM	170–630 nmol/L; 80–410 nmol/L Fraction of 8:00 AM: ≤0.50
Creatine kinase, serum	Male: 25–90 U/L Female: 10–70 U/L	25–90 U/L 10–70 U/L
Creatinine, serum	0.6–1.2 mg/dL	53–106 μmol/L
Electrolytes, serum		
Sodium (Na^+)	136–145 mEq/L	135–145 mmol/L
Chloride (Cl^-)	95–105 mEq/L	95–105 mmol/L
Potassium (K^+)	3.5–5.0 mEq/L	3.5–5.0 mmol/L
Bicarbonate (HCO_3^-)	22–28 mEq/L	22–28 mmol/L
Magnesium (Mg^{2+})	1.5–2.0 mEq/L	1.5–2.0 mmol/L
Estriol, total, serum (in pregnancy)		
24–28 wk; 32–36 wk	30–170 ng/mL; 60–280 ng/mL	104–590 nmol/L; 208–970 nmol/L
28–32 wk; 36–40 wk	40–220 ng/mL; 80–350 ng/mL	140–760 nmol/L; 280–1210 nmol/L
Ferritin, serum	Male: 15–200 ng/mL Female: 12–150 ng/mL	15–200 μg/L 12–150 μg/L
Follicle-stimulating hormone, serum/plasma (FSH)	Male: 4–25 mIU/mL Female:	4–25 U/L
	Premenopause 4–30 mIU/mL	4–30 U/L
	Midcycle peak, 10–90 mIU/mL	10–90 U/L
	Postmenopause, 40–250 mIU/mL	40–250 U/L
Gases, arterial blood (room air)		
pH	7.35–7.45	[H^+] 36–44 nmol/L
P_{CO_2}	33–45 mmHg	4.4–5.9 kPa
P_{O_2}	75–105 mmHg	10.0–14.0 kPa
Glucose, serum	Fasting: 70–110 mg/dL 2 hr postprandial: <120 mg/dL	3.8–6.1 mmol/L <6.6 mmol/L
Growth hormone–arginine stimulation	Fasting: <5 ng/mL Provocative stimuli: >7 ng/mL	<5 μg/L >7 μg/L

Test	Conventional Units	SI Units
Blood, Plasma, Serum—cont'd		
Immunoglobulins, serum		
IgA	76–390 mg/dL	0.76–3.90 g/L
IgE	0–380 IU/mL	0–380 kIU/L
IgG	650–1500 mg/dL	6.5–15 g/L
IgM	40–345 mg/dL	0.4–3.45 g/L
Iron	50–170 µg/dL	9–30 µmol/L
Lactate dehydrogenase, serum	45–90 U/L	45–90 U/L
Luteinizing hormone, serum/	Male: 6–23 mIU/mL	6–23 U/L
plasma (LH)	Female:	
	Follicular phase, 5–30 mIU/mL	5–30 U/L
	Midcycle, 75–150 mIU/mL	75–150 U/L
	Postmenopause, 30–200 mIU/mL	30–200 U/L
Osmolality, serum	275–295 mOsm/kg	275–295 mOsm/kg
Parathyroid hormone, serum,	230–630 pg/mL	230–630 ng/L
N-terminal		
Phosphatase (alkaline), serum	20–70 U/L	20–70 U/L
(p-NPP at 30°C)		
Phosphorus (inorganic), serum	3.0–4.5 mg/dL	1.0–1.5 mmol/L
Prolactin, serum (hPRL)	<20 ng/mL	<20 µg/L
Proteins, serum		
Total (recumbent)	6.0–8.0 g/dL	60–80 g/L
Albumin	3.5–5.5 g/dL	35–55 g/L
Globulin	2.3–3.5 g/dL	23–35 g/L
Thyroid-stimulating hormone,	0.5–5.0 µU/mL	0.5–5.0 mU/L
serum or plasma (TSH)		
Thyroidal iodine (^{123}I) uptake	8–30% of administered dose/24 hr	0.08–0.30/24 hr
Thyroxine (T_4), serum	4.5–12 µg/dL	58–154 nmol/L
Triglycerides, serum	35–160 mg/dL	0.4–1.81 mmol/L
Triiodothyronine (T_3), serum (RIA)	115–190 ng/dL	1.8–2.9 nmol/L
Triiodothyronine (T_3) resin uptake	25–38%	0.25–0.38
Urea nitrogen, serum (BUN)	7–18 mg/dL	1.2–3.0 mmol urea/L
Uric acid, serum	3.0–8.2 mg/dL	0.18–0.48 mmol/L
Cerebrospinal Fluid		
Cell count	0–5 cells/mm^3	0–5 × 10^6/L
Chloride	118–132 mEq/L	118–132 mmol/L
Gamma globulin	3–12% total proteins	0.03–0.12
Glucose	50–75 mg/dL	2.8–4.2 mmol/L
Pressure	70–180 mm H$_2$O	70–180 mm H$_2$O
Proteins, total	<40 mg/dL	<0.40 g/L
Hematology		
Bleeding time (template)	2–7 min	2–7 min
Erythrocyte count	Male: 4.3–5.9 million/mm^3	4.3–5.9 × 10^{12}/L
	Female: 3.5–5.5 million/mm^3	3.5–5.5 × 10^{12}/L
Erythrocyte sedimentation rate	Male: 0–15 mm/hr	0–15 mm/hr
(Westergren)	Female: 0–20 mm/hr	0–20 mm/hr
Hematocrit (Hct)	Male: 40–54%	0.40–0.54
	Female: 37–47%	0.37–0.47

continued

Test	Conventional Units	SI Units
Hematology—cont'd		
Hemoglobin A$_{IC}$	≤6%	≤ 0.06%
Hemoglobin, blood (Hb)	Male: 13.5–17.5 g/dL	2.09–2.71 mmol/L
	Female: 12.0–16.0 g/dL	1.86–2.48 mmol/L
Hemoglobin, plasma	1–4 mg/dL	0.16–0.62 mmol/L
Leukocyte count and differential		
Leukocyte count	4500–11,000/mm^3	4.5–11.0 × 10^9/L
Segmented neutrophils	54–62%	0.54–0.62
Bands	3–5%	0.03–0.05
Eosinophils	1–3%	0.01–0.03
Basophils	0–0.75%	0–0.0075
Lymphocytes	25–33%	0.25–0.33
Monocytes	3–7%	0.03–0.07
Mean corpuscular hemoglobin (MCH)	25.4–34.6 pg/cell	0.39–0.54 fmol/cell
Mean corpuscular hemoglobin concentration (MCHC)	31–37% Hb/cell	4.81–5.74 mmol Hb/L
Mean corpuscular volume (MCV)	80–100 μm^3	80–100 fl
Partial thromboplastin time (activated) (aPTT)	25–40 sec	25–40 sec
Platelet count	150,000–400,000/mm^3	150–400 × 10^9/L
Prothrombin time (PT)	12–14 sec	12–14 sec
Reticulocyte count	0.5–1.5% of red cells	0.005–0.015
Thrombin time	<2 sec deviation from control	<2 sec deviation from control
Volume		
Plasma	Male: 25–43 mL/kg	0.025–0.043 L/kg
	Female: 28–45 mL/kg	0.028–0.045 L/kg
Red cell	Male: 20–36 mL/kg	0.020–0.036 L/kg
	Female: 19–31 mL/kg	0.019–0.031 L/kg
Sweat		
Chloride	0–35 mmol/L	0–35 mmol/L
Urine		
Calcium	100–300 mg/24 hr	2.5–7.5 mmol/24 hr
Creatinine clearance	Male: 97–137 mL/min	
	Female: 88–128 mL/min	
Estriol, total (in pregnancy)		
30 wk	6–18 mg/24 hr	21–62 μmol/24 hr
35 wk	9–28 mg/24 hr	31–97 μmol/24 hr
40 wk	13–42 mg/24 hr	45–146 μmol/24 hr
17-Hydroxycorticosteroids	Male: 3.0–9.0 mg/24 hr	8.2–25.0 μmol/24 hr
	Female: 2.0–8.0 mg/24 hr	5.5–22.0 μmol/24 hr
17-Ketosteroids, total	Male: 8–22 mg/24 hr	28–76 μmol/24 hr
	Female: 6–15 mg/24 hr	21–52 μmol/24 hr
Osmolality	50–1400 mOsm/kg	
Oxalate	8–40 μg/mL	90–445 μmol/L
Proteins, total	<150 mg/24 hr	<0.15 g/24 hr

DIRECTIONS: Each numbered item or incomplete statement is followed by options arranged in alphabetical or logical order. Select the best answer to each question. Some options may be partially correct, but there is only **ONE BEST** answer.

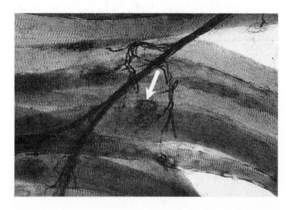

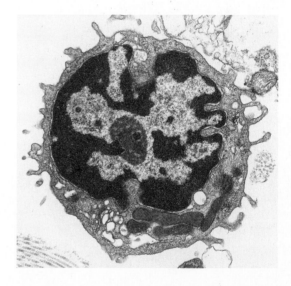

1. The *arrow* in this light micrograph is pointing to a structure that shows a defect that occurs in patients with myasthenia gravis. Which of the following correctly identifies this defect?
A. Decrease in acetylcholine (ACh) receptors
B. Increase in acetylcholinesterase
C. Number of synaptic vesicles
D. Reduction in the junctional folds of the sarcolemma
E. Schwann cell membrane

2. Which of the following is the main activity of the connective tissue cell shown in this transmission electron micrograph?
A. Liberation of pharmacologically active substances
B. Phagocytosis of foreign substances
C. Production of fibers and ground substance
D. Production of immunocompetent cells
E. Release of major basic protein

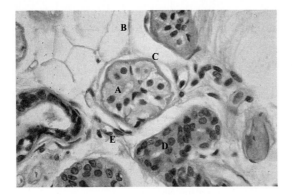

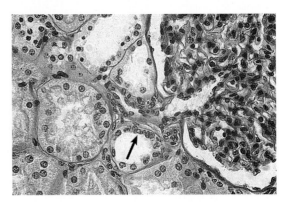

3. Which of the following cells of the dermis shown in this light micrograph fails to reabsorb chloride in patients with cystic fibrosis?
A. Cell at *A*
B. Cell at *B*
C. Cell at *C*
D. Cell at *D*
E. Cell at *E*

5. Which of the following functions is performed by the cells located at the tip of the *arrow* in this light micrograph?
A. Absorption of all glucose
B. Monitoring of chloride content
C. Production of angiotensin-converting enzyme
D. Secretion of erythropoietin
E. Secretion of renin

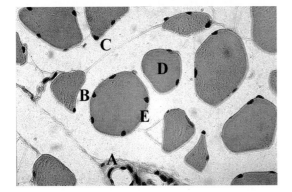

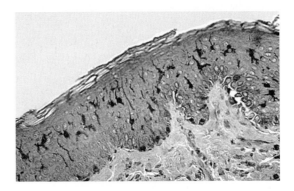

4. Duchenne muscular dystrophy (DMD) is expressed by the defect in which of the following locations shown in this light micrograph?
A. Site *A*
B. Site *B*
C. Site *C* (extracellular protein)
D. Site *D*
E. Site *E*

6. This section of skin has been stained immunohistochemically for S-100 protein, indicated by the dark brown cells showing the location of this cytoplasmic protein. Which of the following is the correct identification of these cells?
A. Keratinocytes and Langerhans cells
B. Melanocytes and Langerhans cells
C. Merkel cells

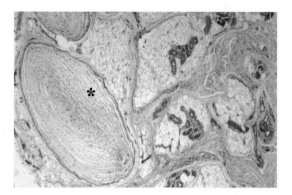

7. Which of the following receptors or nerve endings is indicated by the *asterisk* in this light micrograph of the dermis of the skin?
A. Krause's end bulb
B. Meissner's corpuscle
C. Merkel's ending
D. Pacinian corpuscle
E. Ruffini's corpuscle

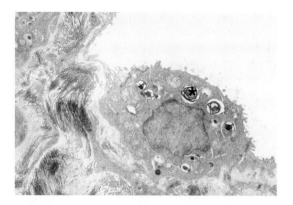

9. The *asterisk* in this electron micrograph indicates an organelle of a cell located in the lung. Which of the following is the correct identity of the characteristic organelle of this cell?
A. Lamellar body
B. Mucous granule
C. Primary lysosome
D. Secondary lysosome

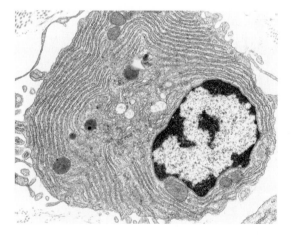

8. The cell shown in the accompanying electron micrograph is best recognized for the production of which of the following substances?
A. Histamine
B. Hydrochloric acid
C. Immunoglobulins
D. Isoenzymes
E. Tropocollagen

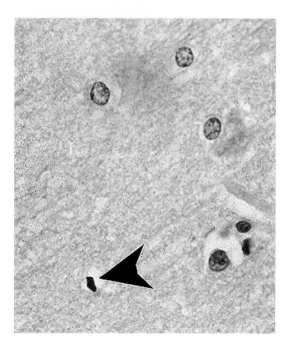

10. In the section of cerebrum shown in this light micrograph, the cell at the tip of the *arrowhead* is responsible for which of the following actions?

A. Destruction of myelin in multiple sclerosis
B. Formation of gemistocytes
C. Formation of gliosis
D. HIV replication
E. Myelin synthesis

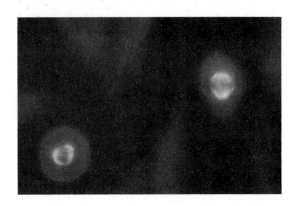

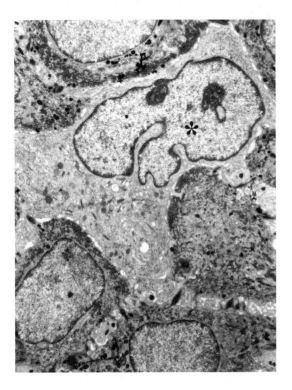

11. The cell located at the *asterisk* in this electron micrograph is positive for CD1 and is involved in the uptake and processing of antigens. Which of the following cells most accurately fits this description?
A. T helper cell
B. Histiocyte
C. Kupffer cell
D. Langerhans cell
E. M cell

12. Which of the following drugs interacts with the fluorescent organelles shown in the accompanying light micrograph and causes a stabilization of microtubules?
A. Bleomycin
B. Cyclosporine
C. Methotrexate
D. Paclitaxel
E. Vinblastine

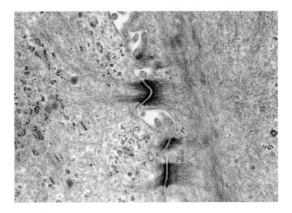

13. This electron micrograph shows several types of junctions and the filaments associated with them. Which of the following is the correct identification of this pair association?
A. Fascia adherens–actin
B. Macula adherens–keratin

C. Macula densa–vimentin
D. Zonula adherens–actin
E. Zonula adherens–vimentin

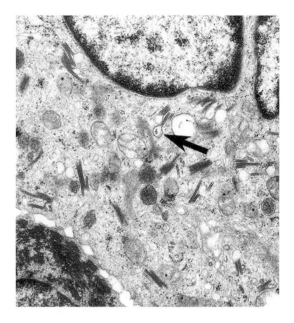

14. The accompanying electron micrograph shows the cytoplasm of an epidermal cell. Which of the following is the correct identification of the characteristic cell-specific organelle indicated by the *arrow?*
A. Beta granule
B. Birbeck granule
C. Melanosome
D. Weibel-Palade granule
E. Zebra body

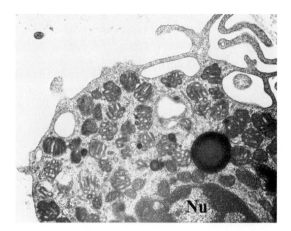

15. Which of the following is the main activity of the connective tissue cell shown in this transmission electron micrograph?
A. Liberation of pharmacologically active substances
B. Phagocytosis of foreign substances
C. Production of fibers and ground substance
D. Production of immunocompetent cells
E. Release of major basic protein

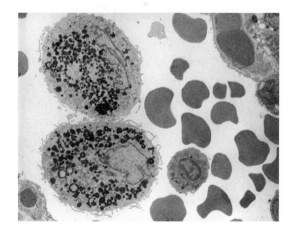

16. This electron micrograph shows a section of lung. Which of the following is the correct identification of the two large cells shown on the left-hand side?
A. Alveolar macrophages
B. Neutrophils
C. Type I pneumocytes
D. Type II pneumocytes

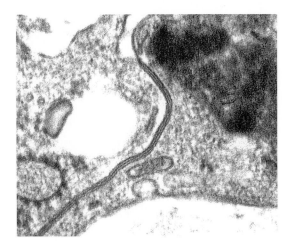

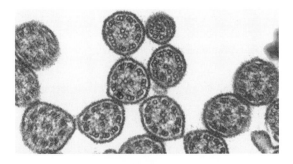

17. Which of the following is the means of communication between the cells seen in this electron micrograph?
A. Gap junction
B. Synapse
C. Zonula adherens
D. Zonula occludens

19. Which of the following is a molecular motor protein present in the structures shown in this electron micrograph?
A. Actinin
B. Clathrin
C. Dynein
D. Kinesin
E. Myosin

20. When stained immunohistochemically, a malignant fibrous histiocytoma of the connective tissue is found to be positive for keratin. Transmission electron microscopy is ordered to confirm the presence of keratin in this tumor of mesodermal origin. Which of the following structures would be seen in or around these tumor cells?
A. Cells arranged like keratinocytes
B. Desmosomes
C. Granules filled with keratin
D. Intracytoplasmic inclusions filled with keratin
E. Tonofilaments

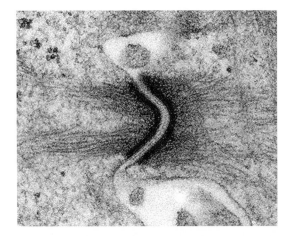

18. This electron micrograph shows a structure that contains a protein against which autoantibodies (IgG) are produced in patients with which of the following dermatologic diseases?
A. Bullous pemphigoid
B. Epidermolysis bullosa simplex
C. Ichthyosis
D. Pemphigus vulgaris
E. Vitiligo

21. Which component of skeletal muscle is missing or abnormal in patients with Duchenne muscular dystrophy?
A. Actin
B. Dystrophin
C. Myosin
D. Tropomyosin
E. Troponin

22. Which of the following hormones causes smooth muscle cells in the gallbladder to contract while concurrently causing the sphincter of Oddi to relax?
A. Cholecystokinin
B. Gastrin
C. Glucagon
D. Motilin
E. Secretin

23. In normal tissue, which of the following types of cellular specialization most effectively provides a permeability seal in the space between cells?
A. Macula adherens
B. Macula occludens
C. Nexus
D. Zonula adherens
E. Zonula occludens

24. At a site of inflammation, digestion of which of the following is considered an autophagic activity in the lysosome of parenchymal cells?
A. Bacteria
B. Centriole
C. Collagen fibers
D. Vesicular contents
E. Viral particle

25. A chromosomal analysis of various tissues taken from a woman shows XO, XX, and XXX. Cells from every tissue type contain 44 autosomes. It is assumed that a single abnormal division accounts for all of these aberrations. Which of the following division processes would account for these chromosome numbers?
A. Meiotic anaphase lagging
B. Meiotic nondisjunction
C. Mitotic anaphase lagging
D. Mitotic deletion
E. Mitotic nondisjunction

26. Under normal conditions, a single secondary spermatocyte that has just completed meiosis I contains which of the following?
A. Either one X chromosome or one Y chromosome

B. Either two X chromosomes or two Y chromosomes
C. One X chromosome and one Y chromosome
D. Two X chromosomes and two Y chromosomes

27. Which cellular organelles are found in excessive amounts in tumor cells specialized to synthesize steroid hormones?
A. Golgi apparatus
B. Nucleus
C. Rough endoplasmic reticulum (RER)
D. Smooth endoplasmic reticulum (SER)

28. In normal stratified epithelia, most of the cells that replace surface cells that are lost through attrition or cell death originate in which of the following?
A. Basal layer
B. Intermediate layer
C. Surface layer
D. Underlying connective tissue

29. Drug X interferes with the cross-linking of tropoelastin but not with the synthesis of tropoelastin. After 2 months of treatment with drug X, which of the following changes is most likely to be seen?
A. Decrease in the amount of tropoelastin in connective tissue
B. Increase in the amount of elastin in connective tissue
C. Increase in the amount of tropoelastin in connective tissue
D. Increase in the elasticity of the tissue

30. A 32-year-old man is undergoing ionizing radiation treatment of a brain tumor. After 2 weeks of treatment, there will most likely be a decrease in the number of which of the following?
A. Astrocytes
B. Microglia
C. Neurons
D. Oligodendrocytes

31. In a surgical biopsy of skeletal muscle, the thick filaments are best described as:
    A. Attached to the Z line
    B. Localized in the A band
    C. Localized in the A and I bands
    D. The same as a single myosin molecule
    E. Shortened during muscle contraction

32. Chloramphenicol is an antibiotic that blocks mitochondrial protein synthesis. In a cell treated with chloramphenicol, synthesis of which of the following proteins will be diminished?
    A. DNA polymerase
    B. Electron transport system subunits
    C. Enzymes of the tricarboxylic acid (TCA) cycle
    D. Permeases of the inner mitochondrial membrane
    E. Structural proteins of the outer mitochondrial membrane

33. Cells may be osmotically coupled when a change in the concentration of an ion in one cell causes a similar change in adjacent cells. Which type of cellular junction would facilitate this phenomenon?
    A. Macula adherens
    B. Macula occludens
    C. Nexus
    D. Zonula adherens
    E. Zonula occludens

34. Nondisjunction of all X chromosomes in a normal oocyte has occurred at the first and second meiotic divisions. During each division, the extra DNA passed to the cell that was to become the egg, which was fertilized by a normal Y-bearing sperm. What is the number of sex chromatin bodies that will be seen in the interphase nuclei in the resulting fetus?
    A. 1
    B. 2
    C. 3
    D. 4
    E. 5

35. A patient with a rapidly growing tumor is treated with nitrogen mustard. Which type of cell will be most depleted 1 month after 1 week of treatment with a sublethal dose of nitrogen mustard?
    A. Continuous replicators
    B. Nonreplicators with no stem cells
    C. Occasional replicators

36. An experimental antifertility drug enables meiotic cells to complete meiosis I but prevents them from entering meiosis II. After treatment with this drug, the blocked cells will contain the same amount of DNA as somatic cells in which stage of the cell cycle?
    A. G_1
    B. G_2
    C. Metaphase of mitosis
    D. Middle of the S phase
    E. Prophase of mitosis

37. Hurler's syndrome is characterized by an accumulation of proteoglycans in connective tissue, macrophage lysosomes, and urine. Which of the following explains this condition?
    A. A proteoglycan-degrading hydrolase is missing
    B. The connective tissue lacks lysosomes
    C. The rate of proteoglycan degradation has increased
    D. The rate of proteoglycan synthesis has increased

38. In normal tissue, what is the function of the zonula adherens?
    A. Allows electronic coupling of adjacent cells
    B. Encircles the cell completely
    C. Fuses the outer leaflets of the plasma membrane
    D. Serves as a barrier to diffusion

39. Which of the following characteristics best describes thick filaments in skeletal muscle?
    A. They are found in the I band
    B. They contain actin
    C. They contain myosin
    D. They contain tropomyosin

40. A 32-year-old man is involved in an industrial accident and severs a peripheral nerve in his forearm. This injury may result in which of the following?
A. Death of neurons in the dorsal horn of the spinal cord
B. Degeneration of nerve processes proximal to the injury
C. Proliferation of Schwann cells proximal to the injury
D. Reactive changes in the lower thoracic dorsal root ganglia cells

41. Zellweger syndrome is characterized by craniofacial abnormalities, hypotonia, hepatomegaly, polycystic kidneys, jaundice, and death in early infancy. The liver, brain, and spleen of patients with this disorder do not produce adequate amounts of catalase and several oxidases. Which cellular organelle is responsible for this disorder?
A. Lysosome
B. Microtubule
C. Mitochondrion
D. Peroxisome

42. Which of the following structures is found on the E face of the plasma membrane?
A. Extrinsic membrane proteins
B. Glycocalyx
C. Nonpolar tails of phospholipids
D. Polar heads of phospholipids

43. The amount of RER exceeds the amount of SER during which of the following cell functions?
A. Contraction of a skeletal muscle fiber
B. Fat absorption in a columnar epithelial cell
C. Peptide hormone production in a glandular cell
D. Steroid hormone production in a glandular cell

44. A characteristic that distinguishes white skeletal muscle fibers from red skeletal muscle fibers is that white fibers
A. Are rich in myoglobin

B. Have the greatest amount of glycogen per fiber
C. Have the greatest number of mitochondria per fiber
D. Have slow contractions and support continuous heavy work

45. Which of the following remains the same during muscle contraction or relaxation?
A. Length of the A band during relaxation
B. Length of the H band during contraction
C. Length of the I band during contraction

46. A 7-year-old boy has purpura and ecchymoses in the oral mucosa and skin, subperiosteal hematomas, and blood in several joints after minimal trauma. The child has a history of impaired wound healing. Which of the following should be considered when making a differential diagnosis?
A. Failure to maintain fully differentiated epithelia
B. Inadequate mineralization of cancellous bone
C. Increased intracellular levels of protein p53
D. Lack of prolyl and lysyl hydroxylase activity

47. Several Volkmann's canals appear in a bone section taken at the autopsy of a 92-year-old woman who died after a serious fall. These structures have which of the following characteristics?
A. They are components of the interstitial lamellae
B. They contain the processes of osteocytes
C. They interconnect haversian canals
D. They interconnect lacunae

48. Hereditary spherocytosis involves a genetic defect that results in which of the following?
A. Change in the structure of spectrin
B. Decrease in the area of hyalomeres
C. Decrease in the diameter of the affected cell
D. Increase in intrinsic cell membrane proteins
E. Increase in the size of the granulomere region of a cell

49. An 8-year-old boy of African American descent is diagnosed with homozygous sickle cell anemia. In which area of the body will the abnormal blood cells resulting from this condition be destroyed by erythrophagocytosis?
A. Cord of Billroth in the spleen
B. Hematopoietic cord in the bone marrow
C. Marginal zone of the spleen
D. Medullary region of the thymus
E. Paratrabecular sinus in a lymph node

50. Many types of neoplasms, such as breast cancer, involve a defect in the ability of a cell to regulate its progression through the cell cycle. Which of the following defects is commonly seen in these types of neoplasms?
A. Lack of cyclin-dependent kinase (CDK) activity
B. Lack of retinoblastoma protein (pRB) phosphorylation
C. Overexpression of D cyclins
D. Underexpression of D cyclins
E. Up-regulation of p53

answers

1. **A** (decrease in acetylcholine receptors) is correct. A reduction in the number of functionally active ACh receptors in the sarcolemma of the myoneural junction leads to myasthenia gravis, an autoimmune disorder characterized by progressive muscular weakness. Antibodies bind to the ACh receptors in the junctional folds and inhibit normal nerve–muscle communication. Cross-linking of the receptors by antibodies increases the rate of endocytosis of the receptors, and they cannot be replaced quickly enough by the muscle. The structure seen at the tip of the arrow is a motor end-plate, or myoneural junction. Branches are seen extending from the axon, and each terminates in a motor end-plate on a muscle fiber.

B (increase in acetylcholinesterase) is incorrect. Acetylcholinesterase breaks down the neurotransmitter ACh, but this enzyme is not affected in myasthenia gravis.

C (number of synaptic vesicles) is incorrect. The number of synaptic vesicles in the terminal bouton of the motor end-plate is not affected in myasthenia gravis.

D (reduction in the junctional folds of the sarcolemma) is incorrect. The junctional folds are the site of ACh binding and of internalization of the receptor–ACh complex, but reduction in the number of folds does not occur in myasthenia gravis.

E (Schwann cell membrane) is incorrect. The Schwann cell membrane wraps around the axon and extends to the muscle cell surface. It is not affected in myasthenia gravis.

2. **D** (production of immunocompetent cells) is correct. This transmission electron micrograph (TEM) shows a lymphocyte, with its characteristic spherical shape, rim of ribosome-filled cytoplasm, spherical nucleus, and microvilli. Some undulation of the nucleus is apparent, and it is not unusual to see a deeply infolded nucleus. Lymphocytes usually contain a considerable amount of heterochromatin. Collagen fibers are visible around the cell, indicating its presence in connective tissue. Transmission electron microscopy cannot determine the type of lymphocyte from its morphologic features; this cell could be a T, B, or null cell. B lymphocytes develop into immunocompetent plasma cells that produce immunoglobulins. T cells can be divided into groups, depending on the expression of receptors, and become immunologically activated as T helper cells, T cytotoxic cells, or T suppressor cells.

A (liberation of pharmacologically active substances) is incorrect. This connective tissue cell does not have organelles that contain pharmacologically active substances. An example of such a connective cell is the mast cell, which would be packed with granules.

B (phagocytosis of foreign substances) is incorrect. This connective tissue cell does not have the features of a macrophage, which phagocytizes foreign substances.

C (production of fibers and ground substance) is incorrect. This connective tissue cell does not produce connective fibers or ground substance components. The fibroblast performs that function, but it would have extensive rough endoplasmic reticulum and a different shape.

E (release of major basic protein) is incorrect. Major basic protein is produced by eosinophils. This connective tissue cell does not have a bilobed nucleus or granules, which are two visible characteristics of the eosinophil.

3. **D** (cell at *D*) is correct. In patients with cystic fibrosis, the sweat gland ducts fail to reabsorb chloride ions, leading to the accumulation of sodium chloride in sweat. This membrane transport failure is caused by a mutation in the cystic fibrosis transmembrane conductance regulator (CFTR). Sweat gland ducts are recognized by their darker-staining characteristics compared with the secretory portions (cell at *A*) of the gland. Secretory cells and duct cells are located close to one another in this area of the dermis because the sweat gland is a simple coiled tubular gland. The coiled termination of the gland presents several profiles of the gland, which appear in cross-section or longitudinal section in a circumscribed area.

A (cell at *A*) is incorrect. The cells at *A* are secretory cells of the sweat gland. The greatest volume of sweat is made by these cells and then modified by the duct cells.

B (cell at *B*) is incorrect. The cell at *B* is an adipocyte, which is not affected in cystic fibrosis.

C (cell at *C*) is incorrect. The cell at *C* is a myoepithelial cell, which has contractile properties and squeezes the secretory portion of the sweat gland. It is recognized by its position near the secretory cells and its eosinophilic or darker-staining properties, indicative of a cytoplasm filled with contractile microfilaments.

E (cell at *E*) is incorrect. The cell at *E* is an endothelial cell; it is not affected in cystic fibrosis.

4. **E** (site *E*) is correct. Site *E* identifies the cell membrane–lamina interactions. DMD is caused by a deficiency of dystrophin, an actin-associated protein. Dystrophin links the cytoplasmic actin filaments with laminin through a transmembrane dystrophin-associated glycoprotein complex. This network helps maintain the structural rigidity of the muscle fiber. It is also thought that the loss of dystrophin leads to sarcolemmal damage and then to necrosis of the muscle cell. Laminin completes the interaction with the extracellular matrix as it becomes associated with collagen in the endomysium. The *DMD* gene is located on the short arm of the X chromosome.

A (site *A*) is incorrect. Vessels such as those seen at site *A* in the connective tissue perimysium are not affected in DMD. Endothelial cells are visible lining the vessel lumen.

B (site *B*) is incorrect. Site *B* represents fibroblasts. Muscle fibers or cells are eventually lost in DMD, and this loss is accompanied by fibrosis and replacement with fat cells. The accumulation of fat cells accounts for the pseudohypertrophy of muscles.

C (site *C*) is incorrect. Site *C* indicates the extracellular protein. Extracellular proteins such as collagen and laminin, seen in this area of the endomysium, are not defective in DMD.

D (site *D*) is incorrect. Site *D* indicates the myofibril filaments. The filaments of actin and myosin are not affected in DMD until the disease progresses and more myocyte necrosis occurs.

5. **B** (monitoring of chloride content) is correct. The tip of the arrow points to the modified cells of the distal convoluted tubule, the macula densa. The section is readily identifiable as kidney because of the presence of the glomerulus at the upper right of the light micrograph. The periodic acid-Schiff stain accentuates the microvillous border of the proximal convoluted tubules and the basal laminae of the tubules and glomerular epithelium. Macula densa cells are noted on light microscopy by their close proximity, shown especially here by the compactness of the nuclei. These cells are able to detect decreases in the filtrate concentration of Na^+ and Cl^- and transfer this information to other cells of the juxtaglomerular apparatus, the renin-containing, or juxtaglomerular (JG), cells. The cells nearest the afferent arteriole within the distal convoluted tubule wall make up the dense spot (macula densa). The JG cells, which are modified smooth muscle cells of the afferent arteriole, respond by secreting renin.

A (absorption of all glucose) is incorrect. As discussed for option B, absorption occurs along the distal convoluted tubule, and the cells located here perform an important function in cooperation with the JG cells and the extraglomerular mesangial cells. However, it is sodium that is absorbed along the distal convoluted tubule. Most glucose is absorbed in the proximal convoluted tubule.

C (production of angiotensin-converting enzyme) is incorrect. Angiotensin-converting enzyme is primarily produced by the endothelial cells of the lung. This enzyme works on the substrate (angiotensin II) produced from the reaction of renin (angiotensinogen) with angiotensin I.

D (secretion of erythropoietin) is incorrect. Erythropoietin is produced by the endothelial cells of the peritubular capillaries in the kidney cortex and perhaps by the extraglomerular mesangial cells.

E (secretion of renin) is incorrect. The cells shown in the light micrograph are located within the wall of the distal convoluted tubule. Renin-secreting cells would be located within the wall of the afferent arteriole.

6. **B** (melanocytes and Langerhans cells) is correct. The darkly stained cells show the positive reaction for S-100 protein. Langerhans cells make up approximately 4% of the epidermal cells and are the cells with long processes distributed through the stratum spinosum layer. Melanocytes are seen along the basal layer of the epidermis. Antibodies to S-100 are used to differentiate neural crest derivatives and their tumors, glial cell and ependymal cell tumors, and tumors of Schwann cells. The pattern of Langerhans cells in the epidermis is especially noticeable in this section of human skin. The cells have long processes that extend through the epidermis and are useful in their function as antigen presenters.

A (keratinocytes and Langerhans cells) is incorrect. Most of the cells seen in the epidermis are keratinocytes, but they do not stain positively for S-100 (as indicated by a dark brown reaction). The nuclei of keratinocytes are visible throughout the stratum spinosum.

C (Merkel cells) is incorrect. Merkel cells are found along the basal surface of the skin and may be modified keratinocytes, which contain neurosecretory granules and may function as mechanoreceptors. Such cells lack processes, unlike those seen in this section of skin.

7. **D** (pacinian corpuscle) is correct. The pacinian corpuscle has the appearance of an onion in cross-section, as seen here in the dermis of the skin. Sweat glands are seen on the right of the light micrograph, visible as tubular structures surrounded by adipose tissue. Pacinian corpuscles are also located in the periosteum and in the connective tissue stroma of some organs; they respond to touch and pressure. An axon is located in the center of the thin sheets of connective tissue lamellae.

A (Krause's end bulb) is incorrect. Krause's end bulbs are smaller than pacinian corpuscles, and the axon within has several branches. Like the pacinian corpuscle, Krause's end bulb is a type of mechanoreceptor.

B (Meissner's corpuscle) is incorrect. Meissner's corpuscles are pear-shaped or tornado-shaped structures located in the dermal papillae. A myelinated nerve fiber zigzags through the middle of this mechanoreceptor, which responds to slight deformation of the skin.

C (Merkel's ending) is incorrect. Merkel's endings are myelinated afferent fibers that terminate in contact with a Merkel cell near the stratum basale.

E (Ruffini's corpuscle) is incorrect. Ruffini's corpuscles are a different type of mechanoreceptor. They are usually oriented parallel to the skin, and bundles of collagen run through their core.

8. **C** (immunoglobulins) is correct. The eccentric nucleus with marginal clumped chromatin, the abundance of RER, and the paranuclear Golgi complex seen in this cell are characteristics of a plasma cell. Mitochondria are randomly distributed through the folds of the RER, and lysosomes make up the organelles. Plasma cells manufacture the antibodies or immunoglobulins in the RER; the Golgi complex cross-links, attaches carbohydrate molecules, and packages the antibody. A directional signal is given to the small secretory vesicle as it travels through the Golgi complex; it then moves to the cell membrane and is released by exocytosis. Some collagen fibrils are seen around the plasma cell.

A (histamine) is incorrect. Histamine is the main product of mast cells, which would not have as much RER as the plasma cell shown in the electron micrograph (EM). Mast cells would also be packed with secretory granules.

B (hydrochloric acid) is incorrect. Hydrochloric acid is produced by parietal cells, which would not have as much RER as the plasma

cell shown in the EM. Also, parietal cells would be packed with mitochondria.

D (isoenzymes) is incorrect. Although cells that secrete isoenzymes would contain the abundance of RER seen in the plasma cell in this EM, they would also contain large secretory granules.

E (tropocollagen) is incorrect. Tropocollagen is secreted by fibroblasts, which are elongated and have a different nuclear shape than the plasma cell seen in this EM. A fibroblast would also be surrounded by collagen, its secretory product.

9. **A** (lamellar body) is correct. The cell seen in this EM is a type II pneumocyte, or great alveolar cell, of the alveolar lining. The lamellar bodies are visible as dark, spherical granules with a concentric lamellar or myelin figure appearance. The cell borders a lumen, which is the alveolar space, and rests on a basal lamina with collagen fibers in the interstitium. The cell is attached to type I pneumocytes, or squamous alveolar cells, on either side by junctions. The lamellar bodies contain surfactant, which relieves surface tension as it spreads out over the surface of the type I cells and becomes a part of the blood–air barrier.

B (mucous granule) is incorrect. Mucous granules would appear as clear or grayish structures on electron microscopy.

C (primary lysosome) is incorrect. Primary lysosomes are homogeneous or contain a crystalline array of material.

D (secondary lysosomes) is incorrect. Secondary lysosomes are heterogeneous. If this were a secondary lysosome, other types of secondary lysosomes would also be present. Although secondary lysosomes may appear as myelin figures and resemble lamellar bodies, the cell shown here is a type II pneumocyte; thus, the organelle is a lamellar body. See the explanation for option A.

10. **D** (HIV replication) is correct. The tip of the arrow points to the small, heterochromatic nucleus of a microglial cell. These cells can be recognized by their dense, irregularly shaped nuclei, compared with the much larger, spherical, euchromatic nuclei of the astrocytes seen elsewhere in the light micrograph. These cells are phagocytic and are derived from precursors in the bone marrow; thus they are considered the macrophage of the central nervous system. In patients infected with HIV-1, the microglia contain the virus and thus assist with its replication.

A (destruction of myelin in multiple sclerosis) is incorrect. The tip of the arrow points to a microglial cell. Destruction of myelin in patients with multiple sclerosis occurs as the result of an autoimmune process. The microglia then move into these areas and phagocytize the degraded myelin; however, they are not responsible for the initial destruction of myelin.

B (formation of gemistocytes) is incorrect. Gemistocytes are astrocytes with a prominent eosinophilic cytoplasm.

C (formation of gliosis) is incorrect. The multiplication of astrocytes around sites of tissue injury is referred to as *gliosis*. Astrocyte nuclei are spherical, euchromatic, and much larger than the nucleus seen at the tip of the arrow, which is a microglial cell.

E (myelin synthesis) is incorrect. Synthesis of myelin in the central nervous system is performed by oligodendrocytes. These cells have a spherical, heterochromatic nucleus that is smaller than the nucleus of astrocytes (seen elsewhere in the light micrograph).

11. **D** (Langerhans cell) is correct. Features of Langerhans cells include a convoluted nucleus with deep infoldings and a clear cytoplasm with scattered organelles. The Langerhans cell is surrounded by keratinocytes with spherical nuclei that are much darker or electron-dense. Most of this dense material consists of bundles of intermediate filaments or tonofibrils. Langerhans cells do not form desmosomes with the keratinocytes but merely make contact with them along their periphery. Thus, no desmosomes would be seen between the Langerhans cell and keratinocytes. The pale cytoplasm indicates the absence of melanosomes. The Langerhans cell plays a significant role in immunologic reactions; is capable of binding, processing, and presenting antigens; and is CD1-positive. The other cells listed in options A, B, C, and E are not CD1-positive. Langerhans cells have dendritic processes, although these cannot be seen in this micrograph.

A (T helper cell) is incorrect. The cell shown is a Langerhans cell. A T helper cell does not have a convoluted nucleus, and it is positive for CD3, CD4, and CD5.

B (histiocyte) is incorrect. A histiocyte is the connective tissue macrophage and would have a more heterogeneous cytoplasm than is seen here. It would also be surrounded by collagen.

C (Kupffer cell) is incorrect. A Kupffer cell is the macrophage of the liver and lines a sinusoid. These features and the sinusoid lumen would be apparent in an EM.

E (M cell) is incorrect. An M cell is associated with lymphocytes in lymphoid aggregates called *Peyer patches*. M cells take up whole particles (bacteria, viruses) but transfer these foreign substances to neighboring lymphocytes. M cells have folds along the intestinal surface that distinguish them from the microvilli-covered enterocytes.

12. **D** (paclitaxel) is correct. The fluorescein-labeled organelles, which appear as bright structures in the center of the cell, are microtubules in the mitotic spindle of metaphase cells. The dark area in the center of the cells represents the chromosomes. Paclitaxel was originally isolated from the bark of the Pacific yew tree. Its mechanism was later found to be stabilization of microtubules, promoting the assembly of tubulin subunits and inhibiting depolymerization. This stabilization prevents chromosome movement and thus mitosis. It is known that microtubules are polar-oriented structures in the mitotic cell, adding tubulin subunits at one end and removing tubulin subunits at the other. Semisynthetic paclitaxel (Taxol) is more commonly used now as an anticancer agent.

A (bleomycin) is incorrect. Bleomycin is a cytostatic antibiotic that inserts into double-stranded DNA, leading to strand breakage.

B (cyclosporine) is incorrect. Cyclosporine inhibits the production of cytotoxic T lymphocytes by inhibiting transcription in precursors to these cells.

C (methotrexate) is incorrect. Methotrexate inhibits the synthesis of DNA and RNA by inhibiting dihydrofolate reductase, an enzyme important in the synthesis of purines and thymidine.

E (vinblastine) is incorrect. Vinblastine, which is derived from the periwinkle plant, acts to prevent the polymerization of tubulin subunits into microtubules. The result, however, is the same as occurs with paclitaxel, which is the prevention of mitosis.

13. B (macula adheren–keratin) is correct. All of the junctions seen are macula adheren junctions or desmosomes joining epithelial cells. They are recognized by a central linear density and by distinct filaments that enter a darker region (intracellular plaque) from the cellular side. Keratin filaments of 10 nm, or intermediate size, are always associated with the macula densa junction. A bundle of

microfilaments or actin filaments is also apparent in the EM, but these microfilaments run at a right angle to the intermediate filaments.

A (fascia adherens–actin) is incorrect. The fascia adherens is a junction found in the transverse portion of the intercalated disk. It is anchored by actin filaments. No sarcomeres or myofibrils are visible in this EM.

C (macula densa–vimentin) is incorrect. Vimentin filaments are characteristic of mesenchymal-derived cells and are not associated with the macula densa or desmosome. Keratin is the characteristic filament of epithelial-derived cells.

D (zonula adherens–actin) and E (zonula adherens–vimentin) are incorrect. The zonula adherens does not have intercellular or transmembrane proteins in the junction. Actin filaments are associated with the zonula adherens, but the filaments seen in this EM are bigger than microfilaments. The filaments can be seen individually at this power; thus, they are intermediate in type (e.g., keratin, vimentin). Vimentin filaments are not associated with any junctional type.

14. B (Birbeck granule) is correct. Birbeck granules, which have a tennis racquet shape, are seen near both the nucleus and the cell membrane of this Langerhans cell. The handle of the racquet has a linear density down the middle that is faintly visible in the EM. It is thought that these structures react with antigen being processed by the Langerhans cell. Note the convoluted nucleus and otherwise lightly staining cytoplasm of this cell. The cell at the lower left is a keratinocyte, which contains darkly stained tonofilaments. The two cells are closely apposed but do not form desmosomes.

A (beta granule) is incorrect. Beta granules of the pancreatic islet contain a characteristic small, round granule that has a crystal (or crystals) lying in a flocculent matrix. They are sometimes called *insulin granules.*

C (melanosome) is incorrect. Melanosomes are ellipsoid organelles that, in the later stages of development, become dense. In the early stages, they have a herringbone appearance. Melanosomes are the characteristic organelle of melanocytes and keratinocytes.

D (Weibel-Palade granule) is incorrect. Weibel-Palade granules are cylindrical structures with tubular inclusions that are characteristic of endothelial cells.

E (zebra body) is incorrect. Zebra bodies are lysosomes with accumulations of glycolipids that appear as stacks of osmiophilic material membranes and are characteristic of Fabry's disease.

15. **A** (liberation of pharmacologically active substances) is correct. This TEM shows a mast cell. The whorled, or scroll-like, arrangement of the granules and their dense numbers are the primary identification factors for this cell at the ultrastructural level. The nucleus is usually centrally located in such a cell, but only a portion of the nucleus (Nu) is seen here. Mast cells often have elaborate cell borders with long microvilli for interaction with the environment. Histamine and other vasoactive mediators are contained in the granules.

B (phagocytosis of foreign substances) is incorrect. The connective tissue cell seen in this TEM does not have the features (secondary lysosomes, heterogeneous cytoplasm) of a macrophage that phagocytizes foreign substances.

C (production of fibers and ground substances) is incorrect. This connective tissue cell does not produce connective fibers or ground substance components. The fibroblast, which performs that function, would have extensive rough endoplasmic reticulum without the large number of granules seen in this TEM.

D (production of immunocompetent cells) is incorrect. This connective tissue cell contains granules, which indicates an end-stage differentiation or a cell other than those associated with the lymphoid cell line.

E (release of major basic protein) is incorrect. Major basic protein is produced by eosinophils. The connective tissue cell shown in this TEM does not have the characteristic crystal-containing granules of an eosinophil.

16. **A** (alveolar macrophages) is correct. These alveolar macrophages appear to be floating in the alveolar space but may be associated with the alveolar epithelium out of the plane. However, alveolar macrophages are free cells that migrate over the luminal surface. The thin alveolar epithelium can be seen at the top right and the bottom left of the electron EM. The ultrastructural features of alveolar macrophages, as seen here, include large size (compared with the red blood cells [RBCs] and neutrophil seen at the right of the center), irregular nuclei, many primary and secondary lysosomes, and a surface with prominent filopodia. Some congestion is present in this lung tissue, as indicated by the large number of RBCs in the alveolar space.

B (neutrophils) is incorrect. These cells are too large to be neutrophils. In addition, they have an irregular, convoluted nucleus instead of the lobed nucleus characteristic of neutrophils.

C (type I pneumocytes) is incorrect. Type I pneumocytes are flat cells, also called *squamous alveolar cells,* associated with the alveolar lining. They are seen lining the lumen at the top right in this EM.

D (type II pneumocytes) is incorrect. Type II pneumocytes are associated with the alveolar wall, forming junctions with type I pneumocytes. They contain lamellar bodies.

17. **A** (gap junction) is correct. The gap junction permits communication between these two cells by allowing passage of small molecules, thus permitting metabolic coupling. Gap junctions are longer than the other types of junctions, and the cell membranes are closely apposed, with gaps along the membranes. The intercellular transmembrane channels, or pores, are made up of a protein called *connexin*. The dotlike connexin can be seen between the cell membranes.

B (synapse) is incorrect. In a synapse, a number of vesicles are associated with one side of the two membranes. The cell membranes are not closely apposed, as seen here; instead, there is a space, or cleft, between the two membranes.

C (zonula adherens) is incorrect. In a zonula adherens, the membranes are not connected with channels between cells.

D (zonula occludens) is incorrect. In a zonula occludens, the membranes fuse; there is no communication between the cells.

18. **D** (pemphigus vulgaris) is correct. In pemphigus vulgaris, the body produces IgG autoantibodies to the transmembrane adhesion protein of the desmosome, desmoglein. The intercellular plaque seen in the micrograph represents desmoglein. Identification of this structure as a desmosome is confirmed by the presence of intermediate filaments entering the cytoplasmic dense plaque on either side. The reaction of the antibody with desmoglein results in dyshesion: The desmosome deteriorates, keratin filaments or tonofilaments are released and clump around the nucleus, and the cells separate. This process leads to intraepidermal vesicle formation, which can contain detached keratinocytes.

A (bullous pemphigoid) is incorrect. Although bullous pemphigoid involves the production of IgG autoantibodies, these autoantibodies

are made against a component of the basal lamina found just beneath the stratum basale.

B (epidermolysis bullosa simplex) is incorrect. In epidermolysis bullosa simplex, a defect in keratin genes occurs. Production of intermediate filaments is responsible for changes in the epidermis.

C (ichthyosis) is incorrect. Ichthyosis is characterized by a thickening of the stratum corneum (external epidermal layer). It can have several causes, but none of them involves the production of autoantibodies.

E (vitiligo) is incorrect. In vitiligo, melanocytes are destroyed by what is thought to be an autoimmune mechanism. Melanocytes are not seen in this EM. Furthermore, melanocytes are not joined by desmosomes, nor are they joined to keratinocytes by desmosomes.

19. **C** (dynein) is correct. These cross-sections of cilia show the characteristic 9 + 2 arrangement of microtubules. Axonemal dynein is the molecular motor protein associated with cilia and flagella. (A flagellum will have the same 9 + 2 arrangement.) Motor proteins generate the sliding, or moving, forces in various cytoskeletal systems. An active ATPase is associated with these motor proteins. Axonemal dynein moves one microtubule across the surface of its neighboring microtubule, resulting in the bending of cilia or flagella.

A (actinin) is incorrect. Actinin is not a molecular motor protein; it is an actin cross-linking protein found in filopodia, lamellipodia (ruffles), stress fibers, and adhesion plaques.

B (clathrin) is incorrect. Clathrin is a protein associated with coated vesicles. It forms a complex on the cytoplasmic side of endocytotic vesicles that lends stability to the vesicle.

D (kinesin) is incorrect. Kinesin is a molecular motor protein, but it is associated with cytoplasmic microtubules and not with axonemal microtubules. Vesicles move along microtubules with the aid of kinesin.

E (myosin) is incorrect. Myosin is a molecular motor protein, but it is not associated with cilia. It is associated with actin in both muscle and nonmuscle filamentous systems.

20. **E** (tonofilaments) is correct. Keratin is an intracellular protein arranged in a fibrillar or filamentous pattern. Keratin filaments are usually bundled into larger groups, which are then referred to as *tonofilaments*. These filaments may extend throughout the cell, giving it structural support and mechanical stability. They may weave close to the nucleus, and they may end in junctions or desmosomes at the cell surface. Desmosomes may not be formed in some tissues, especially tumors.

A (cells arranged like keratinocytes) is incorrect. A cellular arrangement would not necessarily occur in a cell, and the arrangement of the cells does not guarantee the appearance of an intracellular protein.

B (desmosomes) is incorrect. As discussed for option **E,** desmosomes may not be formed in some tissues, even though keratin filaments are present in the cell. Some tumor cells do not make contact and thus do not form desmosomes.

C (granules filled with keratin) and **D** (intracytoplasmic inclusions filled with keratin) are incorrect. Keratin is not packaged into granules, but is arranged as a fibrillar protein in the form of intermediate filaments. If keratin filaments are disrupted, they usually coil throughout the cell in a random arrangement.

21. **B** (dystrophin) is correct. Dystrophin is a structural protein found in striated muscle that binds the cytoplasmic side of the sarcolemma to actin. DMD is characterized by progressive degeneration of skeletal muscle fibers. The severity of the dystrophy depends on the extent of damage to the gene that carries the code for dystrophin. In Duchenne type dystrophy, an X-linked gene results in the absence of dystrophin. In the Becker type of dystrophy, the same X-linked gene is not as severely damaged; as a result, dystrophin is produced by the cell but is abnormal. For this reason, the Becker type is not as severe as DMD.

A (actin) is incorrect. Actin is one of the main components of the thin filaments in muscle fibers. In patients with DMD, dystrophin is absent. This defect contributes to the progressive degeneration of skeletal muscle fibers seen in individuals with this disorder.

C (myosin) is incorrect. Myosin is one of the main components of thick filaments; it is not missing in patients with DMD.

D (tropomyosin) is incorrect. Tropomyosin consists of pencil-shaped molecules that lie in shallow grooves on the surface of the actin filaments. It is not missing in patients with DMD.

E (troponin) is incorrect. A single troponin molecule is bound to tropomyosin by one of its subunits (TnT). TnC, one of the other subunits of troponin, has a great affinity for calcium. The third type of troponin subunit, TnI, binds to actin and prevents an interaction between actin and myosin. When calcium binds to TnC, this subunit undergoes a conformational change that causes tropomyosin to expose previously blocked active sites on actin filaments. This allows myosin heads to bind with actin and allows the thick and thin filaments to slide by each other, shortening the length of the sarcomeres and mediating muscle contraction. These factors are not altered in patients with DMD. Serum troponin levels are increased in patients with an acute myocardial infarction.

22. **A** (cholecystokinin) is correct. Cholecystokinin (CCK) is released by enteroendocrine cells in the small intestine in the presence of lipids. CCK causes smooth muscle in the gallbladder to contract to move bile into the common bile duct to reach the intestine. It has the opposite effect on smooth muscle in the sphincter of Oddi, causing it to relax and allow bile to flow into the duodenum.

B (gastrin) is incorrect. Gastrin is secreted by the enteroendocrine cells of both the stomach and the small intestine. One effect of gastrin is stimulation of the secretion of HCl from the parietal cells in the gastric glands.

C (glucagon) is incorrect. Glucagon is produced by enteroendocrine cells in the stomach and small intestine and by α cells in the pancreas. It primarily stimulates gluconeogenesis in the hepatocytes.

D (motilin) is incorrect. Motilin is synthesized and released by enteroendocrine cells in the small intestine. It increases the peristaltic activity of the intestine.

E (secretin) is incorrect. Secretin is produced by enteroendocrine cells in the small intestine to induce the ductal epithelium of the pancreas to release a bicarbonate-rich watery fluid.

23. **E** (zonula occludens) is correct. The zonula occludens is a beltlike membrane that completely surrounds the cell, forming a permeability seal.

A (macula adherens) is incorrect. A macula adherens joins two cells at a discrete spot on the cell surface. Material can pass between the cells in other areas. Therefore, a macula adherens does not provide a permeability seal around the entire cell.

B (macula occludens) is incorrect. A macula occludens is a beltlike region that does not completely surround the cell. Material can pass between two cells by avoiding this region.

C (nexus) is incorrect. A nexus (gap junction) provides channels that allow ions to flow between adjacent cells. It does not prevent the flow of material between cells.

D (zonula adherens) is incorrect. A zonula adherens is a discrete region in which two cells are held together. Material can pass between the cells by flowing around this zone.

24. **B** (centriole) is correct. Autophagia is the digestion of intracellular constituents by the cell's own lysosomes. The only structure listed that is intrinsic to the cell is the centriole.

A (bacteria) and **E** (viral particle) are incorrect. Bacteria and viruses enter the cell by direct invasion or endocytosis. Because they are not normal components of the cell, their destruction is not considered autophagic activity.

C (collagen fibers) is incorrect. Collagen is found in supporting tissue and hyaline cartilage.

D (vesicular contents) is incorrect. Intracellular vesicles are formed around ingested material, which is not a normal component of the cell. Therefore, the destruction of vesicular contents is not considered autophagic activity.

25. **E** (mitotic nondisjunction) is correct. Changes in the chromosomal constitution of a cell indicate that a mitotic event has occurred. Mitotic nondisjunction is the failure of sister chromatids to separate during anaphase. This process is responsible for a cell containing an extra chromosome.

A (meiotic anaphase lagging) and **C** (mitotic anaphase lagging) are incorrect. Anaphase lagging is the failure of a chromatid to move as quickly as the other chromatids during anaphase. This results in that chromatid (chromosome) being excluded from a daughter cell and in a cell with fewer (not extra) chromosomes.

B (meiotic nondisjunction) is incorrect. Meiotic nondisjunction is the failure of chromatids to separate during meiosis. It results in all cells having the same chromosomal constitution.

D (mitotic deletion) is incorrect. Mitotic deletion is the loss of part of a chromosome during mitosis. It does not change the number of chromosomes in the cell.

26. **A** (either one X chromosome or one Y chromosome) is correct. The normal male gamete (sperm) contains one sex chromosome—either one X or one Y chromosome. When the primary spermatocyte enters meiosis I, the X chromosome and the Y chromosome pair up. At the end of meiosis I, each primary spermatocyte divides, producing two daughter cells, called *secondary spermatocytes*. Each secondary spermatocyte acquires either an X chromosome or a Y chromosome from the primary spermatocyte.

B (either two X chromosomes or two Y chromosomes) is incorrect. When the primary spermatocyte goes through anaphase I, its homologous chromosome pairs separate, so that one sex chromosome ends up at one pole in the cell and the other ends up at the opposite pole. Even if nondisjunction were to occur (i.e., the chromosome pairs failed to separate during anaphase I), neither daughter cell would acquire two of the same chromosomes.

C (one X chromosome and one Y chromosome) is incorrect. During anaphase I, the sex chromosome pair in the primary spermatocyte separates and each member of the pair travels to opposite ends of the cell. After telekinesis, each secondary spermatocyte will contain the single sex chromosome. The only way a single secondary spermatocyte can acquire both chromosomes from a primary spermatocyte is through nondisjunction

(failure of a chromosome pair to separate during anaphase I). This is an abnormal condition, however.

D (two X chromosomes and two Y chromosomes) is incorrect. A primary spermatocyte only inherits a single X chromosome and a single Y chromosome from the spermatogonium. Therefore, a secondary spermatocyte cannot acquire four chromosomes from a primary spermatocyte, especially since the secondary spermatocyte is a product of reductional division of a primary spermatocyte.

27. **D** (smooth endoplasmic reticulum) is correct. SER is a cytoplasmic organelle that contains enzymes required for steroid biosynthesis.

A (Golgi apparatus) is incorrect. The Golgi apparatus is a cytoplasmic organelle in which protein processing takes place.

B (nucleus) is incorrect. The synthesis of steroids takes place in the cytoplasm of the cell.

C (rough endoplasmic reticulum) is incorrect. RER is a cytoplasmic organelle in which protein synthesis takes place.

28. **A** (basal layer) is correct. Cells on the surface of normal stratified epithelia are replaced by continuously replicating vegetative intermitotic cells from the stem cell population in the basal layer.

B (intermediate layer) is incorrect. The intermediate layer in normal stratified epithelia contains differentiating intermitotic cells but no stem cells.

C (surface layer) is incorrect. The surface of normal stratified epithelia contains nonreplicating fixed postmitotic cells.

D (underlying connective tissue) is incorrect. Connective tissue lies beneath the epithelia and does not contribute to the epithelial cell population.

29. **C** (increase in the amount of tropoelastin in connective tissue) is correct. The amount of tropoelastin will increase because the drug does not interfere with tropoelastin synthesis. The elasticity of the tissue may decrease, however, because drug X prevents the cross-linking of tropoelastin fibers that is necessary for the formation of elastin.

A (decrease in the amount of tropoelastin in connective tissue) is incorrect. Tropoelastin continues to be synthesized during treatment with drug X. Therefore, the amount of tropoelastin in connective tissue should increase (not decrease).

B (increase in the amount of elastin in connective tissue) is incorrect. Although tropoelastin continues to be synthesized, drug X prevents it from forming cross-links and thus prevents the formation of elastin.

D (increase in the elasticity of the tissue) is incorrect. Elasticity will decrease because of decreased cross-linking of tropoelastin fibers.

30. **C** (neurons) is correct. Ionizing radiation kills cells in every stage of the cell cycle (i.e., both replicating and nonreplicating cells). Because neurons are fixed postmitotic cells and have no stem cell compartment, they cannot be replaced if they are destroyed.

A (astrocytes), **B** (microglia), and **D** (oligodendrocytes) are incorrect. These central nervous system glial cells are all reverting postmitotic cells. Although they can be damaged by ionizing radiation, they can be replaced.

31. **B** (localized in the A band) is correct. Thick filaments are found only in the A band.

A (attached to the Z line) is incorrect. Thin filaments (rather than thick filaments) are attached to the Z line.

C (localized in the A and I bands) is incorrect. Thin filaments are localized in both the A and the I bands.

D (the same as a single myosin molecule) is incorrect. Thick filaments are composed of hundreds of myosin molecules.

E (shortened during muscle contraction) is incorrect. Thick filaments do not shorten. The length of the sarcomere and the width of the I band shorten.

32. **B** (electron transport system subunits) is correct. Some of the subunits of the electron transport system and certain subunits of adenosine triphosphate (ATP) synthase are transcribed from the mitochondrial genome and translated on mitochondrial ribosomes. The other proteins listed are encoded in nuclear DNA and translated on cytoplasmic ribosomes.

A (DNA polymerase) is incorrect. DNA polymerase catalyzes the polymerization of nucleotides. It is encoded by nuclear (not mitochondrial) DNA.

C (enzymes of the TCA cycle) is incorrect. The TCA cycle is a metabolic pathway that catalyzes the production of ATP. The enzymes in this pathway are encoded by nuclear (not mitochondrial) DNA.

D (permeases of the inner mitochondrial membrane) is incorrect. Permeases are enzymes that enable substances to pass through a cell membrane. These enzymes are encoded by nuclear (not mitochondrial) DNA.

E (structural proteins of the outer mitochondrial membrane) is incorrect. These proteins are encoded by nuclear (not mitochondrial) DNA.

33. **C** (nexus) is correct. A nexus (gap junction) is a bridge between the membranes of adjacent cells. A nexus enables small ions to pass from a cell to an adjacent cell without passing through the extracellular space.

A (macula adherens), **B** (macula occludens), and **D** (zonula adherens) are incorrect. These structures hold cells together mechanically. They do not provide a passageway for communication between adjacent cells.

E (zonula occludens) is incorrect. A zonula occludens creates a permeability seal, which prevents particles from passing between cells.

34. **C** (3) is correct. The number of sex chromatin bodies is equal to the number of X chromosomes minus one. This cell will receive all four X chromatids from the ovum and no X chromosomes from the sperm.

A (1) is incorrect. A single sex chromatin body would be seen during interphase when two X chromosomes are present.

B (2) is incorrect. Two sex chromatin bodies would be seen during interphase when three X chromosomes are present.

D (4) is incorrect. Four sex chromatin bodies would be seen during interphase when five X chromosomes are present.

E (5) is incorrect. Five sex chromatin bodies would be seen during interphase when six X chromosomes are present.

35. **B** (nonreplicators with no stem cells) is correct. Nitrogen mustard is an alkylating agent that kills cells in every stage of the cell cycle. Cells in normal tissues are also affected by this therapy. Nonreplicators with no stem cell compartment will be destroyed and will not be replaced.

A (continuous replicators) is incorrect. Continuous replicators include stem cells for bone marrow and the intestinal epithelium. These cells arrive from a sequence of increasingly differentiated cells. As such, there is a pool of stem cells that can differentiate and replace the continuous replicators when they die or are destroyed.

C (occasional replicators) is incorrect. These cells will be destroyed and replaced.

36. **A** (G_1) is correct. The meiotic cells are blocked after having distributed half of their DNA content to each of two daughter cells. The DNA was previously duplicated during the S phase of the cell cycle. Therefore, the meiotic cells contain the same amount of DNA as a G_1 somatic cell (i.e., before DNA is duplicated).

B (G_2), **C** (metaphase of mitosis), **D** (middle of the S phase), and **E** (prophase of mitosis) are incorrect. A cell that completes meiosis I produces two daughter cells, each of which contains half as much DNA as the parent cell. Thus, each daughter cell contains the same amount of DNA as a somatic cell before it reaches the S phase of the cell cycle. Therefore, these blocked cells will contain less DNA than a somatic cell in the S phase of the subsequent G_2 phase or mitosis.

37. **A** (a proteoglycan-degrading hydrolase is missing) is correct. Patients with Hurler's syndrome lack an enzyme that is necessary for the breakdown of proteoglycans. Proteoglycan synthesis continues, however, and proteoglycans accumulate in body tissues.

B (the connective tissue lacks lysosomes) is incorrect. Lack of a lysosome-specific hydrolase usually means that the lysosomes are not producing the enzyme in adequate amounts. It does not necessarily mean that the lysosomes themselves are in short supply.

C (the rate of proteoglycan degradation has increased) is incorrect. The rate at which proteoglycans break down in patients with Hurler's syndrome is slower that than in normal patients.

D (the rate of proteoglycan synthesis has increased) is incorrect. The rate of proteoglycan synthesis in patients with Hurler's syndrome is the same as that in those who do not have the disease.

38. **B** (encircles the cell completely) is correct. The membranes of adjacent cells bind together within the zonula adherens.

A (allows electronic coupling of adjacent cells) is incorrect. The gap junction (nexus) serves as a means of direct communication between adjacent cells. As a result, electrons flow from cell to cell, resulting in electronic coupling of adjacent cells.

C (fuses the outer leaflets of the plasma membrane) is incorrect. The outer leaflets of the plasma membrane fuse in an occludens junction, not in a zonula adherens.

D (serves as a barrier to diffusion) is incorrect. The zonula occludens provides a permeability seal.

39. **C** (they contain myosin) is correct. The thick filaments contain the contractile protein myosin.

A (they are found in the I band) is incorrect. The thick filaments are found only in the A band.

B (they contain actin) and **D** (they contain tropomyosin) are incorrect. Actin and tropomyosin are found in the thin (not thick) filaments.

40. **C** (proliferation of Schwann cells proximal to the injury) is correct. Injury to a peripheral nerve axon results in a proliferation of Schwann cells, which guide the regenerating axon to its intended target.

A (death of neurons in the dorsal horn of the spinal cord) is incorrect. Injury to a peripheral nerve axon can result in the death of neurons in the dorsal root ganglion of sensory nerve fibers. It does not affect the dorsal horn, which contains the cell bodies of second-order sensory neurons.

B (degeneration of nerve processes proximal to the injury) is incorrect. Injury to a peripheral

nerve axon can result in degeneration of the axon distal to the injury. This suggests that proteins are still being produced in the cell body and transported to the proximal segment of the axon; however, because of the injury, they are not transported to the distal segment of the axon.

D (reactive changes in the lower thoracic dorsal root ganglia cells) is incorrect. Reactive changes associated with damage to a peripheral nerve in the forearm would occur in the dorsal root ganglia located in the lower cervical and upper thoracic regions of the spinal cord, not in the lower thoracic region.

41. **D** (peroxisome) is correct. Peroxisomes contain various oxidative enzymes and catalase. A lack of peroxisomes is responsible for Zellweger syndrome.

A (lysosome) is incorrect. Lysosomes contain hydrolytic (not oxidative) enzymes. When these hydrolytic enzymes are lacking, Tay-Sachs disease or Gaucher's disease may develop. Lysosomes do not play a role in Zellweger syndrome.

B (microtubule) is incorrect. Microtubules are essential for cell movement and maintaining cell shape.

C (mitochondrion) is incorrect. Oxidative phosphorylation occurs in the mitochondria. A defect in the enzymes responsible for oxidative phosphorylation can interfere with the production of adenosine triphosphate.

42. **C** (nonpolar tails of phospholipids) is correct. Nonpolar tails of phospholipids are found on the P and E faces of the plasma membrane.

A (extrinsic membrane proteins), **B** (glycocalyx), and **D** (polar heads of phospholipids) are incorrect. These molecules are found on the extracellular surface of the plasma membrane.

43. **C** (peptide hormone production in a glandular cell) is correct. Cells that are in the process of producing large amounts of protein to export have more RER than SER.

A (contraction of a skeletal muscle fiber) is incorrect. The endoplasmic reticulum is replaced by the sarcoplasmic reticulum (SR) in muscle fibers. Skeletal muscle contains a large amount of SR, which stores much of the calcium that is used during contraction. The amount of SR does not change during contraction.

B (fat absorption in a columnar epithelial cell) is incorrect. Simple columnar epithelium is found along highly absorptive surfaces, including that of the small intestine (where fat is absorbed). Fat is degraded to monoglycerides, cholesterol, and fatty acids, all of which are absorbed. Medium-sized fatty acids are re-esterified to form triglycerides in mucosal cells. This process occurs in the SER. Therefore, the amount of SER will exceed the amount of RER in epithelial cells.

D (steroid hormone production in a glandular cell) is incorrect. Steroid synthesis takes place in the SER. Therefore, this compartment will exceed the RER concentration during this process.

44. **B** (have the greatest amount of glycogen per fiber) is correct. White fibers in skeletal muscle show the greatest amount of glycogen.

A (are rich in myoglobin) is incorrect. Myoglobin is an oxygen-binding molecule. Red muscle fiber is rich in myoglobin.

C (have the greatest number of mitochondria per fiber) is incorrect. The mitochondrion is the "powerhouse" of the cell, generating adenosine triphosphate molecules, which are used for energy. Red skeletal muscle fibers usually contain more mitochondria per fiber than white skeletal muscle fibers.

D (have slow contractions and support continuous heavy work) is incorrect. Red muscle fibers demonstrate slow contractions and support continuous heavy work.

45. **A** (length of the A band during relaxation) is correct. The length of the A band does not change during relaxation.

B (length of the H band during contraction) and **C** (length of the I band during contraction) are incorrect. The length of both the H band and the I band decrease during contraction.

46. **D** (lack of prolyl and lysyl hydroxylase activity) is correct. Ascorbic acid is a cofactor in the catalysis of procollagen hydroxylation. Inadequate hydroxylation of procollagen results in inadequate cross-linking of collagen fibers, and consequently, in weak collagen fibers or an inadequate number of normal collagen fibers. This defect causes weakened capillary and venule walls, which results in leakage of blood and leads to purpura and ecchymosis. It also results in weakened mucosa, which allows oral ulcers to develop. Sharpey's fibers, which attach the periosteum to bone, will also weaken, resulting in subperiosteal hemorrhages.

A (failure to maintain fully differentiated epithelia) is incorrect. Epithelial differentiation is an important function of vitamin A. A deficiency in this vitamin can be ruled out in this patient because his symptoms are not consistent with this problem. Much of the damage observed in the patient (particularly the ecchymoses and purpura) indicates the presence of leaky small blood vessels and suggests that the entire depth of the blood vessel wall has been breached—the endothelium as well as connective tissue surrounding these vessels. Vitamin A deficiency would not be responsible for this type of damage.

B (inadequate mineralization of cancellous bone) is incorrect. The absorption of calcium from the intestine and its uptake into bone is diminished in individuals with hypovitaminosis D. Inadequate mineralization of bone can result in rickets (distortion of muscle-associated bones) or osteomalacia (softening of bone). Neither of these conditions was reported in this patient.

C (increased intracellular levels of protein p53) is incorrect. The intracellular protein p53 accumulates in the cell in response to DNA damage (e.g., as a result of exposure to mutagenic agents or ionizing radiation). This type of exposure was not reported in this patient. Protein p53 causes the cell to arrest in the G_1 phase of the cell cycle, which gives the cell time to attempt to repair the damage before it enters the S phase (when DNA is synthesized).

47. **C** (they interconnect haversian canals) is correct. Volkmann's canals run at various angles to the haversian systems, which run parallel to the long axes of long bones. Thus, they interconnect haversian systems.

A (they are components of the interstitial lamellae) is incorrect. Interstitial lamellae are small chunks of old, remodeled haversian systems. Volkmann's canals are not involved in the remodeling process and are not components of the interstitial lamellae.

B (they contain the processes of osteocytes) is incorrect. Volkmann's canals, like haversian canals, contain blood and lymph vessels. They do not contain the processes of osteocytes.

D (they interconnect lacunae) is incorrect. Lacunae are interconnected by canaliculi, not by Volkmann's canals.

48. **A** (change in the structure of spectrin) is correct. Spectrin is a large, long microfilament with actin-binding sites on each end. These sites allow spectrin molecules to form a dense

cytoskeletal meshwork adjacent to the P surface of the RBC plasmalemma. A defect in the genetic code for spectrin results in a change in spectrin structure and therefore a change in the cytoskeleton of the RBC. Specifically, it causes RBCs to lose their normal biconcavity and take on a spherical shape.

B (decrease in the area of hyalomeres) is incorrect. Spherocytosis affects RBCs. The hyalomere is the peripheral part of platelets (not RBCs).

C (decrease in the diameter of the affected cell) is incorrect. Spherocytosis affects an intracellular structural protein in RBCs. Damage to this protein affects the unique shape of the cell, not its overall diameter.

D (increase in intrinsic cell membrane proteins) is incorrect. Spherocytosis affects the structure of an intracellular protein. It does not affect the intrinsic proteins of the plasmalemma.

E (increase in the size of the granulomere region of a cell) is incorrect. Spherocytosis affects an intercellular protein in RBCs. The granulomere is the granular central region of thrombocytes.

49. **A** (cord of Billroth in the spleen) is correct. The cords of Billroth are oblong aggregations of lymphatic tissue that lie between venous sinusoids in the red pulp of the spleen. Blood entering the spleen from the circulatory system passes through the cords of Billroth, where the formed elements of blood encounter macrophages that reside in these cords. The macrophages destroy damaged erythrocytes, including the sickle-shaped cells in this patient. Because of this activity, splenomegaly is a common finding in African American patients with sickle cell anemia.

B (hematopoietic cord in the bone marrow) is incorrect. The hematopoietic cords of the bone marrow are the areas in which erythrocytopoiesis occurs.

C (marginal zone of the spleen) is incorrect. The marginal zone lies between the red pulp and the white pulp of the spleen. Although it contains macrophages, the primary activity in this region is the presentation of antigens to T cells and B cells by dendritic cells in an attempt to trigger an immune response.

D (medullary region of the thymus) is incorrect. The primary function of the thymus is to produce immunocompetent T cells. The medulla of the thymus contains mature T cells, which leave the thymus via venules and efferent lymphatic vessels to populate other lymphoid organs (e.g., lymph nodes and spleen). Phagocytosis is not carried out by red blood cells.

E (paratrabecular sinus in a lymph node) is incorrect. The subcapsular, medullary, and paratrabecular sinuses of the lymph node are bridged by phagocytic cells. These sinuses contain lymph (not blood).

50. **C** (overexpression of D cyclins) is correct. D cyclins are overexpressed in many types of tumors. An abnormally high level of D cyclins allows the phosphorylation of CDKs, which triggers CDK activity. CDKs then phosphorylate pRBs. Unphosphorylated pRBs block the progression of normal cells from the G_1 phase of the cell cycle (when cell proteins are made) to the S phase (when DNA is duplicated). Phosphorylation of pRBs removes this blockade, allowing the cell to "run" its cell cycle.

A (lack of CDK activity) is incorrect. Nonphosphorylated CDKs are inactive.

B (lack of pRB phosphorylation) is incorrect. Nonphosphorylated pRBs prevent normal cells from progressing from the G_1 to the S phase of the cell cycle. They are part of the cell's intrinsic mechanism for controlling cell growth and preventing the formation of tumors.

D (underexpression of D cyclins) is incorrect. As long as D cyclin levels are not excessive, pRBs will not be phosphorylated. The lack of phosphorylated pRBs prevents normal cells from progressing from the G_1 phase of the cell cycle to the S phase. It is part of the cell's intrinsic mechanism for controlling cell growth.

E (up-regulation of p53) is incorrect. The p53 protein causes the cell to arrest in the G_1 phase of the cell cycle, preventing cell from preparing for replication.

questions

DIRECTIONS: Each numbered item or incomplete statement is followed by options arranged in alphabetical or logical order. Select the best answer to each question. Some options may be partially correct, but there is only **ONE BEST** answer.

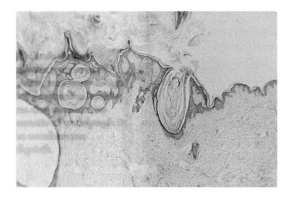

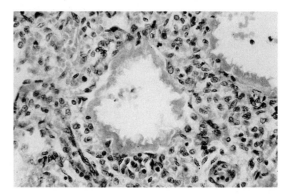

1. The photomicrograph shows tissue obtained by biopsy from a 32-year-old landscaper with a skin lesion in the axilla. Which of the following is the most likely diagnosis?
   A. Basal cell carcinoma
   B. Carcinoma of the sweat gland
   C. Malignant melanoma
   D. Seborrheic keratosis
   E. Squamous cell carcinoma

2. The specimen in this photomicrograph was removed at autopsy from the lung of a neonate who was having difficulty breathing soon after birth. Which of the following is the most likely diagnosis?
   A. Bronchopneumonia
   B. Carcinoma of the lung
   C. Hyaline membrane disease
   D. Interstitial pulmonary fibrosis
   E. Pulmonary edema

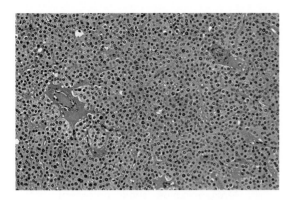

3. The benign tumor shown in the photomicrograph was removed from a 60-year-old woman with a renal calculus. Which of the following changes would you expect to find in the results of this patient's laboratory studies?
   A. Decrease in the blood urea nitrogen (BUN) level
   B. Decrease in the serum calcium level
   C. Decrease in the triiodothyronine (T_3) and thyroxine (T_4) levels
   D. Increase in the serum calcium level
   E. Increase in the T_3 and T_4 levels

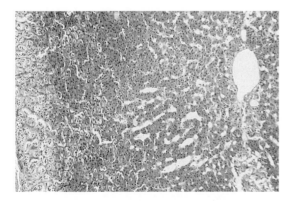

4. The surgical specimen shown here was removed from a young woman with severe cystic acne. Which of the following is the most likely diagnosis?
   A. Adrenogenital syndrome
   B. Alcoholic cirrhosis
   C. Cholangiocarcinoma
   D. Neoplasm of the Leydig cells
   E. Right-sided cardiac failure

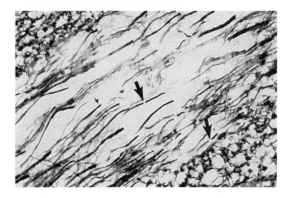

5. The specimen in this photomicrograph was prepared with osmium stain. What do the *arrows* point to?
   A. Adipose cells
   B. The H zone in skeletal muscle
   C. The I band in skeletal muscle
   D. Light collagen bands
   E. The nodes of Ranvier

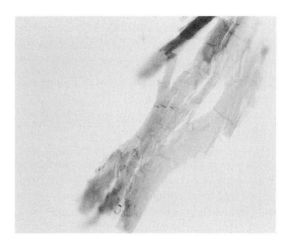

6. The *black bands* crossing at a right angle to the long axis of the fibers in this photomicrograph represent which of the following?
   A. A bands in skeletal muscle
   B. Cross-banding in collagen
   C. I bands in skeletal muscle
   D. Intercalated disks in cardiac muscle
   E. Sarcomeres in cardiac muscle

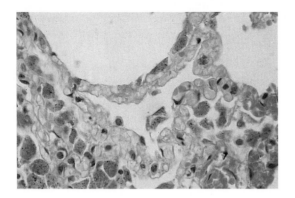

7. This photomicrograph shows a specimen taken from the lung of a 69-year-old man with a lengthy history of ischemic heart disease. The large cells with brown pigment are best classified as which of the following?
   A. Alveolar macrophages with anthracotic pigment
   B. Eosinophils
   C. Hemosiderinophages
   D. Malignant melanoma cells
   E. Type II pneumocytes

8. A 92-year-old woman complains of hearing loss. Which of the following structures in the organ of Corti would be reduced in size in this patient?
   A. Diameter of the inner ear tunnel
   B. Hairs on the surface of the inner hair cells
   C. Thickness of the basilar membrane
   D. Thickness of the tectorial membrane
   E. Thickness of the vestibular membrane

9. Which of the following would correctly describe any B lymphocyte seen in a peripheral blood smear from a 33-year old man?
   A. Actively producing humoral antibody
   B. Differentiated in red bone marrow
   C. Differentiated in the thymus
   D. Well-developed Golgi apparatus
   E. Well-developed rough endoplasmic reticulum (RER)

10. An 18-year-old woman who is undergoing chemotherapy for metastatic melanoma has severe neutropenia. Which of the following agents would most likely be administered to treat this side effect of chemotherapy?
   A. Colony-forming unit–erythrocyte (CFU-E)
   B. Colony-forming unit–granulocyte macrophage (CFU-GM)
   C. Erythropoietin (EPO)
   D. Granulocyte colony-stimulating factor (G-CSF)
   E. Monocyte colony-stimulating factor (M-CSF)

11. A 12-year-old Boy Scout had a painful rash on his lower legs after walking through a patch of poison ivy during a camping trip. Which of the following cells would process and present the antigen introduced by the plant to initiate an immune response in the skin?
   A. CD4 cell
   B. Dendritic reticular cell
   C. Epidermal Langerhans cell
   D. Histiocyte in a cord of Billroth
   E. Kupffer cell

12. A 6-year-old boy who was being treated for otitis media in the pediatric section of a children's hospital acquired a staphylococcal infection. Some staphylococci are phagocytosed by neutrophils (PMNs). Approximately 13 hours later, when the PMNs are no longer viable, viable staphylococci are liberated from these cells. Which disease state is suggested by these findings?
   A. Chédiak-Higashi disease
   B. Chronic granulomatous disease of childhood
   C. Chronic inflammation
   D. Chronic myelogenous leukemia (CML)

13. A 31-year-old man complains of left unilateral ptosis and pupillary constriction in the left eye. Which of the following should be considered when developing a differential diagnosis?
   A. Destruction of the celiac ganglion
   B. Destruction of the postganglionic neurons in the ciliary ganglion

C. Loss of innervation of the superior tarsal muscle (Müller's muscle)

D. Mesothelioma of the diaphragmatic surface of the left lung

E. Papilledema of the left optic disc

14. Electron microscopy of a cell in the bone marrow shows a cell with many channels of smooth endoplasmic reticulum (SER) in the cytoplasm, many electron-dense cytoplasmic granules of uniform size, and a multilobulated nucleus. Which type of cell is being examined?

A. Basophilic erythroblast

B. Developing B lymphocyte

C. Megakaryocyte

D. Neutrophil (PMN)

E. Reticulocyte

15. As a man is walking past a construction site, he is startled by the sudden and repetitive loud noise of a jackhammer nearby. Which structure in the ear protects the inner ear from damage due to exposure to this type of noise?

A. Oval window

B. Round window

C. Stapedius muscle

D. Tectorial membrane

E. Vestibular membrane

16. In a patient with vitamin D deficiency, osteoblasts in the endosteal membrane line which component of a mature spicule of cancellous bone?

A. Calcified cartilage

B. Mineralized osteoid

C. Nonmineralized osteoid

D. Zone of hypertrophied chondrocytes

17. A biopsy specimen of a section of the alveolar septa of the lung of a long-term smoker shows cells containing inhaled tar (carbon) particles. Which of the following cell types is most likely to contain such particles?

A. Ciliated cuboidal cells

B. Endothelial cells

C. Macrophages

D. Type I pneumocytes

E. Type II pneumocytes

18. A 28-year-old technician discovers that the drinking water in his laboratory has been contaminated with tritiated thymidine for the 2 months he worked there around the clock. Almost all of the water he drank during that time was from the laboratory. He is concerned about the effect this exposure may have on his ability to have children. Which of the following would be the most advanced stage of spermatogenesis in which tritiated thymidine would be incorporated into DNA in this person?

A. Early spermatids

B. Fully developed spermatozoa

C. Primary spermatocytes

D. Secondary spermatocytes

E. Spermatogonia

19. A margin of normal tissue and a large, high-grade leiomyosarcoma are removed from the gastrointestinal (GI) tract of a 42-year-old man. The marginal tissue shows an abrupt transition between stratified squamous nonkeratinized or parakeratinized epithelium and simple columnar epithelium. This specimen was obtained from which segment of the GI tract?

A. Gastroduodenal junction

B. Gastroesophageal junction

C. Lip

D. Lower anal canal and skin

E. Oropharynx and esophagus

20. Which of the following cytokines activates macrophages so they can attack and destroy neoplastic cells?

A. Erythropoietin (EPO)

B. Granulocyte colony-stimulating factor (G-CSF)

C. Granulocyte–monocyte colony-stimulating factor (GM-CSF)

D. Thrombopoietin

21. An 81-year-old man complains of difficulty breathing and undergoes a diagnostic bronchopulmonary lavage. Which of the following is removed in large numbers during the lavage of a bronchopulmonary segment?

A. Alveolar macrophages

B. Endothelial cells

C. Goblet cells
D. Type I pneumocytes
E. Type II pneumocytes

22. A B-cell lymphoma typically begins in which of the following sites where B cells are normally found?
A. Deep cortex of the lymph nodes
B. Germinal centers of the lymph nodes
C. Internodular connective tissue in the GI tract
D. Parenchymal elements of the thymus
E. White pulp surrounding a splenic artery

23. During a routine examination, a 43-year-old man is found to have hypermobility of the joints and hyperelasticity of the skin. The patient's medical history includes a corneal rupture. Recent laboratory studies show that the patient has a deficiency of lysyl hydroxylase. Which of the following is the most likely diagnosis?
A. Cystic fibrosis
B. Ehlers-Danlos syndrome
C. Familial hypercholesterolemia
D. Fragile X syndrome
E. Marfan syndrome

24. Which of the following is a physiologic feature of every endocrine gland?
A. Dependence on autonomic innervation
B. Dependence on pituitary stimulation
C. Extensive local blood supply
D. Extensive SER
E. Intracellular storage of large amounts of hormone

25. A 29-year-old woman bruises easily and has slight mucosal bleeding. The results of laboratory studies are as follows:

Complete Blood Count (CBC)
White blood cells (WBCs), 6300/mm³
Red blood cells (RBCs), 4.8 million/mm³
Platelet count, 92,000/mm³

Differential Count
Lymphocytes, 23%
Neutrophils, 67%
Basophils, 0.5%
Monocytes, 8%
Eosinophils, 1.5%

Which of the following is the most likely diagnosis?
A. Leukocytosis
B. Neutropenia
C. Poikilocytosis
D. Polycythemia
E. Thrombocytopenia

26. Which of the following is responsible for maintaining the normal discoid shape of thrombocytes?
A. Fibrinogen
B. Glycogen
C. Hyalomere microfilaments
D. An open canalicular system
E. Serotonin in the granulomere

27. An analysis of the karyotype of a pediatric patient shows two cell populations, both of which are aneuploid. One has $2n + 1$ chromosomes; the other has $2n - 1$. Which single event is responsible for both types of aneuploidy seen in this patient?
A. Nondisjunction of a homologous pair of chromosomes (total of four chromatids) during anaphase I of meiosis
B. Nondisjunction of a sister pair of chromatids at anaphase II of meiosis
C. Nondisjunction of a sister pair of chromatids during a mitotic anaphase of embryogenesis
D. Polygyny
E. Polyspermy

28. Microscopic examination of a surgical specimen taken from a small bowel resection shows varying degrees of pyknosis, karyorrhexis, and karyolysis in enterocytes located on the tips of the intestinal villi. Which of the following conditions is suggested by these findings?
A. Anaplasia
B. Apoptosis
C. Dysplasia
D. Inflammation

29. A 43-year-old man is diagnosed with poikilocytosis. Which of the following is an example of a poikilocyte?
A. Erythrocyte < 6 μm in diameter
B. Erythrocyte > 9 μm in diameter
C. Erythrocyte in a rouleau formation
D. Spherocyte
E. Stab (band) eosinophil

30. A bronchopulmonary lavage produces a normal amount of surfactant. Which type of cell in the lung is the primary source of surfactant?
A. Bronchiolar gland cell
B. Dust cell
C. Goblet cell
D. Type I pneumocyte
E. Type II pneumocyte

31. Approximately 3 minutes after blood is drawn from a patient during a routine physical examination, it is placed in a 0.9% NaCl solution. Which of the following changes may take place?
A. Crenation
B. Hemolysis
C. Increase in oxyhemoglobin content
D. Spherocytosis
E. No change

32. Which of the following cell types is an important direct target for HIV?
A. CD4 T cell
B. CD8 T cell
C. CD20 B cell
D. Natural killer (NK) cell
E. Plasma cell

33. Cancer is 25 times more likely to develop in renal allograft recipients who use immunosuppressive therapy than in healthy people due to the suppression of which of the following?
A. Basophils
B. Dendritic reticular cells
C. NK cells
D. Plasma cells
E. T suppressor cells

34. If the life span of osteoclasts remains constant with aging but the life span of osteoblasts is progressively shortened, which disease process is most likely to develop?
A. Osteoclastoma
B. Osteomalacia
C. Osteopetrosis
D. Osteoporosis
E. Scurvy

35. Two weeks after being tackled during football practice, a 20-year-old college student complains of frequent, severe headaches. A neuroradiologic examination shows several small, radiopaque specks near the center of the brain, suggesting calcification. Which of the following is most likely responsible for this finding?
A. Corpora amylacea in the pineal gland
B. Corpora arenacea in the pineal gland
C. Cupula of the crista ampullaris
D. Otoliths in the macula of the saccule
E. Otoliths in the macula of the utricle

36. A 29-year-old woman has been exposed to a large number of endotoxin-producing gram-negative bacteria, resulting in a large concentration of bacterial lipopolysaccharides in her blood. Which type of cell will respond to these changes by producing tumor necrosis factor (TNF)?
A. Basophil
B. Endothelial
C. Eosinophil
D. Monocyte
E. Platelet

37. A blood smear is prepared using a sample taken from a 12-year-old girl with chronic myelogenous leukemia (CML). Which of the following cell types will show the most prominent or largest nucleoli?
A. Basophilic myelocyte
B. Mature neutrophil (PMN)
C. Myeloblast
D. Neutrophilic metamyelocyte
E. Polychromatophilic normoblast

38. Assuming that a normal gamete contains 100 copies of ribosomal genes, how many copies of these genes are in a diploid cell during the G_2 phase of the intermitotic cell cycle?
   A. 100
   B. 200
   C. 300
   D. 400

39. Lipid-soluble high–molecular-weight alcohols readily enter the cell without using an energy-dependent process. When the alcohol concentration outside the cell increases, the rate at which it enters the cell increases; however, the concentration of alcohol inside the cell never exceeds the concentration of alcohol outside the cell. This indicates that these alcohols are transported across the cell membrane by which of the following?
   A. Active transport
   B. Carrier-facilitated diffusion
   C. Exocytosis
   D. Non–carrier-mediated transport

40. Which of the following best describes a cardiac muscle fiber?
   A. A nexus is found in the intercalated disk
   B. Each fiber is innervated by an individual nerve ending
   C. It lacks myofibrils
   D. T tubules are found at the A–I intercept

41. Which of the following best describes the development of skeletal muscle?
   A. A multinucleated cell is formed by repeated nuclear divisions in the absence of cytoplasmic division
   B. A multinucleated cell results from the fusion of many single cells
   C. After puberty, muscle mass grows by an increase in cell number
   D. Skeletal muscle is derived from the epithelial ectodermal and endodermal layers

42. A high–molecular-weight protein (500 amino acids) enters the cell without first being degraded by which mechanism?

   A. Active transport
   B. Carrier-facilitated diffusion
   C. Endocytosis
   D. Exocytosis
   E. Non–carrier-mediated transport

43. In a particular organism, the nucleolar organizer is located on the short arm of a single chromosome pair. Deletion of both members of the chromosome pair would result in which of the following effects?
   A. Increased hybridization of DNA with 18S and 28S recombinant ribonucleic acid (rRNA)
   B. Increased number of nucleoli
   C. Increased synthesis of 45S RNA
   D. Loss of secondary constrictions

44. Which of the following is a distinguishing characteristic of synapses?
   A. A myelin sheath must be present if synaptic transmission is to occur
   B. Mitochondria and vesicles containing neurotransmitters accumulate in the presynaptic area
   C. Most synapses exist between two dendritic processes
   D. Occluding junctions hold the two neuronal processes together
   E. Satellite cells intervene between the neuronal processes

45. The blood–brain barrier prevents certain substances from passing from the blood into the central nervous system. This function is primarily the responsibility of which of the following?
   A. Accumulation of reactive astrocytes at the site of injury
   B. Association of the choroid plexus with pia mater cells
   C. Maintenance of the resting membrane potential
   D. Presence of occluding junctions between capillary endothelial cells

46. The hypertonic quality of the interstitium of the renal medulla affects which of the following?
A. Resorption of water from the proximal convoluted tubule
B. Resorption of water from the straight collecting tubules
C. Resorption of water from the thick ascending portion of Henle's loop

47. Microscopic evaluation of a biopsy specimen taken from the femur of a 3-year-old girl shows interstitial lamellae that appear on the most radiolucent areas of a photomicrograph. Interstitial lamellae are a consequence of which of the following events?
A. Failure of haversian systems to form correctly
B. Inadequate intake of vitamin C
C. Partial resorption of haversian systems by osteoclasts
D. Pulling apart of haversian systems by Sharpey's fibers
E. Stimulation of the periosteum by parathyroid hormone (PTH)

48. Removal of the anterior lobe of the pituitary gland would have which of the following effects on the male reproductive system?
A. Decreased synthesis of androgen-binding protein
B. Increased production of testosterone
C. Increased spermatogenesis

49. Specimens taken from several parts of the GI tract of a patient with cystic fibrosis are being prepared for microscopic study. In which structure will an epithelium be seen in which every surface cell is capable of secreting mucus?
A. Duodenum
B. Esophagus
C. Lower anal canal
D. Stomach
E. Transverse colon

50. A blood smear prepared from a sample obtained from a patient with leukemia contains many large cells. Each of the cells has a round nucleus containing several prominent nucleoli and a cytoplasm filled with small azurophilic granules. Using the description of the cells, which of the following is the most likely diagnosis?
A. Acute lymphoblastic leukemia (ALL)
B. Basophilic leukemia
C. Monoblastic leukemia
D. Promyelocytic leukemia
E. Stem cell leukemia

answers

1. **D** (seborrheic keratosis) is correct. Normal epidermis can be seen to the right and hyperkeratosis to the left in the photomicrograph. Excessive keratin formation (entrapped in the epidermis) can also be seen. Seborrheic keratoses are benign lesions; however, when they suddenly increase in number, the patient may have an underlying stomach cancer (Leser-Trélat sign).

    A (basal cell carcinoma) is incorrect. Basal cell carcinoma normally arises from cells in the stratum basale layer of the epidermis. It invades the dermis but usually does not affect the superficial layers of the epidermis.

    B (carcinoma of the sweat gland) is incorrect. Carcinoma of the sweat gland is a rare adenocarcinoma. It has a glandular appearance, not the sheetlike appearance of the tissue seen in this photomicrograph.

    C (malignant melanoma) is incorrect. Malignant melanoma arises from melanocytes, which usually are most easily seen near the border between the epidermis and the dermis. It is not characterized by excessive keratin production (as shown), which normally occurs on the epidermal surface.

    E (squamous cell carcinoma) is incorrect. Squamous cell carcinoma is characterized by nests of squamous cells similar to those found in the stratum spinosum of the epidermis. Squamous pearls consisting of keratin may appear in the center of these nests. However, the excessive amounts of keratin on the epidermal surface that appear in the photomicrograph are not associated with this type of cancer.

2. **C** (hyaline membrane disease) is correct. An amorphous eosinophilic hyaline material lines the alveoli and bronchioles in the photomicrograph and forms a barrier between blood and air (diffusion defect). Hyaline membrane disease is due to a lack of surfactant, which leads to collapse of the alveoli and massive intrapulmonary shunting of blood.

    A (bronchopneumonia) is incorrect. Bronchopneumonia involves a suppurative inflammation that can fill the alveoli, bronchioles, and bronchi. Note that most of the nuclei in the photomicrograph are round to ovoid rather than multilobulated like neutrophils. Due to a lack of surfactant, the alveoli are collapsed; hence, the nuclei are primarily those of type I pneumocytes.

    B (carcinoma of the lung) is incorrect. Several types of carcinomas arise in the lung, including squamous cell carcinoma, adenocarcinoma, small cell carcinoma, and mesothelioma. These tumors contain pleomorphic cells. Thus, if a carcinoma were shown in the photomicrograph, discrete areas of the specimen would contain cells of the same type, but with variations in their appearance.

    D (interstitial pulmonary fibrosis) is incorrect. Interstitial pulmonary fibrosis results in widespread fibrosis but with few inflammatory cells. It can be ruled out in this case because of the extensive number of inflammatory cells. There are no areas of fibrosis.

E (pulmonary edema) is incorrect. Pulmonary edema results in the alveoli being filled with fluid, which is usually a transudate (low protein and cell content). Pulmonary edema can be ruled out in this case because the alveoli are collapsed and do not contain fluid.

3.   **D** (increase in the serum calcium level) is correct. The field of view in this photomicrograph is dominated by well-differentiated cells containing a prominent nucleus and a limited cytoplasm. These are characteristics of the chief cell, which is the dominant cell type in parathyroid tissue. The excessive number of chief cells without intervening adipose cells suggests an adenoma, which is a benign neoplasm. Chief cells produce parathyroid hormone, which increases calcium levels in the blood. Increased calcium in the urine predisposes an individual to calculus formation.

A (decrease in the BUN level) is incorrect. The BUN level is an indication of the rate at which amino acids are metabolized in the liver. A decrease in BUN levels may indicate reduced activity of the liver enzymes in the urea cycle that convert toxic ammonia (a byproduct of deamination) into urea. This occurs in cirrhosis of the liver. The photomicrograph shows parathyroid tissue, which is not associated with urea metabolism.

B (decrease in the serum calcium level) is incorrect. The photomicrograph shows an overgrowth of chief cells, which indicates a parathyroid tumor. Chief cells secrete parathyroid hormone, which promotes the absorption of calcium from the kidneys and the resorption of bone from increased osteoclastic activity. When the tumor is removed, the calcium levels will fall into the normal range.

C (decrease in the T_3 and T_4 levels) and **E** (increase in the T_3 and T_4 levels) are incorrect. The dominant cell in the photomicrograph is the chief cell of the parathyroid gland, which

is identified by its prominent nucleus and limited cytoplasm. The overgrowth of these cells suggests a parathyroid adenoma. T_3 and T_4 are produced by the thyroid gland, not the parathyroid gland. Removal of the parathyroid tumor will not affect the production of thyroid hormones.

4.   **A** (adrenogenital syndrome) is correct. The photomicrograph shows the three layers of the adrenal cortex; the vein to the right is in the adrenal medulla. The zona glomerulosa is the most lightly stained region (far left). This zone primarily synthesizes mineralocorticoids. Deep to the zona glomerulosa is the zona fasciculata. This zone primarily synthesizes cortisol. Deep to the zona fasciculata is an area of hyperplasia in the zona reticularis. In females, overproduction of androgens by the zona reticularis may result in a virilism syndrome (female pseudohermaphroditism) if the patient has classic 21- or 11-hydroxylase enzyme deficiency. This patient most likely has the nonclassic type of 21-hydroxylase deficiency, which usually causes severe acne.

B (alcoholic cirrhosis) is incorrect. The left half of the photomicrograph clearly shows three layers of tissue. In cirrhosis of the liver, sheets of hepatocytes are surrounded by bands of fibrous tissue, which are not evident in the photomicrograph.

C (cholangiocarcinoma) is incorrect. Cholangiocarcinomas arise from the epithelial lining of the bile ducts. The structure of the epithelium lining the lumen of structures in the biliary tree ranges from a layer of hepatocyte plasma membranes lining the bile canaliculi to the highly twisted mucosa lining the cystic duct. None of the characteristic biliary lumina appear in the photomicrograph. The majority of cases of cholangiocarcinoma in the United States arise from primary sclerosing cholangitis associated with ulcerative colitis.

D (neoplasm of the Leydig cells) is incorrect. The Leydig cell has a large nucleus and is found alone or with a few other Leydig cells within the supporting tissue of the seminiferous tubules (i.e., along the periphery of the tubules) in the testis. Neither tubular cells nor tissue with a histology resembling that of Leydig cells appears in the photomicrograph. Also, the patient was female.

E (right-sided cardiac failure) is incorrect. Right-sided cardiac failure produces an increase in venous hydrostatic pressure. Increased pressure in the vena cava is transmitted back into the hepatic vein and eventually into the central veins of the liver. Congestion of blood in these veins gives the liver surface a "nutmeg" appearance. Note that the vein in this photomicrograph is not congested.

5. **E** (the nodes of Ranvier) is correct. The photomicrograph shows a segment of a peripheral nerve stained with osmium, which stains myelin black. The nodes of Ranvier are discrete regions along the axon that are not covered by myelin. These unmyelinated regions serve as the anatomic basis for saltatory conduction.

   A (adipose cells) is incorrect. The adipose cell is round and filled with a lipid droplet that often presses the nucleus against the periphery of the cell. Adipose cells also react to the special stain (osmium) that was used to prepare the specimen in the photomicrograph; their characteristic appearance is not seen here.

   B (the H zone in skeletal muscle) is incorrect. The H zone is the region within the sarcomere of skeletal muscle fibers where the thick and thin myofilaments overlap. It can be viewed under relatively high magnification ($\times1000$). It would not be seen under the low-power magnification used in the photomicrograph.

   C (the I band in skeletal tissue) is incorrect. The I band is the light area, or isotropic band, in the sarcomere of skeletal muscle. The Z line inserts into it. Much higher resolution is needed to see the I band than was used in the photomicrograph.

   D (light collagen bands) is incorrect. The light bands in collagen fibers alternate with dark bands. However, they can only be seen with the high resolution of an electron microscope.

6. **D** (intercalated disks in cardiac muscle) is correct. The photomicrograph shows cardiac muscle that has been teased to demonstrate how the cardiac muscle cells anastomose and branch with one another. The dark bands are intercalated disks. Adjacent cardiac muscle cells are held together in this region by various types of cell-to-cell junctions. Gap junctions allow intercellular ionic (electrical) communication.

   A (A bands in skeletal muscle) is incorrect. The A (anisotropic) band consists of the thick, myosin-rich myofilaments of the sarcomere. Although A bands cross the muscle fiber in skeletal and cardiac tissue, they are much thinner than intercalated disks. Also, thousands of A bands would be seen instead of the dozen or so intercalated disks shown in this preparation.

   B (cross-banding in collagen) is incorrect. The alternating light–dark band pattern in collagen is an ultrastructural feature. It cannot be seen using light microscopy.

   C (I bands in skeletal muscle) is incorrect. The I bands in skeletal muscle are so called because they are isotropic (i.e., they allow light to pass through). Because they cannot appear as dark bands, they are ruled out in this preparation. As with A bands, I bands are much smaller than the intercalated disks seen here.

   E (sarcomeres in cardiac muscle) is incorrect. A sarcomere extends from one Z line to the next in both cardiac and skeletal muscle.

Furthermore, it is much smaller than the intercalated disks shown in this preparation.

7. **C** (hemosiderinophages) is correct. Under certain circumstances, such as intra-alveolar hemorrhage in chronic heart failure, alveolar macrophages phagocytose red blood cells. One of the products of hemoglobin catabolism is hemosiderin, a substance that is stored within the macrophage, where it appears as brown pigment. This most often occurs in patients with chronic passive congestion of the lung due to a heart problem, as seen in this patient. Because these macrophages store hemosiderin, they are often referred to as *hemosiderinophages* or *heart-failure cells.*

A (alveolar macrophages with anthracotic pigment) is incorrect. Anthracosis is a form of pneumoconiosis that is induced by coal dust deposits in the lungs. It can result in anthracotic pigment filling the alveoli and alveolar macrophages (black lung disease).

B (eosinophils) is incorrect. Eosinophils contain granules that stain pink.

D (malignant melanoma cells) is incorrect. Malignant melanoma arises from melanocytes. Melanin granules are black.

E (type II pneumonocytes) is incorrect. Type II pneumonocytes (also known as *greater alveolar cells*) are found in the alveolar epithelium and secrete surfactant. These cells have large, round nuclei and a vacuolated cytoplasm that does not contain granules. Electron microscopy may show structures (lamellar bodies) indicating intracellular storage surfactant. Such cells do not appear in the photomicrograph.

8. **B** (hairs on the surface of the inner hair cells) is correct. The term *hairs* refers to stereocilia, which are microvilli, not cilia. The core of the stereocilium contains actin filaments cross-linked with fimbrin near the apical plasmalemma of the hair cell; this arrangement is responsible for its rigidity. When sound waves move the basilar membrane in the cochlea, the stereocilia are bent, causing release of the content of the stereocilia into synaptic-like structures. This release excites the afferent nerve fibers that are closely associated with each hair cell. The hairs (stereocilia) on the surface of the inner and outer hair cells decrease in number and size during the aging process, thereby reducing the ability to hear.

A (diameter of the inner ear tunnel) is incorrect. The inner ear tunnel is filled with endolymph. The diameter of this tunnel has nothing to do with the process of hearing.

C (thickness of the basilar membrane) is incorrect. The basilar membrane supports the organ of Corti in the inner ear. Vibrations in the basilar membrane cause the organ of Corti to move in relation to the overlying tectorial membrane. Hair cells (stereocilia) in the organ of Corti project into the tectorial membrane. The first step in the neurophysiology of hearing is movement of the basilar membrane, which causes the stereocilia to bend. The thickness of the basilar membrane is not as important in the hearing process as a decrease in the number of hairs on the hair cells.

D (thickness of the tectorial membrane) is incorrect. The tectorial membrane overlies the organ of Corti in the inner ear. Hair cells (stereocilia) in the organ of Corti project their hairs into the tectorial membrane. When the organ of Corti moves (as occurs when the underlying basilar membrane "vibrates"), causing these hairs to bend. The thickness of the tectorial membrane is not as important in the hearing process as a decrease in the number of hairs on the hair cells.

E (thickness of the vestibular membrane) is incorrect. The vestibular membrane is the part of the cochlear duct that faces the scala vestibuli. It does not play a role in the process of hearing. Furthermore, this membrane is two cells thick throughout life.

9. **B** (differentiated in red bone marrow) is correct. B lymphocytes undergo differentiation from precursor cells in red bone marrow.

   A (actively producing humoral antibody) is incorrect. Active production of humoral antibody is a function of plasma cells, which are terminally differentiated B cells.

   C (differentiated in the thymus) is incorrect. T cells (not B cells) differentiate in the thymus gland.

   D (well-developed Golgi apparatus) is incorrect. A well-developed Golgi apparatus would be found in the terminally differentiated descendant of a B lymphocyte (the plasma cell), but not in the B cell itself.

   E (well-developed RER) is incorrect. A well-developed RER would be found in terminally differentiated descendants of B lymphocytes (plasma cells) but not in the B cell itself.

10. **D** (G-CSF) is correct. G-CSF stimulates granulocytopoiesis (production of granulocytes), especially the production of neutrophils (PMNs). Thus, it can cause the number of PMNs in the blood to increase from neutropenic to normal levels.

   A (CFU-E) is incorrect. Neutropenia is an abnormally low number of neutrophils in the blood. Patients with neutropenia require a factor that stimulates the production of neutrophils. CFU-E is a cell, not a growth factor.

   B (CFU-GM) is incorrect. Neutropenia is an abnormally low number of neutrophils in the blood. Patients with neutropenia require a factor that stimulates the production of neutrophils. CFU-GM is a cell, not a growth factor.

   C (EPO) is incorrect. Neutropenia is an abnormally low number of neutrophils in the blood. EPO stimulates erythrocytopoiesis, not granulocytopoiesis.

   E (M-CSF) is incorrect. Neutropenia is an abnormally low number of neutrophils in the blood. M-CSF stimulates the production of monocytes, not neutrophils.

11. **C** (epidermal Langerhans cell) is correct. Poison ivy introduces a foreign antigen to the skin. Langerhans cells function as the epidermal counterpart to the dendritic reticular cells in the germinal centers of lymph nodules because they are able to take up an antigen, process it, and present it to immunocompetent cells.

   A (CD4 cell) is incorrect. The CD4 cell (T helper cell) can up-regulate antibody production by B cells by means of cytokine secretion. It participates in a secondary response to antigen exposure rather than the primary response that occurs in the skin.

   B (dendritic reticular cell) is incorrect. The dendritic reticular cell is found in the lymph nodes and can trap, process, and present antigens to immunocompetent cells. Because it is not found in the epidermis, it is not likely to participate in an immune response to poison ivy.

   D (histiocytes in a cord of Billroth) is incorrect. Tissue macrophages or histiocytes can present an antigen after it has been phagocytosed and processed. A histiocyte in the spleen is not likely to be involved in an immune response to poison ivy exposure on the skin.

   E (Kupffer cell) is incorrect. Kupffer cells are fixed macrophages (histiocytes) that line or bridge the hepatic sinusoids. Because they are not found in the skin, they would not participate in an immune response to poison ivy.

12. **B** (chronic granulomatous disease of childhood) is correct. Chronic granulomatous disease of childhood is associated with a genetic defect that results in the failure of PMNs to produce hydrogen peroxide. As a result, bacteria that enter these cells are not killed by the cell. Instead, when the PMN dies, viable bacteria are released.

A (Chédiak-Higashi disease) is incorrect. Chédiak-Higashi disease is characterized by a lag in the initiation of the fusion of lysosomes with ingested bacteria (microbicidal defect). In this case, the cell is capable of destroying ingested bacteria but may take longer to do so.

C (chronic inflammation) is incorrect. The term *chronic inflammation* is usually applied to a long-standing infection in connective tissue.

D (CML) is incorrect. CML is characterized by the appearance of undifferentiated hematopoietic cells in the peripheral blood. In contrast, this patient's PMNs are fully functional (i.e., capable of killing phagocytosed bacteria). CML is more likely to occur in adults between the ages of 39 and 60 years.

13. **C** (loss of innervation of the superior tarsal muscle) is correct. Carcinoma in the apex of the left lung can destroy the superior cervical sympathetic ganglion, whose postganglionic sympathetic fibers innervate both the dilator muscle of the iris and Müller's muscle (the smooth muscle component of the levator palpebrae superioris muscle). Contraction of Müller's muscle raises the upper eyelid. Its function is overruled by contraction of the orbicularis oculi muscle. The activity of both muscles is seen during a blink.

A (destruction of the celiac ganglion) is incorrect. The celiac ganglion is a sympathetic ganglion located in the abdomen. Its postganglionic fibers do not innervate the eye.

B (destruction of the postganglionic neurons in the ciliary ganglion) is incorrect. The ciliary ganglion is a parasympathetic ganglion. The clinical signs described for this patient strongly suggest a defect in sympathetic innervation of the eye, not parasympathetic innervation.

D (mesothelioma of the diaphragmatic surface of the left lung) is incorrect. Mesothelioma is a neoplasm that arises from the pleural mesothelium. A mesothelioma on the diaphragmatic surface of the lung would not be positioned correctly to destroy the superior sympathetic ganglion.

E (papilledema of the left optic disc) is incorrect. Papilledema of the optic disc indicates increased intracranial pressure, not a loss of sympathetic innervation to the dilator muscle and Müller's muscle of the eye.

14. **C** (megakaryocyte) is correct. The DNA in megakaryocytes undergoes several rounds of endoreduplication, which result in a cell with a multilobulated nucleus containing 16C, 32C, or 64C DNA and a cytoplasm full of granules. Small islands of granule-containing cytoplasm are surrounded by membranes of the SER, often referred to as *platelet demarcation membranes.* Each island separates from the megakaryocyte to exist independently as a platelet.

A (basophilic erythroblast) is incorrect. Basophilic erythroblasts do not have a multilobulated nucleus. Also, their cytoplasm is full of free polysomes, not granules.

B (developing B lymphocyte) is incorrect. A developing B lymphocyte does not have a multilobulated nucleus. It has a small amount of cytoplasm that does not contain an SER or cytoplasmic granules.

D (PMN) is incorrect. Each PMN has a multilobulated nucleus and many cytoplasmic granules. However, these granules are of two distinct sizes (400 nm and 700 nm), unlike the uniform granules seen in platelets. Furthermore, a PMN would not show SER channels.

E (reticulocyte) is incorrect. Reticulocytes do not have a nucleus, and their cytoplasm contains only a few free polysomes.

15. C (stapedius muscle) is correct. The stapedius muscle controls the oscillatory stroke of the footplate of the stapes. Innervated by the facial nerve (cranial nerve VII), this muscle contracts in response to sudden, repetitive, loud noise and reduces the oscillatory response of the stapes. The stapedius muscle protects the structures of the inner ear from damage due to repetitive, loud noises.

A (oval window) is incorrect. The oval window passively responds to insult and has no protective mechanism of its own.

B (round window) is incorrect. The round window responds passively to insult by bulging outward to relieve the pressure transferred to it by perilymph, which responds to the pressure induced by the movement of the footplate of the stapes against the oval window.

D (tectorial membrane) is incorrect. The tectorial membrane passively responds to insult. It does not have a protective mechanism of its own.

E (vestibular membrane) is incorrect. The vestibular membrane passively responds to insult; it does not have a protective mechanism of its own.

16. C (nonmineralized osteoid) is correct. The youngest part of a developing spicule of cancellous bone is along its outermost edge, which is composed of the fresh (nonmineralized) osteoid most recently synthesized by the layer of osteoblasts of the endosteum. Because vitamin D ensures an adequate supply of calcium to mineralize osteoid, this nonmineralized zone would be relatively thick in a patient lacking vitamin D.

A (calcified cartilage) is incorrect. Calcified cartilage can be found in the center of the spicules of bone formed by means of endochondral ossification. This would place the calcified cartilage farthest from the endosteal membrane.

B (mineralized osteoid) is incorrect. Mineralized osteoid is the older osteoid in the bone spicule. It lies deep in the spicule, not close to the endosteal membrane.

D (zone of hypertrophied chondrocytes) is incorrect. Hypertrophied chondrocytes are found in a specific layer of the epiphyseal plate. This layer does not have an endosteal surface.

17. C (macrophages) is correct. The alveolar macrophage ("dust" cell) wanders over the alveolar surface, phagocytosing bacteria and other inhaled particles, including particles released from inhaled cigarette smoke. These cells digest the phagocytosed bacteria using lysosomal enzymes. Because there is no enzyme "carbonase," the undigested particles of tar remain in the cells for life.

A (ciliated cuboidal cells) is incorrect. Ciliated cuboidal cells are found in higher (wider) segments of the respiratory tree (not in the alveoli).

B (endothelial cells) is incorrect. Endothelial cells line the alveolar capillaries. Although they reside within the alveolar septum (respiratory membrane), they are not phagocytes. Therefore, they are unlikely to contain lung contaminants (including those introduced by inhaled cigarette smoke).

D (type I pneumocytes) is incorrect. Type I pneumocytes lie within the alveolar septum and face the air in the alveolus. Because they are extremely thin structures, they are able to facilitate the passage of gas between air and blood. They are not phagocytes; therefore, they are unlikely to contain any lung contaminants (including those introduced by inhaled cigarette smoke).

E (type II pneumocytes) is incorrect. Type II pneumocytes reside within the alveolar septum, where they synthesize and release surfactant. These are not phagocytic cells, and they are unlikely to contain any lung contaminants (including those introduced by inhaled cigarette smoke).

18. **B** (fully developed spermatozoa) is correct. The most advanced stage of spermatogenesis involves the production of mature spermatozoa. It takes approximately 62 days for spermatogonia to become spermatozoa. Spermatogenesis would result in the uptake of radioactive thymidine, and it would be found in all cells derived from exposed spermatogonia.

A (early spermatids), **C** (primary sperma-tocytes), **D** (secondary spermatocytes), and **E** (spermatogonia) are incorrect. The normal sequence of steps in spermatogenesis is spermatogonia, primary spermatocyte, secondary spermatocyte, and spermatid, which undergoes morphologic changes to become the mature sperm. The DNA of early spermatids, primary and secondary spermatocytes, and spermatogonia contain labeled thymidine.

19. **B** (gastroesophageal junction) is correct. The stratified squamous wet epithelium of the esophagus changes abruptly to a simple columnar epithelium (as seen in the upper gastric region) at the gastroesophageal junction.

A (gastroduodenal junction) is incorrect. Both the stomach and the duodenum are lined with a simple columnar epithelium.

C (lip) and **D** (lower anal canal and skin) are incorrect. The junction between the lip and the surrounding skin marks a sharp transition from a stratified squamous wet epithelium to

a stratified squamous dry epithelium. The same type of epithelial junction is seen between the lower anal canal and the surrounding skin. Neither junction contains a simple epithelium.

E (oropharynx and esophagus) is incorrect. Both of these structures are lined with a stratified squamous nonkeratinized epithelium.

20. **C** (GM-CSF) is correct. GM-CSF facilitates the differentiation of a hematopoietic stem cell into the precursor of both the granulocyte and the monocyte lines of cytodifferentiation, and it activates macrophages. GM-CSF has been used in clinical trials of patients with advanced-stage malignant melanoma, with encouraging results.

A (EPO) is incorrect. EPO is produced by the kidney in response to low oxygen levels in the blood. Its target is the red blood cell precursor in bone marrow, which causes it to become committed to erythrocytopoiesis.

B (G-CSF) is incorrect. G-CSF enhances only granulocytopoiesis (not monocytopoiesis).

D (thrombopoietin) is incorrect. Thrombo-poietin enhances thrombocytopoiesis. It does not induce monocytopoiesis or macrophage activity.

21. **A** (alveolar macrophages) is correct. The alveolar macrophage (dust cell) wanders over the alveolar surface, phagocytosing inhaled particles. This is the only place in the body where macrophages migrate over a surface area; elsewhere, they migrate within connective tissue. These cells are "free" and are located on the air surface of the respiratory membrane. As a result, they are easily captured by saline lavage of a pulmonary lobule or bronchopulmonary segment.

B (endothelial cells) is incorrect. Endothelial cells line the walls of capillaries; they would not be exposed to the saline solution.

C (goblet cells) is incorrect. Few, if any, goblet cells would appear in a lavage of a bronchopulmonary segment because these cells are attached to their basal lamina.

D (type I pneumocytes) and E (type II pneumocyte) are incorrect. Few (if any) type I and type II pneumocytes would appear in a lavage of a bronchopulmonary segment because these cells are attached to their basal lamina.

22. **B** (germinal centers of the lymph nodes) is correct. The germinal centers in all lymph nodes are composed almost exclusively of B cells.

A (deep cortex of the lymph nodes) is incorrect. The deep cortex of a lymph node is composed mainly of T cells, not B cells.

C (internodular connective tissue in the GI tract) is incorrect. The connective tissue that lies between the lymph nodules in the GI tract is composed mostly of T cells.

D (parenchymal elements of the thymus) is incorrect. The parenchymal elements of the thymus are composed of T cells.

E (white pulp surrounding a splenic artery) is incorrect. The white pulp that surrounds arteries in the spleen is composed mostly of T cells.

23. **B** (Ehlers-Danlos syndrome) is correct. Ehlers-Danlos syndrome is a multitude of disorders caused by a defect in an autosomal recessive gene involved in the synthesis of collagen or collagen cross-linking events. At least 10 varieties of this disorder are known. This patient may have variant VI, which is characterized by decreased hydroxylation of lysyl residues in type I and type III collagen.

A (cystic fibrosis) is incorrect. Cystic fibrosis is the most common lethal genetic disease affecting white children. It is caused by a defect in the function of all exocrine glands.

The organs most likely to be seriously affected are the lungs and pancreas because this disorder results in abnormally viscous secretions that block the airways and pancreatic ducts.

C (familial hypercholesterolemia) is incorrect. Familial hypercholesterolemia is a genetic disease caused by mutations in the gene for receptor proteins. It results in defective catabolism and excessive biosynthesis of cholesterol. This patient's symptoms suggest abnormal collagen formation; familial hyper-cholesterolemia does not play a role in collagen formation.

D (fragile X syndrome) is incorrect. Fragile X syndrome occurs in males and is characterized by mental retardation and macro-orchidism. It is identified by an abnormal banding pattern on the affected X chromosome, which represents the amplification of sets of three nucleotides and which disrupts the normal function of the gene.

E (Marfan syndrome) is incorrect. Marfan syndrome is an autosomal dominant disorder that results in a defect in the production of fibril, a structural glycoprotein secreted by fibroblasts that forms microfibrillar aggregates in the extracellular matrix. These aggregates serve as scaffolds for normal elastic fibers. The most serious clinical sign of Marfan syndrome is loss of elasticity in the tunica media of the aorta. This defect is the pathologic basis for aortic aneurysm, which can result in aortic dissection or rupture.

24. **C** (extensive local blood supply) is correct. Endocrine glands have no duct system and secrete their product directly into the blood vessels that serve them. All endocrine glands are highly vascularized.

A (dependence on autonomic innervation) is incorrect. Most endocrine glands are influenced by pituitary factors or blood levels of the product they regulate. An exception is the adrenal medulla, which is influenced through direct innervation by the sympathetic division of the autonomic nervous system.

B (dependence on pituitary stimulation) is incorrect. The activity of many endocrine glands is induced by factors released by the pituitary gland. Exceptions include the parathyroid gland (which is directly influenced by serum calcium levels) and the islets of Langerhans in the pancreas (which are directly influenced by the level of glucose in the blood).

D (extensive SER) is incorrect. Only endocrine cells that produce steroid hormones contain a well-developed SER.

E (intracellular storage of large amounts of hormone) is incorrect. Most endocrine glands store relatively small amounts of hormone; however, the thyroid gland stores large amounts of hormone extracellularly in colloid-filled follicles.

25. **E** (thrombocytopenia) is correct: Thrombocytopenia is characterized by a thrombocyte count of ≤100,000 platelets/mm³. Clinically significant thrombocytopenia is the result of inadequate thrombocyte production in the red bone marrow or decreased thrombocyte survival in the blood. Thrombocytopenia is one of the most common findings in patients with AIDS.

A (leukocytosis) is incorrect. Leukocytosis is characterized by an abnormal increase in the white WBC concentration in the blood. The WBC concentration for this patient is within normal limits.

B (neutropenia) is incorrect. Neutropenia is characterized by an abnormally low PMN count. The PMN concentration for this patient is within normal limits.

C (poikilocytosis) is incorrect. Poikilocytosis is characterized by RBCs with abnormal shapes but not necessarily by an abnormal number of RBCs.

D (polycythemia) is incorrect. Polycythemia is characterized by an abnormal increase in the RBC concentration in blood. The RBC concentration for this patient is within normal limits.

26. **C** (hyalomere microfilaments) is correct. The cytoskeleton of the thrombocyte is composed of microfilaments and microtubules. Most of these are found in the peripheral hyalomere (clear zone) of the platelet.

A (fibrinogen) is incorrect. Fibrinogen is a protein produced in the liver and is critical for blood clotting. It is not a component of the cytoskeleton of platelets and thus does not contribute to the structural integrity of the platelet.

B (glycogen) is incorrect. Glycogen is the intracellular storage form of glucose. It does not contribute to the structural integrity of the platelet.

D (an open canalicular system) is incorrect. The canalicular system is a set of cytoplasmic canaliculi that communicates with the exterior of the platelet. It is not a component of the cytoskeleton of the platelet; therefore, it does not contribute to the structural integrity of the platelet.

E (serotonin in the granulomere) is incorrect. Serotonin is stored in granules in the more centrally located granulomere region of a platelet. It does not play a role in maintaining the discoid shape of platelets.

27. **C** (nondisjunction of a sister pair of chromatids during a mitotic anaphase of embryogenesis) is correct. The failure of sister chromatids in a single chromosome to separate during early anaphase of mitosis results in one line of cells missing one chromosome and another line of cells having one extra chromosome.

A (nondisjunction of a homologous pair of chromosomes [total of four chromatids] during anaphase I of meiosis) is incorrect. Nondisjunction during meiosis I can result in two different kinds of gametes: one with n + 1 chromosomes and the other with n − 1 chromosomes. However, only one of these gametes would participate in fertilization with another normal (haploid) gamete. This would result in trisomy or monosomy, but not both.

B (nondisjunction of a sister pair of chromatids at anaphase II of meiosis) is incorrect. When a pair of sister chromatids fails to separate during meiosis II, the result is two different kinds of gametes: one containing n + 1 chromosomes and the other containing n − 1 chromosomes. Therefore, fertilization of one of the abnormal gametes with a normal gamete would result in either trisomy or monosomy, but not both.

D (polygyny) is incorrect. Polygyny involving fertilization with a normal sperm results in triploidy (not aneuploidy).

E (polyspermy) is incorrect. Polyspermy involving fertilization with a normal oocyte results in triploidy.

28. **B** (apoptosis) is correct. Apoptosis (programmed cell death) occurs in several stages, which can be identified by light microscopy. During the first stage, pyknotic changes are indicated by the presence of one or more dark-staining masses on the inside of the nuclear membrane. During the second stage (karyorrhexis), nuclear material breaks into fragments. During the third stage (karyolysis), the nucleus breaks up into smaller, membrane-bound bodies (apoptotic bodies), each of which contains some nuclear material. Eventually, this apoptotic debris is scavenged by macrophages and lost to the luminal contents.

A (anaplasia) is incorrect. Anaplasia is a severe type of dysplasia characterized by marked pleomorphism, extreme hyperchromaticity of the nucleus, and a nucleus-to-cytoplasm ratio closer to 1:1 than the normal 1:5. It is not characterized by the changes described for this specimen.

C (dysplasia) is incorrect. Dysplasia is characterized by a loss of uniformity in cell size and a change in the shape and orientation of cells (pleomorphism). It does not result in degradation of the nucleus.

D (inflammation) is incorrect. Inflammation is characterized by a proliferation of immune cells: neutrophils (PMNs) during the acute phase and lymphocytes, macrophages, and plasma cells during the chronic phase. It is not characterized by the changes described for this specimen.

29. **D** (spherocyte) is correct. Poikilocytes are abnormally shaped red blood cells (RBCs). An example of a poikilocyte is a spherocyte, which is an RBC with an abnormal shape that is most likely due to a defect in the cytoskeletal protein spectrin. Lack of spectrin makes it impossible for the cell to maintain its normally biconcave shape.

A (erythrocyte <6 μm in diameter) is incorrect. A RBC <6 μm in diameter is a microcyte. Because it has a normal biconcave shape, it is not considered a poikilocyte.

B (erythrocyte >9 μm in diameter) is incorrect. An RBC >9 μm in diameter is a macrocyte. Macrocytes have a normal biconcave shape; thus, they are not considered poikilocytes.

C (erythrocyte in a rouleau formation) is incorrect. RBCs normally stack, forming a rouleau; they must have a normal (biconcave) shape to do so.

E (stab [band] eosinophil) is incorrect. The appearance of stab, or band, forms of neutrophils, basophils, and eosinophils is normal during the last step of cytodifferentiation, before the mature granulocyte is produced.

30. **E** (type II pneumocyte) is correct. Type II pneumocytes (great alveolar cells) are located in the alveolar wall. They are large cells with myelin-like figures in their cytoplasm, and they produce surfactant in the alveolus.

A (bronchiolar gland cell) is incorrect. Bronchiolar glands produce mucus, not surfactant.

B (dust cell) is incorrect. Dust cells (alveolar macrophages with phagocytosed anthracotic pigment) are not involved in the production of surfactant.

C (goblet cell) is incorrect. Goblet cells produce mucus, not surfactant.

D (type I pneumocyte) is incorrect. Type I pneumocytes comprise the very thin surface lining of the alveolus. They are covered with surfactant but do not manufacture it.

31. **E** (no change) is correct. A 0.9% NaCl solution is isotonic to red blood cells (RBCs). Therefore, the cell will neither swell nor shrink, and nothing will happen to its intracellular contents.

A (crenation) is incorrect. Crenation is the loss of water from the cell to the surrounding fluid. It occurs when a cell is placed in a hypertonic solution, such as 1.5% NaCl. The solution would draw water out of the cell, leaving it dehydrated and shrunken (or crenated).

B (hemolysis) is incorrect. Hemolysis of RBCs occurs when RBCs are placed in a hypotonic solution (e.g., 0.02% NaCl), which causes them to swell and burst.

C (increase in oxyhemoglobin content) is incorrect. The blood sample being placed in a saline solution will have little or no effect on the oxyhemoglobin content of RBCs. If anything, the RBCs in solution would gradually lose oxygen and become progressively deoxygenated.

D (spherocytosis) is incorrect. Spherocytosis is characterized by the presence of RBCs with an abnormal shape (round, not concave) due to a genetic defect in the cytoskeletal protein spectrin.

32. **A** (CD4 T cell) is correct. The CD4 T cell (T helper cell) is one of the major targets for HIV (macrophages are also major HIV targets). Several years after the initial infection, the number of CD4 T cells declines. This results in the loss of a multitude of helper functions, which take place by means of the lymphokines that are normally secreted by these cells to enhance the activity of other immune cells. The patient then becomes increasingly susceptible to infection by other organisms (opportunistic infections).

B (CD8 T cell) is incorrect. The CD8 T cell is not a direct target of HIV infection. However, its ability to function is adversely affected when lymphokine production decreases as the number of CD4 cells decreases after an individual is infected with HIV.

C (CD20 B cell) is incorrect. CD20 is a nonpolymorphic molecule expressed only on B cells. It can be used as a marker to classify lymphoid neoplasms immunologically. The B cell is not a common target of HIV.

D (NK cell) is incorrect. The NK cell is not a direct target of the HIV virus. However, its ability to function is adversely affected by the decrease in lymphokine production that results from the loss of CD4 cells in individuals with HIV.

E (plasma cell) is incorrect. Plasma cells are terminally differentiated B lymphocytes. They are not direct targets of HIV.

33. **C** (NK cells) is correct. NK cells normally provide surveillance for the immune system. Their cytotoxic activity is triggered by exposure to transformed cells, including neoplastic cells. Immunosuppressive therapy, such as cyclosporine therapy, selectively suppresses NK cell activity, thereby increasing the patient's risk of cancer.

A (basophils) is incorrect. The basophil is a granulocyte that takes part in immediate hypersensitivity reactions. Suppressing the hypersensitivity reaction does not induce cellular transformations that can result in a neoplasm.

B (dendritic reticular cells) is incorrect. Dendritic reticular cells are found in the germinal centers of lymph nodules. These cells trap and present antigens to immunocompetent cells. Suppressing these normal functions does not induce cellular transformations that can result in a neoplasm.

D (plasma cells) is incorrect. The plasma cell is a terminally differentiated B cell. It synthesizes antibodies, which target specific non-self entities and mark them for extinction. Suppressing plasma cell activity does not induce cellular transformations that can result in a neoplasm.

E (T suppressor cells) is incorrect. T suppressor cells (CD8 T cells) down-regulate antibody production. Suppressing their activity does not induce cellular transformations that can result in a neoplasm.

34. **D** (osteoporosis) is correct. Osteoporosis is a reduction in bone mass, which increases the risk of fracture after minimal trauma. Osteoporosis develops as a result of an imbalance between bone deposition and bone resorption. Women tend to be at greater risk for this condition as they age because the life span and activity of osteoblasts decreases with the loss of estrogen after menopause. If the loss of osteoblast activity is not accompanied by a change in osteoclast activity, bone loss will continue, resulting in a detectable loss of bone mass over time.

A (osteoclastoma) is incorrect. Osteoclastoma (giant cell neoplasm in bone) is a relatively common benign bone neoplasm and comprises 20% of benign bone neoplasms. It usually arises in the epiphyseal regions of the long bones of the extremities, and it is characterized by the presence of a large number of osteoclast-like cells. It has no effect on the life span of osteoblasts.

B (osteomalacia) is incorrect. Osteomalacia is characterized by inadequate mineralization of bone matrix. It is associated with vitamin D deficiency, which reduces the rate of absorption of calcium across the lining of the intestines; this then reduces the amount of calcium available to mineralize the bone matrix.

C (osteopetrosis) is incorrect. Osteopetrosis is characterized by the production of excessive amounts of bone matrix. Patients with this condition have brittle bones.

E (scurvy) is incorrect. Scurvy is characterized by the inability of osteoblasts to manufacture normal amounts of bone matrix (collagen). Scurvy is often associated with hypovitaminosis C.

35. **B** (corpora arenacea in the pineal gland) is correct. Calcified corpora arenacea (brain sand) is found in the normal pineal gland, which is located in the midline of the posterior portion of the third ventricle. It is often used as a marker for the midline of the brain.

A (corpora amylacea in the pineal gland) is incorrect. Corpora amylacea are not found in the center of the brain.

C (cupula of the crista ampullaris) is incorrect. The cupula of the crista ampullaris in the semicircular canal does not contain any material that would appear as radiopaque specks on an x-ray film.

D (otoliths in the macula of the saccule) and **E** (otoliths in the macula of the utricle) are incorrect. Otoliths (ear stones) are found in the gelatinous mass in the macula of the utricle or the saccule of the inner ear. They are too small to be detected by an x-ray film. Furthermore, they are components of the vestibular system in the ear; they are not located in the center of the brain.

36. **D** (monocyte) is correct. Mononuclear phagocytes (monocytes and macrophages) respond to liposaccharides by releasing TNF, which causes endothelial cells to release interleukin 6 (IL-6) and IL-8.

   A (basophil) is incorrect. Basophils induce type I hypersensitivity reactions (anaphylaxis) by releasing a variety of vasoactive substances (e.g., histamine) and chemotactic factors for PMNs and eosinophils.

   B (endothelial) is incorrect. Endothelial cells respond to increased levels of TNF by releasing IL-6 and IL-8.

   C (eosinophil) is incorrect. Eosinophils play a role in immune responses to parasitic infections and immune responses mediated by immunoglobulin E.

   E (platelet) is incorrect. Platelets are involved in homeostasis and in the production of platelet-derived growth factor, which induces the proliferation or migration of monocytes, fibroblasts, and smooth muscle cells.

37. **C** (myeloblast) is correct. CML is characterized by the presence of granulocytic and erythroid cells at various stages of differentiation in the peripheral blood. In general, the younger (less differentiated) the cell, the larger its size and the more prominent its nucleoli. The myeloblast is the least differentiated of all the cell types listed. Therefore, it would have the most prominent, or largest, nucleoli.

   A (basophilic myelocyte) is incorrect. The myelocyte is the next to the least mature cell listed. Myelocytes usually show their nucleoli, but not as prominently as a promyelocyte or myeloblast.

B (mature PMN) is incorrect. Mature PMNs do not show nucleoli.

   D (neutrophilic metamyelocyte) is incorrect. As a moderately differentiated cell with a bean-shaped nucleus, the metamyelocyte may or may not contain highly distinct nucleoli.

   E (polychromatophilic normoblast) is incorrect. In the polychromatophilic normoblast, most of the nucleus is heterochromatized or pyknotic. As a result, its nucleoli would not be seen.

38. **D** (400) is correct. During the G_2 phase, the cell contains four times the amount of deoxyribonucleic acid as the gamete. Therefore, it will contain 400 copies of the ribosomal genes.

   A (100) is incorrect. There are 100 ribosomal genes in a gamete.

   B (200) is incorrect. There are 200 ribosomal genes present during the G_1 phase of the cell cycle.

   C (300) is incorrect. There are 300 ribosomal genes in some cells during the early part of the S phase of the cell cycle.

39. **D** (non–carrier-mediated transport) is correct. When molecules cross the cell membrane without a carrier, they cannot move against their concentration gradient and energy is not required for their movement. Non–carrier-mediated movement is restricted to a class of molecules with similar physical properties (e.g., high molecular weight).

   A (active transport) is incorrect. Active transport requires energy.

   B (carrier-facilitated diffusion) is incorrect. Carrier-facilitated diffusion involves the use of molecule-specific carriers.

   C (exocytosis) is incorrect. Exocytosis is used to transport material in bulk out of the cell.

40. **A** (a nexus is found in the intercalated disk) is correct. A nexus (gap junction) in the intercalated disk plays an important role in the transmission of stimuli from one cardiac muscle fiber to the next.

 B (each fiber is innervated by an individual nerve ending) is incorrect. Cardiac muscle fibers are not innervated separately.

 C (it lacks myofibrils) is incorrect. Cardiac muscle fibers contain striated myofibrils.

 D (T tubules are found at the A–I intercept) is incorrect. T tubules are located at the Z line.

41. **B** (a multinucleated cell results from the fusion of many single cells) is correct. The skeletal muscle cell is the result of the fusion of many myoblasts into a myotube.

 A (a multinucleated cell is formed by repeated nuclear divisions in the absence of cytoplasmic division) is incorrect. The skeletal muscle cell is a result of the fusion of many myoblasts.

 C (after puberty, muscle mass grows by an increase in cell number) is incorrect. Muscle grows in mass by an increase in cell size (hypertrophy), not cell number.

 D (skeletal muscle is derived from the epithelial ectodermal and endodermal layers) is incorrect. Skeletal muscle is derived from the mesoderm.

42. **C** (endocytosis) is correct. Endocytosis is a mechanism for the cellular uptake of macromolecules.

 A (active transport) is incorrect. Active transport is a mechanism for carrying small molecules across a plasma cell membrane.

 B (carrier-facilitated diffusion) is incorrect. Carrier-facilitated diffusion is a mechanism for the uptake of small molecules into the cell.

 D (exocytosis) is incorrect. Exocytosis is a mechanism for moving material out of the cell.

 E (non–carrier-mediated transport) is incorrect. Non–carrier-mediated transport is a mechanism for the uptake of small, uncharged molecules and lipid-soluble material into the cell.

43. **D** (loss of secondary constrictions) is correct. The nucleolar organizer contains the secondary constriction region. If the organizer is completely deleted, the secondary constriction region is also removed from the chromosome.

 A (increased hybridization of DNA with 18S and 28S rRNA) is incorrect. If the nucleolar organizer is completely deleted from the cell, the genes that code for rRNA will be lost.

 B (increased number of nucleoli) is incorrect. If the nucleolar organizer is completely deleted from the cell, no nucleoli will be formed in the cell.

 C (increased synthesis of 45S RNA) is incorrect. If the nucleolar organizer is completely deleted, the cell will not be able to synthesize 45S (a precursor to rRNA).

44. **B** (mitochondria and vesicles containing neurotransmitters accumulate in the presynaptic area) is correct. Mitochondria and synaptic vesicles containing neurotransmitters are found in the presynaptic area of the neuron.

 A (a myelin sheath must be present if synaptic transmission is to occur) is incorrect. Synapses occur between myelinated and nonmyelinated axons.

 C (most synapses exist between two dendritic processes) is incorrect. Most synapses occur between axons and dendrites.

 D (occluding junctions hold the two neuronal processes together) is incorrect. Synapses do not contain occludens junctions.

E (satellite cells intervene between the neuronal processes) is incorrect. There are no intervening cells in a synapse.

45. **D** (presence of occluding junctions between capillary endothelial cells) is correct. The zona occludens is found between adjacent endothelial cells, and it plays a major role in the function of the blood–brain barrier.

A (accumulation of reactive astrocytes at the site of injury) is incorrect. Reactive astrocytes form at sites of injury. The blood–brain barrier is active in the uninjured brain.

B (association of the choroid plexus with pia mater cells) is incorrect. The choroid plexus plays an important role in the production of cerebrospinal fluid.

C (maintenance of the resting membrane potential) is incorrect. Membrane potentials are determined by the overall charge across the membrane of the nerve cell. They do not affect the blood–brain barrier.

46. **B** (resorption of water from the straight collecting tubules) is correct. A hypertonic interstitium in the area of the straight collecting tubules enhances the resorption of water in response to antidiuretic hormone.

A (resorption of water from the proximal convoluted tubule) and **C** (resorption of water from the thick ascending portion of Henle's loop) are incorrect. Resorption of water from these segments of the nephron is more strongly influenced by the movement of sodium, which is actively pumped out of each segment.

47. **C** (partial resorption of haversian systems by osteoclasts) is correct. During the remodeling of compact bone, osteoclasts resorb major regions of existing haversian systems, leaving some of the lamellae of these systems in place.

Thus, the resulting interstitial lamellae are the oldest lamellae in compact bone and have the highest degree of mineralization.

A (failure of haversian systems to form correctly) is incorrect. Interstitial lamellae are found in the remnants of remodeled haversian systems. After osteoclasts have ceased creating tunnels during the resorption process, the tunnels are filled by means of osteoblast activity to create a new haversian system. The haversian system must be normal for the remodeling process to occur.

B (inadequate intake of vitamin C) is incorrect. Vitamin C is necessary for the osteoblast to synthesize the collagen component of osteoid. Hypovitaminosis C results in scurvy, which is characterized by thin spicules of bone, indicating that little or no collagen synthesis is occurring.

D (pulling apart of haversian systems by Sharpey's fibers) is incorrect. Sharpey's fibers are collagen fibers that run from the periosteum into compact bone, anchoring the periosteum firmly to the bone. Sharpey's fibers do not hold haversian systems together.

E (stimulation of the periosteum by PTH) is incorrect. PTH enhances the production and activity of osteoclasts. If anything, PTH activity would reduce the number of interstitial lamellae in compact bone.

48. **A** (decreased synthesis of androgen-binding protein) is correct. Removal of the anterior lobe of the pituitary would remove follicle-stimulating hormone (FSH) and luteinizing hormone (LH) and lead to decreased synthesis of androgen-binding protein by the Sertoli cells. Antigen-binding protein is the binding protein for sex hormones and has a higher binding affinity for testosterone than for estrogen.

B (increased production of testosterone) is incorrect. Removal of the anterior lobe of the pituitary would end FSH and LH production and lead to a decrease in testosterone production.

C (increased spermatogenesis) is incorrect. Removal of the anterior lobe of the pituitary would eliminate FSH and LH and lead to decreased spermatogenesis.

49. **D** (stomach) is correct. Every columnar cell on the surface of the gastric epithelium secretes an insoluble mucus, which plays an important role in protecting the stomach wall from being digested by its own highly acidic secretions.

A (duodenum) is incorrect. The duodenum is lined with both simple columnar absorptive cells (enterocytes) and goblet cells, which produce mucus. However, the goblet cells are interspersed among the duodenal enterocytes; therefore, mucus is not produced by every surface cell.

B (esophagus) is incorrect. The esophagus is lined with a stratified squamous wet-type epithelium that does not manufacture mucus.

C (lower anal canal) is incorrect. The lower anal canal is lined with stratified squamous wet-type epithelium that does not secrete mucus.

E (transverse colon) is incorrect. Although the colonic epithelium contains a large number of goblet cells (which secrete mucus), these cells are interspersed among colonic enterocytes (water-absorbing cells). As a result, mucus is not secreted by every surface cell.

50. **D** (promyelocytic leukemia) is correct. The cell is a promyelocyte, which has a round nucleus containing several prominent nucleoli and a cytoplasm filled with small azurophilic granules. Dominance of this type of cell in the blood smear suggests promyelocytic leukemia. This type of leukemia is a distinctive variant of chronic lymphocytic leukemia (CLL) of B-cell lineage, or B-CLL. It is characterized by massive splenomegaly and a markedly elevated leukocyte count. The disease is most common in elderly men; it is aggressive, with a survival rate of 2 to 3 years.

A (ALL) is incorrect. ALL is characterized by a large number of lymphoblasts or immature lymphocytes. The cytoplasm of these cells is not filled with azurophilic granules. The peak age of incidence is childhood, and it occurs twice as often in white patients as in black patients.

B (basophilic leukemia) is incorrect. Basophilic leukemia is a rare form of leukemia characterized by the presence of basophils in various stages of differentiation.

C (monoblastic leukemia) is incorrect. Monoblastic leukemia is characterized by an abundance of agranular monoblasts.

E (stem cell leukemia) is incorrect. Stem cell leukemia is characterized by an abundance of very immature cells. These cells have prominent nucleoli, but they are not differentiated well enough to show cytoplasmic granules. This type of leukemia is also known as *acute undifferentiated leukemia*.

Index

Note: Page numbers followed by f indicate figures; those followed by t indicate tables; and those followed by b indicated boxed material.

Henle's loop
thick ascending segment of, 179f, 183, 184f
thick descending limb of, 179f, 180f, 181, 182f, 184f
thin segment of, 179f, 182–183, 184f
Heparan sulfate, 56
Heparin
as anticoagulant, 134
in hypersensitivity reaction, 152f
Hepatic acinus(i), 171f, 172
metabolic zones of, 172
Hepatic artery, common, 172
Hepatic lobule, 171–172, 171f
Hepatic metastases, 174
Hepatic sinusoids, 172, 173f
Hepatic vein, 172
Hepatitis, viral, 174
Hepatocellular carcinoma, 174
Hepatocytes, 173, 173f
Hepatolenticular degeneration, 228
Hereditary hypercholesterolemia, defective transport in, 8
Hereditary spherocytosis, 133t, 249, 266
Herpetic stomatitis, 163
Herring body, 217f
Heterochromatin, 30f, 32
Heterophagic function, of lysosomes, 16
Heterophagosome, 18f
Hirschsprung's disease, 169
Histamine
in hypersensitivity reaction, 151, 152f
in inflammation, 136
production of, 254
Histiocytes, 147, 255, 280
Histones, reversible modifications to, 33
HIV (human immunodeficiency virus)
CD4 T cells in, 273, 287
replication of, 243–244, 255
Hodgkin's disease, 158
Hofbauer cells, 209
Holocrine secretion, 48
Homocystinuria, 62
Hordeolum, 232
Horizontal cells, of retina, 230f, 231
Hormone(s), 214–215
abbreviations for, 216b
Hormone secretion, regulation of, 215
Horner's ptosis, 232
Horner's syndrome, 232
Howship's lacunae, 103
Human chorionic gonadotropin (hCG), 200–201, 203f, 204, 209
Human immunodeficiency virus (HIV)
CD4 T cells in, 273, 287
replication of, 243–244, 255
Human papilloma virus (HPV16, HPV18), 205
Human placental lactogen, 209
Humoral immunodeficiency diseases, 151
Humoral immunologic response, 149–151, 150f, 152f

Hunter's syndrome, 57b
Huntington's chorea, 74b
Hurler's syndrome, 57b, 248, 263
Hyaline arteriolosclerosis, 123
Hyaline cartilage(s), 101t
C-shaped, 115
Hyaline cartilage model, 106, 107f
Hyaline membrane disease, 268, 276
Hyalomere, 133
Hyalomere microfilaments, 272, 285
Hyaluronic acid, 55–56, 56f
Hyaluronidase, 56
Hydatidiform mole, 211
Hydrocele, 195–196
Hydrocephalus, 73
Hydrochloric acid (HCl), 166, 254
Hydropic degeneration, 6
Hydroxyapatite crystals, 102
21-Hydroxylase deficiency, 277
Hypercholesterolemia
familial, 284
hereditary, 8
Hyperopia, 229
Hyperplastic arteriolosclerosis, 123
Hypersensitivity reactions, 151, 152f
Hypertrophy, zone of, in epiphyseal plate, 109, 109f
Hypodermis, 90
Hyponychium, 98
Hypophyseal portal system, 125, 215–216, 217f
Hypophysis, 215–218, 217f, 218f, 219t
Hypothalamo-hypophyseal portal veins, 217f
Hypothalamo-hypophyseal tract, 217f
Hypothalamo-hypophyseal-adrenal axis, 222f
Hypothalamo-hypophyseal-thyroid axis, 216, 218f
Hypothalamus, regulation of anterior pituitary by, 216, 218f
Hypovitaminosis A, 265
Hypovitaminosis C, 249, 265, 291
Hypovitaminosis D, 266
and bone growth, 110, 271, 282

I

I (isotropic) band, 79, 80f, 278
during muscle contraction and relaxation, 83f, 265
I-cell disease, 19t
Ichthyosis, 258
vulgaris, 92, 94
ICSH (interstitial cell–stimulating hormone), 194, 195f
Identical twins, 210–211
IF(s) (intermediate filaments)
in cytoskeleton, 26f, 27–28, 27t
in intestinal lining, 47f
IFN-γ (interferon-γ), 148f, 149t
Igs. *See* Immunoglobulin(s) (Igs).
IL. *See* Interleukin (IL).
Immotile cilia syndrome, 26, 47b, 193
Immune responses. *See* Immunologic response(s).